VASCULAR MEDICINE – FROM ENDOTHELIUM TO MYOCARDIUM

VASCULAR MEDICINE
FROM ENDOTHELIUM TO
MYOCARDIUM

Edited by

ERNST E. VAN DER WALL

Department of Cardiology,
Leiden University Medical Centre,
Leiden, The Netherlands

VOLKERT MANGER CATS

Department of Cardiology,
Leiden University Medical Centre,
Leiden, The Netherlands

and

JAN BAAN

Department of Cardiology,
Leiden University Medical Centre,
Leiden, The Netherlands

KLUWER ACADEMIC PUBLISHERS
DORDRECHT / BOSTON / LONDON

A C.I.P. Catalogue record for this book is available from the Library of Congress.

ISBN-13: 978-94-010-6505-4   e-ISBN-13: 978-94-009-0037-0
DOI: 10.1007/ 978-94-009-0037-0

Published by Kluwer Academic Publishers,
P.O. Box 17, 3300 AA Dordrecht, The Netherlands.

Sold and distributed in the U.S.A. and Canada
by Kluwer Academic Publishers,
101 Philip Drive, Norwell, MA 02061, U.S.A.

In all other countries, sold and distributed
by Kluwer Academic Publishers,
P.O. Box 322, 3300 AH Dordrecht, The Netherlands.

Cover photo: Theo J.C. van Berkel

Printed on acid-free paper

This publication has been made possible with educational grants from:

Lorex Synthélabo

&

Bristol-Myers Squibb
Guidant
Medtronic

We acknowledge greatly the assistance of our secretary Anneke van der Mey in preparing and editing this book manuscript.

TABLE OF CONTENTS

Albert V.G. Bruschke

In September 1997 a Symposium was organized to celebrate the 50th anniversary of the Department of Cardiology of the Leiden University Hospital.

Looking backwards it is interesting to observe how in this half century the focus of patient care and research in cardiology has moved away from congenital and rheumatic heart disease towards the area of coronary heart disease and even in this field there have been continuous shifts of the focus of interest which for many years appeared to pendulate between the myocardium and the coronary arteries. Ischemic heart disease had been known or at least suspected to originate in the coronary arteries for more than two centuries as testified in 1778 by a letter of E. Jenner to Heberden: "The importance of the coronary arteries, and how much the heart must suffer from their not being able duly to perform their functions, (we cannot be surprised at the painful spasms) is a subject I need not enlarge upon, therefore shall only just remark that it is possible that all the symptoms may arise from this one circumstance."[1] However, to quote Proudfit, "Coronary disease is an arterial abnormality in which the clinical manifestations are myocardial"[2] and until the introduction of coronary arteriography by F. Mason Sones in the early sixties the arterial abnormalities themselves

Quoted from "A disorder of the breast" collection of original texts on ischemic heart disease, selected and commented upon by H.A. Snellen. Kooyker Scientific Publications, Rotterdam, 1976.

Proudfit WL, Bruschke AVG, Sones FM Jr. Natural history of obstructive coronary artery disease: Ten-year study of 601 nonsurgical cases. Progress Cardiovasc Dis 1978;21:53-78.

escaped entirely clinical recognition by available diagnostic techniques. Furthermore, interventions like mechanical desobstruction or bypass surgery of the coronary arteries were not even thought of. This may explain why even after perfection of coronary arteriography to a safe and reliable diagnostic technique it still took some time before, often somewhat reluctantly, not only serious consideration was given to the myocardium but also or mainly to its supplying arteries.

In the last two decades our understanding of the pathogenesis of coronary atherosclerosis and development of therapeutic modalities has gained enormous momentum and today we may witness breakthroughs in many areas occurring with breathtaking speed. One of the most fascinating developments is the changing concept of the coronary arterial system which until recently was regarded as a simple conduit for blood but now appears to be a complex organ system governed by numerous internal and external controlling mechanisms which are gradually being unraveled.

Compared to the revolutionary developments in basic research the progress made in therapeutic possibilities is still relatively modest. Remembering that it took about a decade before the introduction of coronary arteriography, the most significant clinical breakthrough in coronary artery disease in the last 50 years, began to bear fruit by making bypass surgery possible, this should be no reason for concern. On the other hand, current scientific developments are of a highly complex nature and consequently more than ever before a multidisciplinary approach is required to use new insights to the benefit of patients. Basic researchers, clinical investigators and practicing clinicians should endeavour to understand each other and maintain a meaningful dialogue. Due to the speed and diversity of current developments this is a difficult task; many clinicians are confronted with new scientific insights in areas they are not familiar with while basic scientists often are unaware of new diagnostic and therapeutic potential. At Leiden University this problem was recognized a long time ago and therefore the "Working Group of Cardiovascular Research Leiden" was established. From the beginning this was intended to be a platform for active scientists and clinicians who wished to explore the possibilities provided by intensive cooperation. This formula has proved to be extremely successful and it has been the basis of this multidisciplinary symposium.

This book discusses recent developments and insights in fields which are familiar to most of us as well as new developments in areas of research, clinical diagnosis and therapeutic options which have not yet, or barely, reached the stage of clinical applicability but are destined to play a major role in the near future. Therefore this book should be of interest to anyone who wishes to update his or her knowledge in (cardio)vascular medicine and is highly recommended to anyone who wishes to get prepared for tomorrow.

Jan Baan, Department of Cardiology, Leiden University Medical Centre, Albinusdreef 2, 2333 ZA LEIDEN, The Netherlands
Co-authors: Paul Steendijk, Jan Baan Jr.

Jeroen J. Bax, Department of Cardiology, Leiden University Medical Centre, Albinusdreef 2, 2333 ZA LEIDEN, The Netherlands
Co-author: Ernst E. van der Wall

Theo J.C. Van Berkel, From the Division of Biopharmaceutics, Leiden/Amsterdam Center for Drug Research, Sylvius Laboratories, Leiden University, Leiden, The Netherlands (M.V.E., N.H., Th.J.C.V.B.); SmithKline Beecham Research and Development, The Frythe, Welwyn, United Kingdom (P.H.E.G.); and Department of Pediatrics, University Hospital, Leiden, The Netherlands (P.M.H.).
Co-authors: Miranda Van Eck, Nicole Herijgers, Peter M. Hoogerbrugge, Pieter H.E. Groot.

Albert V.G. Bruschke, Department of Cardiology, Leiden University Medical Centre, Albinusdreef 2, 2333 ZA LEIDEN, The Netherlands

Louis Havekes, TNO-PG, Gaubius Laboratory and MGC-Department of Human Genetics, P.O. Box 2215, 2301 CE Leiden, The Netherlands
Co-authors: Bart J.M. van Vlijmen, Miek C. Jong, Pieter H.E. Groot, Ko Willems van Dijk, Marten H. Hofker

Frits Haverkate, Division of Vascular and Connective Tissue Research, TNO-PG Gaubius Laboratory, P.O. Box 2215, 2301 CE LEIDEN, The Netherlands

Frits H.A.F. de Man, Department of Cardiology, Leiden University Medical Centre, Albinusdreef 2, 2333 ZA LEIDEN, The Netherlands
Co-authors: Mariëtte J.V. Hoffer#, Augustinus H.M. Smelt*, Jan A. Gevers Leuven*+, Arnoud van der Laarse
#Department of Human Genetics, Leiden University Medical Centre, Albinusdreef 2, 2333 ZA LEIDEN, The Netherlands
*Department of Internal Medicine, Leiden University Medical Centre, Albinusdreef 2, 2333 ZA LEIDEN, The Netherlands

[+]TNO-PG, Gaubius Laboratory, Zernikedreef 9, 2333 CK Leiden, The Netherlands

Han J.G.H. Mulder, Department of Cardiology, Leiden University Medical Centre, Albinusdreef 2, 2333 ZA LEIDEN, The Netherlands
Co-author: Martin J. Schalij

Johan H.C. Reiber, Division of Image Processing, Department of Radiology and Cardiology[*], Leiden University Medical Centre, Albinusdreef 2, 2333 ZA LEIDEN, The Netherlands
Co-authors: Bob Goedhart, Hans G. Bosch, Rob J. van der Geest, Jouke Dijkstra, Gerhard Koning, Mahmoud Ramze Rezaee, Boudewijn P.F. Lelieveldt, Albert de Roos[#], Ernst E. van der Wall[*#], Albert V.G. Bruschke[*]
[#]Interuniversity Cardiology Institute of The Netherlands, Catharijnesingel 52, 3511 GC Utrecht, The Netherlands

Tjeerd J. Römer, Department of Cardiology, Leiden University Medical Centre Albinusdreef 2, 2333 ZA Leiden, The Netherlands
Co-author: James F. Brennan III[*]
[*]3M Austin Sector Laboratory, A03-1N-05, 11705 Research Blvd., Austin, TX 78759, U.S.A.

Johan J. Schipperheijn, Department of Cardiology, Leiden University Medical Centre, Albinusdreef 2, 2333 ZA LEIDEN, The Netherlands

Peter W.H.M. Verheggen, Department of Cardiology, Leiden University Medical Centre, Albinusdreef 2, 2333 ZA LEIDEN, The Netherlands
Co-author: Volkert Manger Cats

Hubert W. Vliegen, Department of Cardiology, Leiden University Medical Centre, Albinusdreef 2, 2333 ZA LEIDEN, The Netherlands
Co-authors: J. Wouter Jukema, Arnoud van der Laarse, Hermann Haller[*]
[*]Department of Medicine, Franz-Volhard-Klinik, Universitatsklinikum Rudolf Virchow, Wiltbergstrasse 50, 13125 Berlin, Germany

'CARDIOLOGY LEIDEN', THE FIRST 40 YEARS

Johan J. Schipperheijn

The founding, 1947 - 1957

In Internal Medicine, the diagnosis of heart disease has always been regarded as difficult and it requiered highly technical skills. This was especially true at the Leiden University Hospital, because this the place where electrocardiography, developed by Einthoven at the Physiology Laboratory of the University, was first applied in clinical practice. Congenital or valvular disease of the heart is easily detected because of the murmurs and clicks that it causes, but it requires great experience and skill to diagnose the underlying disorder properly by auscultation; a skill that many experienced and highly qualified internists never developed. Arrhythmias of the heart were elusive and practically impossible to diagnose without proper equipment, same was true for angina the diagnosis of which was based solely on the patient's history. To aid in the diagnosis, clinical electrocardiography and fluoroscopy of the chest was introduced in the thirties; examining patients and interpreting the recordings and images was so difficult that it inevitably became the domain of specialists in cardiology. In this role Dr. Herman Snellen was appointed in 1937 as a consultant in Cardiology at the Department of Internal Medicine by Kuenen, professor of Internal Medicine and in 1934 one of the founders and the first president of the Dutch Society of Cardiology. Snellen's task was to examine patients on request of the internist, and, in particularly, to study patients using electro-cardiography, fluoroscopy and X-ray photography. He passed his thesis in 1939 on X-ray diagnosis of sclerosis of the heart and the aorta. During the

1

E.E. van der Wall et al. (eds.), Vascular Medicine, 1-11.
© 1997 *Kluwer Academic Publishers.*

Second World War the University was closed; the University Hospital continued its task as the main hospital of the city of Leiden, but development in the diagnosis and treatment of heart disease came to a halt. As far as treatment was concerned, the hospital at that time had little to offer anyhow, since there was no cardiac surgery and the only effective drugs available for the treatment of heart failure were digitalis and mercury diuretics. For the treatment of arrhythmias, there were chinidine and digitalis, while for coronary artery disease short-acting nitrates were the only remedy.

The restoration of the University and its Hospital after the war coincided with a break-through in the treatment of congenital and later acquired valvular disease of the heart. In 1944 Blalock carried out the shunt operation, that still carries his name, in a child with Fallot's tetralogy. He performed the operation on a request from Helen Taussig, the paediatrician who did so much for the development of electrocardiographic and X-ray diagnosis of congenital heart disease in the thirties and forties. When surgery of the heart and the great vessels developed, it became clear that for a proper planning of the operation noninvasive diagnostic techniques were insufficient. X-ray diagnosis was first boosted by intravenous injection of iodine salts. The catheterization of the heart, its feasibility demonstrated when Forsmann in 1929 bravely passed a catheter into his own pulmonary artery, was soon used not only to measure pressure and oxygen saturation in the different compartments of the heart, but also to inject contrast material selectively. It adds to the credits of Mulder, professor of Internal Medicine at Leiden, that he recognized the importance of the new developments in the United States and Great Britain and in 1947 asked Snellen to found a Department of Cardiology not only to continue noninvasive techniques, but also to develop catheterization in adults as well as children necessary for the new surgical treatment.

In 1949 the new departments of Cardiology and Paediatric Cardiology fused and formed a 'Thorax Centre', be it a very small one according to present day standards, a form of organisation that was later also adopted in Rotterdam. In 1952 the thoracic surgeon Brom came to Leiden. Brom pioneered open heart surgery in Utrecht together with Jongbloed, the physiologist who worked on heart-lung machines. When Brom came to Leiden he founded the first Department of Thoracic Surgery in the Netherlands. On his instigation, the Thorax Centre was divided into three separate departments under the competency of the Departments of Internal Medicine, Paediatrics and Surgery. The weekly rounds along the paediatric beds together continued and the catheterization laboratory was developed jointly, but Paediatric Cardiology became a separate department with, of course, its main interest in congenital heart disease. Dr Caro Bruins became head of the department.

It took some time before thorax surgery in post-war European countries reached the standards of the centres in the United States, but Brom managed to do this in only a few years. Snellen at the Cardiology Department in the same short period of time developed the necessary catheterization techniques and started with phonocardiography. The high speed photographical recorders, a legacy of the war industry, that became available in the early fifties allowed for faithful recording of heart sounds and external pulsations of the heart and large blood vessels. This soon developed into a clinical diagnostic technique that under Hartman became the corner stone of noninvasive diagnosis of valvular heart disease. It was used to select patients for catheterization, and became indispensable for the follow-up after surgery.

In 1955 the Department had fully developed into a 'centre of reference'. Patients were referred by cardiologists and internists only, for diagnosis and to pose an indication for surgical treatment. A visit to the outpatient clinic implied for the patient a full round along electrocardiography, phonocardiography and fluoroscopy and of course history taking, physical examination and blood tests as usual in Internal Medicine. Patients with serious valvular disease were admitted to the ward for catheterization. The presentation of cases to the surgeon once a week became the most important activity of the department.

In recognition of the maturity reached by the Department, Snellen was appointed professor in Cardiology in 1955. First as an extracurricular professor, in 1956 as a part-time, extraordinary professor and in 1959 as a full professor.

The second phase, 1960 - 1970

In the late fifties, the possibilities of cardiac surgery were still limited. Equipment for extracorporeal circulation during surgery was available, but could be used only for children weighing less than 35 kg. The only operations performed 'on perfusion' were closure of a ventricular or atrial septal defects of the primum type, occasionally a widening of the pulmonary outflow tract. All other more simple operations were performed on the beating heart, often after cooling the patient in ice. Correction of complicated vitia like Fallot's tetralogy and implantation of artificial valves was not yet possible at that time. As soon as the first artificial valves became available around 1960, it triggered a rapid development of diagnostic techniques. Research efforts in the department were primarily aimed at further refinement of phonocardiography. Recordings of heart sounds, of the apex beat and arterial and venous pulsations were used to diagnose valvular lesions and to estimate their severity. An attempt was made to develop ballistocardiography into a useful diagnostic tool, with little success. Indications for catheterization and subsequent surgical treatment were based primarily on phonographic signs. Hartman who had acquired remarkably extensive, encyclopedic knowledge on phonocardiography became an internationally recognized expert in the field. In 1964 he passed his doctoral thesis on phonocardiographic signs in patients with aortic stenosis. Electrophysiology was no longer a field of interest at the department. Electrocardiography was of course used as a clinical tool, but the main centre for research on the electrical activation of the heart at that time was in Amsterdam, where Durrer published in the late fifties and early sixties a series of important papers on that subject and became an authority in the field. Durrer's basic research on electrical activation triggered a great interest in electrophysiology in his clinic, and made it the centre for diagnosis and treatment of arrhythmias in the Netherlands. At Leiden, research in electrophysiology of the heart remained restricted to the development of artificial pacemakers. A prototype of an external pacemaker was built and tested in dogs, but research in this filed was discontinued when implantable pacemakers came available commercially. Research on the properties of the electrode-tissue interface continued and methods were developed to detect changes of the electrical impedance of the electrodes that are still being used today.

From the early days, a close cooperation existed with the Anatomy Department where an active working group studied the embryology of the heart. When Cardiology and Paediatric Cardiology became separate departments, the contacts between Anatomy and Cardiology waned and ceased to be stimulating. Other contacts within the Medical Faculty waxed, however, and in the late sixties Hemker, at that time already an established investigator in the field of coagulation of the blood, joined the department and started a laboratory for Cardiobiochemistry. A pilot study was done on the preservation of myocardium, but the main topic became enzyme release from the infarcted myocardium. The first major paper on this subject appeared in 1970 in Circulation. It led to the development of a new method for the quantitation of infarct size, based on consecutive measurements of enzyme concentration in the blood. The enzyme α-hydroxy butyrate dehydrogenase was used, which was found to have several advantages over enzymes used elsewhere for the same purpose. The method was developed into a reliable tool for clinical research, still used today to independently measure infarct size in intervention studies.

Major developments in Cardiac Surgery and Cardiology in the United States in the sixties had profound influences on the department. The heart-lung machines were improved and, later in the sixties, could be used in adults, which allowed for complicated surgical procedures. Replacement of diseased valves with artificial valves became possible. The expertise in phonocardiography in the department was extended to artificial valves and early signs of dysfunction were studied. Catheterization techniques were improved and in cooperation with Philips Röntgen factories an excellent quality of angiograms and ventriculograms was achieved.

In the early days of valve replacement surgery, perioperative mortality was alarmingly high. This was partly due to the preservation technique of intermittent cross-clamping and coronary perfusion used at that time. Perfusion failed occasionally and especially patients with an already compromised pump function were serious at risk of incurring perioperative ischemic damage. A poor condition of the myocardium was considered a contraindication for cardiac surgery. This kindled an interest in measuring pump function, preferably from the ventriculogram and pressure measurements at the catheterization laboratory only. At that time, knowledge on heart muscle contraction was limited and understanding of the causes of mechanical dysfunction was rudimentary. Snellen asked ter Keurs and the author (JJS), both physiologists who had worked in the field of Neurophysiology at the Physiology Laboratory, to join the Cardiology Department and to do experimental work on heart muscle contraction. The Department of Paediatric Cardiology did the same, where Versprille, a physiologist from the University of Utrecht, started working on pump function of the heart in new-born animals. The sixties were the advent of modern treatment of coronary artery disease. Attempts to improve blood supply to the heart surgically, in case of severe occlusive disease of the coronary arteries, date as far back as 1935, but the first successful revascularizations by interposition or bypass grafting date from the mid sixties. In 1970 the first bypass operation was performed at the Leiden University Hospital and in the Cardiology Department the necessary angiographic skills were developed to diagnose the patients. Buis, head of the catheterization laboratory, developed coronary angiography using the Judkins' percutaneous technique that became available in 1967. In cooperation with Philips Röntgen factories he reached a high quality of angiography that allowed later for participation in international studies on the results of coronary surgery.

In Leiden, treatment of patients with an acute myocardial infarction was still in its infancy up to the late sixties. Till 1973, patients with an acute infarction were admitted, for severe cases, to a general Intensive Care Unit, but mostly to a small unit at the Internal Medicine Department. Cardiologists became involved only in case of serious arrhythmias or valvular complications. In 1970, two beds at the Intensive Care Unit were placed under supervision of a cardiologist and were used for patients with a large myocardial infarction. At that time, in other University Hospitals in the Netherlands, the care for patients with an acute infarction occurred already completely under supervision of cardiologists of a Cardiology Department and in most places specially equipped Coronary Care Units were available. Interventions in the coronary circulation were not possible yet, but patient management in Coronary Care Units was aimed at treating serious and potentially lethal arrhythmias. Treatment and prevention of arrhythmias prompted research activities in which the Cardiology Department in Amsterdam played a leading role. Because of the relatively late introduction of Coronary Care facilities in Leiden very little research was done in this field.

For the Department the late sixties were a transition phase in which the interest and research activities shifted from noninvasive diagnostic techniques in valvular heart disease to invasive diagnostic and later interventional techniques in coronary artery disease. Research was aimed at mechanical performance of the heart, heart muscle function and the pathological processes underlying coronary artery disease and consequently the prevention of that disease. Snellen initiated the transition, but he approached the retirement age of sixty five. Although professors at that time were allowed to stay until they were seventy years old, Snellen wanted to retire at the age of sixty five and, of course, did not want to restrict his successor in further developing the research of the department. His decision to attach a biochemist and physiologists to the department, however, had a decisive influence on future developments.

The third phase, 1970 - 1987

In the early seventies, the Medical Faculty carefully selected a successor for Snellen as head of the department. Late 1972, Dr. Varnauskas from Göteborg Sweden became the second professor in Cardiology. His main field of interest was the diagnosis and treatment of coronary artery disease and he was well known internationally for organising follow-up studies of coronary artery surgery. One of the conditions for his coming to Leiden was the founding of a Coronary Care Unit with modern facilities like central supervision, monitoring equipment visible from every room in the unit and primarily a specially trained nursing staff. A temporary building in the inner courtyard of the Internal Medicine Department was soon to house the new CCU. Varnauskas stimulated the development of coronary angiography. He prompted Buis, head of the catheterization laboratory, to write his doctoral thesis on angiographic follow-up of bypass surgery. Buis passed his thesis in 1974.

Hemker, who had founded the Cardiobiochemistry laboratory, accepted a professorship at the new Medical Faculty in Maastricht. Witteveen, who had passed his thesis on assessment of infarct size in 1972, became the new head of the lab and continued the work. The newly developed method for determining infarct size was applied in the Coronary Care Unit. In 1976 Van der Laarse, a biochemist from Amsterdam, became the head of the Laboratory. He continued research on enzyme release, but extended the research into the field of ischemia and myocardial function.

Research on pump function of the heart was developing slowly. Facilities for experimental studies were set up in the Physiology Laboratory and some experimental work, initiated by Varnauskas, was done on the influence of antiarrhythmic drugs on heart muscle action potential. Facilities for studies in large animals came available and were used to build and test a thermodilution cardiac output meter designed in Göteborg. It would be the last time that an effort was made to develop medical technological devices; commercial industrial companies took over in that field. Within a period of ten years scientists and technicians of the Cardiology Department and the Physiology Laboratory had developed and constructed prototypes of artificial heart valves, heart lung machines, artificial pacemakers, special purpose amplifiers and pulse generators. All in the tradition of Einthoven, whose major contribution to Cardiology and Physiology was also based on development and construction of a special research tool, the string galvanometer.

In the Department of Paediatric Cardiology a study was completed on postnatal development of innervation of the AV-node and Rohmer, who later succeeded Caro Bruins as head of the department, passed his thesis on insufficiency of the pulmonary valve after surgical correction of Fallot's tetralogy, applying a new method for intravascular electromagnetic flow measurements.

The reorientation of the department of Cardiology towards coronary artery disease kindled interest in prevention of the disease. The early publications from the Framingham study, which dated from the late fifties, received little attention, but in the early seventies when the Seven Countries Study was published the importance of dietary advice for infarct survivors and patients after bypass surgery became apparent. Bonjer published guidelines for the detection and prevention of ischemic heart disease and Weeda organised the rehabilitation after infarction or cardiac surgery.

After little more than a year Varnauskas laid down his professorship and returned to Sweden. Snellen temporarily returned as head of the department, until in 1975 Dr. Alex Arntzenius became the new professor in Cardiology and head of the department. Arntzenius, who was trained as a cardiologist by Snellen, had studied vectorcardiography and had produced a thesis on that subject, was working as an associate professor at Rotterdam at the Thorax Centre under Hugenholtz. In Rotterdam he was involved in programs for the detection of coronary artery disease and in prevention. With his arrival, the course set by Varnauskas was maintained. The coronary angiography and the follow-up after bypass operations became the domain of Buis, but Arntzenius devoted himself to epidemiology and preventive cardiology. He participated in epidemiological studies like the Westland Project, an early risk factor survey in the Netherlands.

Arntzenius had also great interest in physiology of the heart, mechanical function and pump function, but also electrical activation of the heart. During his stay at Rotterdam, he had an original idea based on earlier experience with ballistocardiography. By rapid downward displacements of the body synchronous with the heart beat, he thought he could support the heart mechanically, in fact by mimicking the movement of the body due to ejection of blood from the ventricles as recorded in ballistocardiography. A high-powered actuator at the Physiology Laboratory, developed for the study of skeletal muscle function, was used to test his theory in a series of animal experiments. The results were promising enough to draw the attention of a large industry as American Optical and it led to the construction of three large actuators for use in patients in cardiogenic shock. One of the machines was already placed in Leiden, when Arntzenius was still working at Rotterdam. It was used in a small series of patients in cardiogenic shock. Arntzenius showed that rapid downward movement of the patient indeed raised blood pressure and improved the circulation. Despite the promising result, the development of the method was discontinued, because slightly later, in the United States, the intraaortic balloon pump was developed as a cardiac support device. The pump required the introduction of a large catheter into the aorta, but it was at least as effective, and it could be operated at the bedside. Moreover, it was less expensive and far less bulky and noisy than Arntzenius' 'shaking bed'. All work on the development was already stopped soon, when Arntzenius became the head of the department. From the days of his thesis on vectorcardiography Arntzenius was interested in electrical activation of the ventricles. He had used a crude electrical model of the heart to predict changes in the vectorcardiogram caused by infarctions. When at Rotterdam he joined a research group that developed more sophisticated discrete element models implemented on the computers of the Thorax Centre. Data published by Durrer on the activation of the ventricles were used to initiate activation in the model. When Arntzenius came to Leiden, he used part of his research development fund to bye equipment for the perfusion of large hearts. It was used in a series of validation experiments of the model. Arntzenius wanted to use the computer model to solve first the 'forward' and subsequently the 'backward' problem. The forward problem is the exact prediction of the shape of the vectorcardiogram using data on the geometry, including infarct localisation, if appropriate, and onset of activation. The backward problem is the exact estimation of infarct size and localisation from the vectorcardiogram. The research on the perfused heart showed that both the forward and the backward problem could be solved, but also that the solution required very exact data on the geometry of the heart, as well as exact data on the activation pattern of the heart, in fact a complete lay-out of the Purkinje network was needed. It was obvious from the results, that it would never be possible to estimate infarct size and localisation in a clinical situation from clinically available data only, at least not with a reasonable degree of precision. The set-up for the perfusion of large hearts was later used to study the mechanics of artificial valves in situ. Pig hearts with an artificial valve implanted in advance pumped a crystalline solution into an artificial circulation, while the coronary vessels were perfused with blood. Valve motion was viewed through an endoscope inserted into the apex or left atrium. This work was done by Gerda van Rijk, a thorax surgeon.

Contractility of the heart remained an area of interest in clinical cardiology. Indices of contractility were used to characterize pump function that were based on intraventricular pressure measurements. Clinicians were not satisfied, however, and considered them unsatisfactory. At the Department of Paediatric Cardiology, Baan began a study on contractility based on pressure volume relations. He experimented with magnetic fluids to measure volume, but later adapted a method based on measurement of electrical conductance, originally developed at the Cardiology Department by Koops and Corten to measure volume changes in the aorta, and developed it into a practical tool for estimating ventricular volume that could even be used in patients. With the use of the method he studied load dependency of the endsystolic pressure-volume relation, the contractility index that at that time had replaced earlier indices based on pressure measurements alone. The conductance catheter method is presently used in over 100 institutes.

The measurement of contractility remained a challenging problem in cardiac physiology, because the contractile properties of single cardiac muscle fibres were at that time only poorly understood. The force-length and the force-velocity relation were measured earlier, but the work was done in papillary muscle preparations that were inevitably partly damaged. The crushed end of the muscle added a series elastic element to the contracting part, the properties of which added to the properties of the contracting muscle. At the Department of Cardiology, ter Keurs was among the first in the world who managed to perform laser diffraction measurements of sarcomere length in cardiac muscle. By applying an ingenious feed back control of sarcomere length he was the first to measure a true isosarcometric' force-length relation in trabecula of the right ventricle of the rat. This breakthrough in cardiac muscle physiology was widely recognized. The Dutch Heart Foundation appointed ter Keurs to the position of Established Investigator and generously subsidized the work. He subsequently studied restoring forces in cardiac muscle and force-velocity relations. The results of his studies strongly influenced views on contractility of the heart, world wide. In the early eighties, when insight into the contractility problem had widened considerably, the need for complete and accurate studies of contractility in patients had subsided, ironaically. The protection of the heart during surgery greatly improved when in 1977 cold cardioplegia was introduced. It became possible to operate safely even on hearts with severe ischemic damage. After 1977 the number of operations peformed at Leiden rapidly increased from around 50 to over 200 per year and mortality fell to a low level. Quality of coronary angiography was maintained at a high level. After the attempts to treat patients in cardiogenic shock with counterpulsations, the intraaortic balloon pump was introduced in 1974 and clinical experience with this cardiac assist device was gathered. Buis participated in the European Study on Coronary Surgery.

Arntzenius started a large clinical intervention study on prevention of coronary artery disease in 1981. It was at that time well recognized that a high serum cholesterol level is a risk factor for coronary artery disease. Proof that reduction of serum cholesterol levels could slow down or even reverse progression of arteriosclerosis was not available. In the Leiden Intervention Trial patients who underwent coronary angiography were carefully instructed to follow a dietary regimen. After two years the angiography was repeated and angiograms were compared. Results, published in the New England Journal of Medicine in 1985, showed that in patients in whom serum cholesterol fell, coronary sclerosis had progressed more slowly than in patients whose cholesterol levels did not fall; and occasionally their lesions showed more regression.

When the Leiden Intervention Trial was finished, Arntzenius retired. It took more than a year before the Medical Faculty appointed Dr. Albert Bruschke as the new head of the Department. Bruschke had been the head of the Cardiology Department of the Antonius Hospital in Nieuwegein, and was an expert in coronary angiography; he had published outstanding papers on the natural course of coronary artery disease, documented angiographically. Trained in the Cleveland Clinics, he introduced coronary angiography into the Netherlands. When he became head of the Cardiology Department in Leiden in 1986 he continued the line of research. In 1985 ter Keurs accepted a professorship in Calgary, Canada, and the studies on the physiology of cardiac muscle fibres in Leiden were terminated. Baan at the Department of

Paediatric Cardiology later joined the Department of Cardiology and continued studies on pressure volume relations. At the Cardiobiochemistry Laboratory the field of interest was extended into endothelial function and arteriosclerosis. These changes set the stage for present day experimental and clinical research in the Department of Cardiology.

ARE C-REACTIVE PROTEIN AND FIBRINOGEN RISK FACTORS?

Frits Haverkate

Summary

The function of haemostasis components in the cause and progression of atherosclerosis gained considerable interest since a study by de Wood et al.[1] who showed the importance of coronary obstruction by thrombi and an epidemiological study by Meade et al.[2] who found that fibrinogen and a few other haemostasis parameters indicated the risk of a coronary event in a healthy population. In the years which followed several haemostasis components in blood, including platelet, coagulation and fibrinolysis factors, were found to have a different concentration from normals in individuals at cardiovascular risk. As most, if not all, changes of levels pointed towards a hypercoagulable state in stroke, coronary disease or peripheral atherosclerosis, the rationale of the association between haemostasis and cardiovascular disease in prospective studies seems to be obvious: a change in levels of a haemostatic parameter triggers arterial thrombosis, a key factor in the etiology of cardiovascular disease. Out of all the haemostatic risk factors, fibrinogen has a dominant place. It has been repeatedly found to be a risk factor in stroke, coronary heart disease and peripheral atherosclerosis.[3] Moreover, in contrast to other haemostatic risk factors, it is gradually correlated to the extent of the atherosclerosis as determined by coronary angiography[4] or ultrasound techniques.[5]

E.E. van der Wall et al. (eds.), Vascular Medicine, 13-21.
© 1997 *Kluwer Academic Publishers.*

Fibrinogen and the acute-phase response

Fibrinogen, like many other plasma proteins, is known as an acute-phase reactant. These reactants are mainly produced by hepatocytes and the increased expression of the acute-phase protein genes is driven by cytokines, which are produced by activated macrophages and other cells. During inflammation, infection or tissue damage, the plasma concentrations of some of the acute-phase reactants can rise by up to 10,000-fold.

The increase of fibrinogen levels in patients with cardiovascular disease, whether or not clinically manifest, may be associated with the intrinsic inflammation and tissue damage within the arterial lesions with extensive and severe atheroma resulting in raised concentrations of acute-phase reactants. This hypothesis presumes a continuous, low-grade acute-phase response in atherosclerosis.

To test this hypothesis, we compared increased fibrinogen levels in patients at coronary risk with levels of C-Reactive Protein (CRP), known as one of the most sensitive acute-phase proteins in human beings, in a prospective study, the ECAT (European Concerted Action on Thrombosis and Disabilities) Angina Pectoris (AP) study.

Results of the ECAT angina pectoris study

Fibrinogen

We conducted a prospective multicentre study of 3043 patients with non-severe angina pectoris who were followed up for two years.[6] Baseline measurements included the concentrations of plasma fibrinogen as derived from the clotting time according to the method of von Clauss.[7] Results were analysed in relation to the subsequent incidence of myocardial infarction or sudden coronary death. Baseline characteristics of the patients included are shown in Table 1. Of the 3043 patients enrolled in the study, 2960 were followed for two years. During this period 837 patients underwent coronary artery by-pass surgery, 223 coronary angioplasty, and 49 both interventions. A total of 106 definite coronary events was reported in the 2-year follow-up, 40 of which occurred in patients undergoing one of the above interventions just before or after the clinical event. An additional 154 major events did not fulfill the criteria for study end-points.

Multiple regression techniques indicated significant positive correlations between the concentration of fibrinogen and the incidence of coronary events. After adjustment for age, sex, centre and confounding factors including smoking status, body mass index, and the extent of coronary artery disease, fibrinogen concentrations in the group with events were, on

Table 1. Baseline characteristics of patients enrolled in the ECAT AP Study

	Cases n = 106	Controls n = 2700	P-value
Sex			0.18
Male (%)	90	85	
Age (yr)			0.02
<45	12	11	
45-69	78	85	
>69	9	4	
Smoking Status			0.60
Current smokers	24	20	
Ex-smokers	54	52	
Non smokers	23	29	
Type of Angina			0.06
Unstable*	58	48	
Stable	36	37	
Without typical chest pain	7	15	
Medications			
Aspirin	32	25	0.08
β-blockers	37	36	0.61
Calcium	69	66	0.59
Nitrates	73	65	0.11

* Either worsening of angina within the previous 4 weeks or angina at rest

the average, 6.5 % higher than those in the event-free group (P = 0.01).The risk for patients in the bottom fifth of the sample in terms of fibrinogen levels was nearly three times greater than for those in the top fifth (Table 2). The strength of this association in the patients with angina pectoris is similar in magnitude to that in healthy subjects.[6]
The baseline measurements of the acute-phase proteins fibrinogen and CRP were strongly correlated (r=0.49; P<0.001). This indicates that the fibrinogen level in the group of patients with angina pectoris is highly determined by the acute-phase response.

Table 2. Relative risk of coronary events according to the level of fibrinogen of patients enrolled in the ECAT AP Study (n = 2838)*

Quintile					Standardized Relative Risk**
1	2	3	4	5	(95% CI)
1.0	1.89	2.33	2.56	2.89	1.31 (1.07-1.61)

* The relative risk adjusted for all conforming factors. The group of patients with the lowest value (quintile 1) serves as the reference group
** The standardized relative risk is defined as the risk for each increase of one SD in fibrinogen concentration. CI Confidence Interval

The association of fibrinogen levels with the coronary risk was no longer significant after adjustment for confounding factors plus CRP. It strongly indicates that the acute-phase response contributes to the increase of fibrinogen in patients at risk.

C-Reactive protein
A surprising result was that CRP is a coronary risk factor itself. An ultrasensitive assay performed in Professor MB Pepys' laboratory (an automated microparticle enzyme immunoassay, Imx, Abbott Lab, Abbott Park, Illinois, USA), was used to determine CRP in a subgroup of 2121 patients of the ECAT AP study.[8] There was a positive and significant correlation between the CRP concentration and the incidence of coronary events, after adjustment for age, gender, centre, and other confounding factors, including smoking status, body mass index, and ejection fraction. The relative risk of a coronary event appeared to be about two times greater in the fifth quintile of CRP concentration than in the first four quintiles, irrespective of adjustment for other coronary risk factors (Table 3). Approximately one third of the coronary events during the 2 year follow-up were among patients with CRP concentrations of more than 3.6 mg/L at entry to the study.
This is the first time that CRP has been shown to be a risk factor in cardiovascular disease.[9] Thereupon, other studies extended this observation to healthy populations where CRP was a risk factor for myocardial infarction[10,11] and stroke.[10] Moreover, Ridker et al.[10] found that aspirin assignment was associated with a reduction in the risk of MI among men with baseline levels of CRP in the highest quartile. It suggests that aspirin may be effective in cardiovascular disease by virtue of its antiinflammatory

Table 3. Relative risk of coronary events by CRP concentrations of patients enrolled in the ECAT AP study (n = 2121)

Factors adjusted for		Relative Risk (95% CI)	Relative risk by quintiles* of CRP concentration (number of events)	
			quintile (1-4)	quintile 5
1. Age, centre		1.45(1.15-1.83)	1.0(48)	2.25(27)
2. As 1	+ medication	1.36(1.07-1.71)	1.0(48)	2.25(27)
3. As 2	+ smoking	1.27(1.00-1.60)	1.0(51)	1.89(24)
	+ body mass index			
	+ tryglycerides			

* Highest quintile CRP concentration (>3.6 mg/L) relative to those in quintiles 1-4 as reference group

action instead of its antiplatelet action. Liuzzo et al.[12] found that CRP predicted a poor outcome in patients with unstable angina.

Cardiovascular disease and acute-phase response

The acute-phase response observed in cardiovascular disease may simply reflect the intrinsic inflammation and tissue damage within the arterial lesions, with extensive and severe atheroma resulting in raised concentrations of fibrinogen and CRP. This hypothesis could explain the association of both acute-phase proteins with known risk factors for atherosclerosis. In this respect fibrinogen and CRP show a number of similarities; both are positively associated with age, smoking status, and body mass index. CRP, not fibrinogen, is negatively correlated with the angiographically determined ejection fraction (Table 4). Alternatively, or additionally, raised concentrations of fibrinogen and CRP may reflect inflammation, infection, or tissue damage elsewhere in the body that somehow promotes atherogenesis. For example, Helicobacter pylori,[13] Chlamydia pneumoniae infections[13] and bronchitis[14] are associated with

Table 4. Association of fibrinogen and CRP with known cardiovascular risk factors as determined in the ECAT AP Study

	Fibrinogen P-value*	CRP P-value*
Increased Age	< 0.001	< 0.001
Inreased Smoking Status	< 0.0001	< 0.0001
Increased Body Mass Index	0.003	< 0.001
Increased Triglycerides	NS**	< 0.001
Increased History of MI	NS	0.01
Decreased Ejection Fraction	NS	< 0.001

* The accociations with age were adjusted for gender and centre, the associations with other risk factors for age, gender and centre
** NS = non-significant (P > 0.01)

coronary heart disease.

Results obtained with CRP may not be extrapolated to all acute-phase reactants. For instance, Serum Amyloid A (SAA) Protein was not associated in the ECAT study with the risk of coronary events in patients with non-severe angina,[8] but it was so in severe unstable angina.[12] Apparently, either the regulation of its production, or the function of the acute-phase reactant is essential in this respect. Indeed, each acute-phase protein has its own specific function which may even contribute to the risk in cardiovascular disease. Raised fibrinogen levels may trigger coagulation, platelet aggregation, migration of smooth muscle cells and increase blood viscosity.[3] CRP stimulates the production by mononuclear cells of tissue factor,[15] the main initiator of blood coagulation. It interacts with LDL[16] and damaged cell membranes[17] and can activate the complement system.[18]

As a consequence, the causal role of the proteins cannot be excluded. They may contribute causally to the risk of a coronary event by virtue of their specific functions.

CRP, fibrinogen and cholesterol

An interesting, new aspect of the results of the ECAT AP study is that the predictive values of fibrinogen and CRP are independent of total cholesterol levels in blood.[6] Apparently, cholesterol levels are regulated by mechanisms completely different from those which regulate fibrinogen or CRP. This has important implications for the risk factor control. Assays of these proteins in plasma are, therefore, promising in addition to the determination of the cholesterol level.

Figure 1 shows that
- high concentrations of fibrinogen (> 3.31 g/L) and CRP (> 2.17 g/L) combined with hyper-cholesterolemia identify patients at particularly high risk for coronary events
- low concentrations of fibrinogen (< 2.71 g/L) and CRP (< 0.88 mg/L) indicates a low risk of new coronary events, even in patients with high serum cholesterol levels (> 6.8 mMol/L).

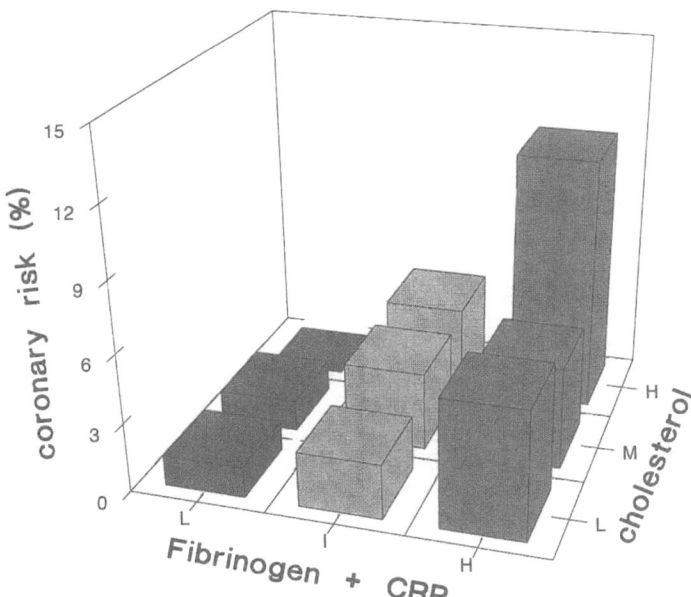

Figure 1. Incidence of coronary events during two years of follow-up according to concentrations of total cholesterol, and of the combined concentrations of fibrinogen and CRP. The concentrations of the variables are divided into three categories, L = Lower; M = middle for cholesterol; I (= intermediate) refers to all combinations of fibrinogen and CRP concentrations other than lower-lower or higher-higher; H = higher. Each category contains a third of the sample. The values of the tertiles are 2.71 and 3.31 g/L for fibrinogen, 5.79 and 6.80 mmol/L for cholesterol and 0.88 and 2.17 mg/L for CRP.

Conclusions

1. Fibrinogen is a strong and independent cardiovascular risk factor not only in apparently healthy people, but also in patients with manifest coronary artery disease. Its increase in patients at risk is associated with an acute-phase response.
2. CRP is an independent risk factor in cardiovascular disease, both in patients with angina and in apparently healthy people.
3. As increase of fibrinogen and CRP in individuals at risk is associated with the acute-phase response, they may reflect inflammation and tissue damage within the arterial lesions, or infection such as bronchitis which has been shown to be a risk factor for coronary events.
4. Causal effects of fibrinogen or CRP cannot be excluded. Each of them may contribute to a coronary event through their specific functions.
5. Both fibrinogen and CRP predict coronary events independent of cholesterol. Assays of fibrinogen and CRP may be highly useful in identifying patients with a low risk despite high cholesterol, and patients with a higher risk based not only on high cholesterol levels.

References

1. De Wood MA, Spores J, Notske R et al. Prevalence of total coronary occlusion during the early hours of transmural myocardial infarction. N Engl J Med 1980;303:897-902.
2. Meade TW, North WRS, Chakrabarti R, Stirling Y, Haines AP, Thompson SG. Haemostatic function and cardiovascular death: early results of a prospective study. Lancet 1980;i:1050-54.
3. Koenig W, Ernst E. Fibrinogen and artherothrombogenesis. Current Opinion Lipidol 1993;4:471-76.
4. Bolibar I, Kienast J, Thompson SG, Matthias R, Niessner H, Fechtrup C on behalf of the ECAT Angina Pectoris Study Group. Relation of fibrinogen to presence and severity of coronary artery disease is independent of other coexisting heart disease. Am Heart J 1993;125:1601-5.
5. Folsom AR, Wu KK, Shakar E, Davis CE for the Atherosclerosis Risk in Communities (ARIC) Study Investigators. Arterioscler Thromb 1993;13:1829-36.
6. Thompson SG, Kienast J, Pyke SDM, Haverkate F, Loo JCW van de, for the European Concerted Action on Thrombosis and Disabilities Angina Pectoris Study Group. Hemostatic factors and the risk of myocardial infarction or sudden death in patients with angina pectoris. N Engl J Med 1995;332:635-41.
7. Clauss von A. Gerinnungsphysiologische Schnellmethode zur Bestimmung des Fibrinogens. Acta Haematol 1957;17:237-46.
8. Haverkate F, Thompson SG, Pyke SDM, Gallimore JR, Pepys MB for the European Concerted Action on Thrombosis and Disabilities Angina Pectoris Study Group. Lancet 1997;349:462-66.
9. Haverkate F. Low-grade acute-phase reactions in arteriosclerosis and the

consequences for haemostatic risk factors. Fibrinolysis 1992;6(Suppl.3):17-18.

10. Ridker PM, Cushman M, Stampfer MJ, Tracy RP, Hennekens CH. Inflammation, aspirin, and the risk of cardiovascular disease in apparently healthy men. N Engl J Med 1997;336:973-9.

11. Kuller LH, Tracy RP, Shaten J, Meilahn EN, for the MRFIT Research Group. Relation of C-reactive Protein and Coronary Heart Disease in the MRFIT nested case-control study. Am J Epidemiol 1996;144:537-47.

12. Liuzzo G, Biasucci LM, Gallimore JR et al. The prognostic value of C-Reactive Protein and Serum Amyloid A Protein in severe unstable angina. N Engl J Med 1994;331:417-24.

13. Patel P, Mendall MA, Carrington D et al. Association of Helicobactor pylori and Chlamydia pneumoniae infections with coronary heart disease and cardiovascular risk factors. Br Med J 1995;311:711-4.

14. Jousilahti P, Vartiainen E, Tuomilehto J, Puska P. Symptoms of chronic bronchitis and risk of coronary disease. Lancet 1996;348:567-72.

15. Cermak J, Key NS, Bach RR, Balla J, Jacob HS, Vercellotti GM. C-Reactive Protein induces human peripheral blood monocytes to synthesize tissue factor. Blood 1993;82:513-520.

16. Pepys MB, Rowe IF, Baltz ML. C-Reactive Protein: binding to lipids and lipoproteins. Int Rev Exp Pathol 1985;27:83-111.

17. Volanakis JE, Narkas AJ. Interaction of C-Reactive protein with artificial phosphatidyl-choline bilayers and complement. J Immunol 1981;126:1820-25.

18. Volanakis JE. Complement activation by C-Reactive Protein complexes. Ann N Y Acad Sci 1982;389:235-50.

INFLAMMATORY ACTIVITY IN THE PATHOGENESIS OF UNSTABLE ANGINA

Peter W.H.M. Verheggen, Volkert Manger Cats

Summary

Unstable angina, non-Q wave and Q-wave myocardial infarction are collectively known as the acute coronary syndromes as they share a common pathophysiology. In contrast with the reversible syndrome of stable angina, the acute coronary syndromes occur unpredictably, most often without provocation by activity. Unstable angina is thought to be the result of plaque rupture, ulceration or erosion complicated by intracoronary thrombus formation restricting coronary flow with subsequent myocardial ischemia.[1]

Since the introduction of coronary arteriography, cardiologists have judged the severity of atherosclerotic lesions by anatomical standards such as lumen diameter stenosis. This approach still holds for exercise-induced stable angina. In unstable angina, however, it could be argued that for reasons of pathophysiology, coronary lesions could better be classified as biologically active or inactive. Presently, a low-grade, chronic inflammatory response is central in the most cohesive theory of atherogenesis, the "response to injury" hypothesis.[2] If atherosclerosis is viewed as chronic inflammation, the conversion of a lesion from inactive to active could result from activation of the inflammatory process. This chapter deals with various aspects of inflammation related to the pathogenesis of the acute coronary syndromes, in particular unstable angina.

E.E. van der Wall et al. (eds.), Vascular Medicine, 23-31.
© 1997 *Kluwer Academic Publishers.*

Inflammation in coronary plaque disruption

The atherosclerotic plaque contains monocytes, macrophages and T-lymphocytes. However, these cell types are much more abundant in unstable than stable coronary plaques, suggesting that an inflammatory process and recruitment of additional cells precedes clinical manifestations. This finding has been documented in histopathologic studies both at autopsy and in living patients.

Sato et al.[3] found significant monocellular infiltrates in 30% of patients dying within one month of an episode of unstable angina, compared with 8% of patients dying due to coronary artery disease but without unstable angina. Moreno et al.[4] designed a study to identify and quantify the macrophage content of human coronary plaque tissue from patients with well defined ischemic coronary syndromes. They examined atherectomy specimens from patients with unstable angina, non-Q-wave infarction, and stable angina. Plaque area was similar in the three groups, but the proportion of plaque containing macrophages was 13% in unstable angina, 14% in non-Q-wave infarction and only 3% in stable angina. Van der Wal et al.[5] studied the cellular characteristics of coronary plaques in 20 patients who died from acute myocardial infarction. Macrophages were the predominant cells at the immediate site of either rupture or superficial erosion of the fibrous cap. These cells expressed the HLA-DR antigens, indicating that they were in an activated state. HLA-DR activity was low in other areas of the plaque.

Relation between inflammatory cell function and thrombosis

In patients with unstable angina, monocytes express thrombogenic substances that may directly affect the balance between thrombolytic and thrombotic activity at the culprit lesion. Activated lymphocytes are present in patients with unstable angina. Pure monocyte cultures from patients with unstable angina do not express procoagulant activity until they are exposed to lymphocytes from patients with unstable angina. Monocytes isolated from the peripheral blood of patients with unstable angina express increased levels of tissue factor, a membrane glycoprotein that initiates the extrinsic coagulation cascade, and possibly are able to contribute to an enhanced thrombotic state.[6] This activity is high when measured in monocytes from peripheral blood of patients with unstable angina but is low in monocytes from patients with stable angina, noncardiac chest pain or normal subjects. Fibrinopeptide A, a marker of thrombin formation, and monocyte procoagulant activity move together, being elevated in the active phase but returning to normal in the inactive state in coronary artery disease.[7]

Lymphocyte activation and the expression of monocyte procoagulant activity do not appear to be an epiphenomenon of myocardial ischemia, because they are not found in patients with stable angina.[7]

Effects of circulating inflammatory cells in unstable angina

Leukocytes and their products can activate many processes at the culprit lesion of acute coronary syndromes. Recent studies have examined leukocyte membrane markers in patients with unstable angina. Among these markers are the CD11/CD18 glycoproteins, of which the CD11b/CD18 category is functionally the most important. Expression of this marker is induced by inflammation.[8]

The CD11/CD18 molecule on granulocyte and monocyte membranes facilitates the adhesion of these cells to endothelium. Adhesion occurs early in any inflammatory response and is probably a crucial step in the pathogenesis of vascular injury as observed in acute coronary syndromes. Mazzone et al.[9] measured CD11b/CD18 expression on granulocytes and monocytes obtained from the coronary sinus and aorta during cardiac catheterization in patients with non-cardiac chest pain and stable and unstable angina. No gradient across the coronary circulation was detected in patients with non-cardiac chest pain or stable angina. However, in patients with unstable angina, CD11b/CD18 expression was higher on granulocytes and monocytes from the coronary sinus. Rab et al.[10] documented an increase in monocyte-macrophage HLA-DR surface antigens, indicative of activation of the cell, in patients with unstable angina but not in normal subjects or in control subjects with cardiomyopathy. These results indicate that an inflammatory process is taking place within the coronary circulation of patients with unstable angina.

Not only leukocyte surface markers are activated in unstable angina. Studies demonstrated that neutrophil function and secretion have changed as well. During chest pain in unstable angina, neutrophils release the enzyme elastase which can damage endothelium and basement membranes.[11,12]

Leukotrienes are substances released by leukocytes that cause a variety of deleterious effects on granulocytes in contact with endothelium and damage endothelial structure. Urinary excretion of leukotrienes has been reported to be higher in patients with unstable coronary syndromes when compared with normal subjects or patients with stable angina.[13] Vaddi et al.[14] investigated cytokine production by mononuclear leukocytes from patients with ischemic heart disease. They measured kinetics of secretion of tumor necrosis factor-α and interferon-γ by mononuclear leukocytes from 8 control subjects, 10 patients with stable angina, and 10 patients with unstable angina pectoris. Secretion of both tumor necrosis factor-α and interferon-γ by mononuclear cells was consistently higher in patients compared to control subjects. The authors concluded that increased cytokine secretion is associated with ischemic heart disease.[14]

Circulating inflammatory markers and prognosis in unstable angina

Markers of inflammation might reflect the intensity of the underlying inflammatory process in coronary artery disease. Similarly, levels of inflammatory markers might predict short and long term course and clinical events. Haverkate et al.[15] investigated the existence and possible significance of the acute phase response as reflected in C-reactive protein (CRP) levels in patients with stable angina. They used a highly sensitive immunoassay to measure CRP in 2121 patients with stable angina. All patients underwent coronary angiography and extensive clinical and laboratory assessment at study entry, and were then followed for 2 years. Concentrations of CRP at study entrance were associated with the occurrence of coronary events. There was a two-fold increase in the risk of a coronary event in patients whose CRP concentration was in the fifth quintile (>3.6 mg/L), compared with the first four quintiles. A third of the events occurred among patients who had a CRP concentration of more than 3.6 mg/l.

Mendall et al.[16] studied 303 men aged 50-69 years selected from general practice registers and found that the prevalence of indirect evidence of ischemic heart disease increased progressively as blood concentration of CRP rose. In a recently published report of a longitudinal follow-up study in apparently healthy men participating in the Physicians Health Study, plasma CRP concentrations among 543 men who went on to have myocardial infarction or ischemic stroke were higher than among 543 men without vascular events. The use of aspirin in this study group was associated with significant reductions in the risk of myocardial infarction among men in the highest quartile of CRP concentration, but with only small, nonsignificant reductions among those in the lowest quartile.[17]

Other studies have demonstrated systemic evidence of acute inflammation in unstable angina. Berk et al.[18] found elevated levels of CRP in 90% of patients with unstable angina, compared with 13% of stable angina patients. Serial CRP levels correlated with clinical outcome.

In a study of Liuzzo et al.[19], CRP, serum amyloid A protein and troponin-T was measured in 32 patients with chronic stable angina, 31 with severe unstable angina, and 29 with acute myocardial infarction. Sixty-five percent of patients with unstable angina had elevations of both CRP and serum amyloid A protein levels compared to 13% of patients with stable angina. Patients with unstable angina and elevations of these inflammatory markers were more likely to experience recurrent chest pain and had more ischemia during Holter monitoring. Sixty percent of them required revascularization compared with 18% of patients with unstable angina without elevated levels of these markers. Coronary events were much more common in patients with unstable angina and elevated CRP and serum amyloid A protein levels. Troponin-T levels were normal in all included patients, ruling out myocardial necrosis as a cause of elevated levels of markers of inflammation. The increased concentrations of CRP in patients with unstable angina remain unexplained. No correlation was found between CRP level and the extent of coronary atherosclerosis in patients with stable angina, and neither was it related to minor degrees of myocardial necrosis or to prolonged ischemic episodes in patients with variant angina.[20]

CRP is synthesized and secreted by the liver after stimulation by inflammatory mediators such as interleukin-6 (IL-6). IL-6 is a cytokine with proinflammatory and procoagulant activity. Biasucci et al.[21] measured levels of IL-6 and CRP in 38 patients with unstable angina at the time of their admission to the coronary care unit and in 29 patients with stable angina. They hypothesized that if IL-6 is involved directly in the mechanisms that lead to instability, it should be elevated in unstable angina and should be related to levels of CRP and therefore to prognosis. Median IL-6 levels were 5.25 pg/ml in patients with unstable angina but were below the detection limit of the assay in patients with stable angina. A significant correlation was observed between IL-6 en CRP levels. This study strengthens the importance of IL-6 in the pathophysiology of unstable angina and supports the hypothetical assumption that elevated levels of acute phase proteins result from activation of the cytokine-inflammatory pathway.

Fibrinogen, also an acute phase protein, has been identified in several large-scale epidemiological studies as an independent predictor of thrombotic cardiovascular events. And, because it is a pivotal component of the coagulation cascade, it may be more directly involved in the clinical expression of atherosclerotic coronary artery disease than non-specific markers of inflammation. The hepatic synthesis of fibrinogen is regulated primarily by IL-6 released from activated monocytes. In patients with unstable angina, monocyte tissue factor expression and plasma fibrinogen correlated closely; both correlated directly with the degree of activation of the coagulation system and with fibrin formation.[22] In the TIMI IIIB trial the prognostic value of fibrinogen was studied in 1473 patients with unstable angina and non-Q-wave infarction.[23] Overall, no association was found between baseline fibrinogen and the occurrence of myocardial infarction or cardiac death during hospital stay (≤10 days). However, patients with spontaneous ischemia had higher fibrinogen concentrations than those without this event. A baseline fibrinogen concentration $\geq$ 3 g/l was associated with a modest trend toward an increased risk of death, myocardial infarction or spontaneous ischemia.

These results strengthen the pathobiologic link between atherosclerosis, inflammation, thrombosis, and coronary events.

Infectious agents related to the pathogenesis of coronary artery disease

Knowledge regarding the mechanisms by which the various established risk factors may contribute to the development of an inflammatory process in coronary artery disease is incomplete. This has led investigators to pursue other possible etiologies and factors that may be involved. An alternate explanation that recently has received considerable attention is the infectious theory of atherosclerosis. In particular Chlamydia pneumoniae, Helicobacter pylori, Herpes simplex virus, and Cytomegalovirus have been implicated as possible primary etiologic factors or cofactors in the pathogenesis of atherosclerosis, including the acute coronary syndromes. However, the results of different studies are not unequivocal and more research is needed to elucidate the role for infectious agents in atherosclerotic heart disease.

Clinical implications

Although the factors involved in the transition from stable to unstable coronary artery disease are incompletely understood, the evidence reviewed clearly supports a role for an inflammatory process in the pathogenesis of unstable angina. Stimulation of lymphocytes and macrophages within the plaque, secretion of chemotactic factors and lysosomal enzymes, breakdown of the connective tissue skeleton of the plaque predisposing it to fissure, exposure of thrombogenic material inside the plaque, platelet activation, thrombosis, and recruitment of large numbers of white cells with secretion of enzymes and inflammatory mediators, are factors involved in the development of instability.

However, most plaque ruptures do not precipitate a coronary event. The formation of a thrombus large enough to impede flow is an exceptional rather than a usual consequence of plaque rupture. It can be postulated that the acute inflammatory process is an important factor promoting thrombus formation in acute coronary syndromes, but the fibrinolytic system as a rule prevents the development of significant thrombus. Therefore, should the inflammatory process be a target of therapy in acute coronary syndromes?

In contrast to antianginal, antiplatelet, and antithrombotic drugs that interfere with late events in the pathophysiologic cascade of unstable angina, antiinflammatory drugs would be directed at an earlier component of the cascade. Attenuation of the inflammatory response in the arterial wall by statins may be associated with a decreased risk of subsequent acute events, even without substantial reduction in the degree of obstruction. This view may explain the provocative observations in recent trials of lipid-lowering therapy for regression of coronary artery disease.

Conclusion

The data presented strongly suggest that an acute inflammatory process is an early component in the pathophysiology of unstable angina. The culprit atherosclerotic plaque in patients with unstable angina contains many activated macrophages and lymphocytes, particularly at the site of plaque rupture. Leukocyte membrane markers of activation such as the CD11b/CD18 glycoprotein are present at higher levels in coronary sinus effluent than in peripheral blood in patients with unstable angina. Activated leukocytes secrete leukotrienes, cytokines, metalloproteinases and procoagulant factors, which may cause a variety of deleterious effects at the culprit lesion. Markers of systemic inflammation such as CRP, interleukin-6 and fibrinogen are elevated in unstable angina and increased levels are associated with short-term outcome.

The phenomenon of infiltration of the coronary arteries by inflammatory mononuclear cells is particularly important, since atherosclerosis is increasingly thought to be a chronic inflammatory disease that develops in response to metabolic, physical, or environmental injuries such as hypercholesterolemia, hypertension, or cigarette smoking. One of the characteristic features of active inflammatory responses is the capacity of secreted lytic enzymes to break down connective tissue, causing tissue destruction and compromising structural integrity. These local cellular actions probably account for the local weakening of the plaque that results in rupture. In this context, the biologic (inflammatory) state of a coronary lesion may be a more important determinant of the clinical outcome than, for example, the degree of stenosis.

The actual chain of events involved in this process is still not known and research must continue in this important field of the pathogenesis of atherosclerosis.

References

1. Fuster V, Badimon L, Badimon JJ, Chesebro JH. The pathogenesis of coronary artery disease and the acute coronary syndromes: Part 1 and 2. N Engl J Med 1992;326:242-50 and 310-8.
2. Ross R. The pathogenesis of atherosclerosis: a perspective for the 1990s. Nature 1993;362:801-9.
3. Sato T, Takebayashi S, Kohchi K. Increased subendothelial infiltration of the coronary arteries with monocytes/macrophages in patients with unstable angina: Histological data on 14 autopsied patients. Atherosclerosis 1987;68:191-7.
4. Moreno PR, Falk E, Palacios IF, Nervell JB, Fuster V, Fallon JT. Macrophage infiltration in acute coronary syndromes: implication for plaque rupture. Circulation 1994;90:775-8.
5. van der Wal AC, Becker AE, van de Loos CM, Das PK. Site of intimal rupture or erosion of thrombosed coronary atherosclerotic plaques is characterized by an inflammatory process irrespective of the dominant plaque morphology. Circulation 1994;89:36-44.
6. Serneri GG, Abbate R, Gori AM et al. Transient intermittent lymphocyte activation is responsible for the unstability of angina. Circulation 1992;86:790-7.
7. Jude B, Agraou B, McFadden EP et al. Evidence for time-dependent activation of monocytes in the systemic circulation in unstable angina but not in acute myocardial infarction or in stable angina. Circulation 1994;90:1662-8.
8. Smith CW, Rothlein R, Hughes BJ et al. Recognition of an endothelial determinant of CD18-dependent human neutrophil adherence and transendothelial migration. J Clin Invest 1988;82:1746-56.
9. Mazzone A, de Servi B, Ricevuti G et al. Increased expression of neutrophil and monocyte adhesion molecules in unstable coronary artery disease. Circulation 1993;88:358-63.
10. Rab ST, Alexander RW, Ansari AA. Evidence for activated circulating macrophages/monocytes in unstable angina. J Am Coll Cardiol 1990;15:168A.
11. Mehta J, Dinerman J, Mehta P et al. Neutrophil function in ischemic heart disease. Circulation 1989;79:549-56.
12. Dinerman JL, Mehta JL, Saldeen TGP et al. Increased neutrophil elastase release in unstable angina pectoris and acute myocardial infarction. J Am Coll Cardiol 1990;15:1559-63.
13. Carry M, Korley V, Willerson J, Weigelt T, Ford-Hutchinson A, Tagari P. Increased urinary leukotrine excretion in patients with cardiac ischemia.Circulation 1992;85:230-6.
14. Vaddi K, Nicolini FA, Mehta P, Mehta JL. Increased secretion of tumor necrosis factor-α and interferon-γ by mononuclear leukocytes in patients with ischemic heart disease. Circulation 1994;90:694-9.
15. Haverkate F, Thompson SG, Pyke SDM, Gallimore JR, Pepys MB, for the European Concerted Action on Thrombosis and Disabilities Angina Pectoris Study Group. Production of C-reactive protein and risk of coronary events in stable and unstable angina. Lancet 1997;349:462-6.
16. Mendall MA, Patel P, Ballam L, Strachan D, Northfield TC. C-reactive protein and its relation to cardiovascular risk factors: a population based cross sectional study. BMJ 1996;312:1061-5.
17. Ridker PM, Cushman M, Stampfer MJ, Tracey RP, Hennekens CH. Inflammation,

aspirin, and the risk of cardiovascular disease in apparently healthy men. N Engl J Med 1997;336:973-9.

18. Berk BC, Weintraub WS, Alexander RW. Elevation of C-reactive Protein in "active" coronary artery disease. Am J Cardiol 1990;65:168-72.

19. Liuzzo G, Biasucci LM, Gallimore JR et al. The prognostic value of C-reactive protein and Serum Amyloid A Protein in severe unstable angina. N Engl J Med 1994;331:417-24.

20. Liuzzo G, Biasucci LM, Rebuzzi AG et al. Plasma protein acute-phase response in unstable angina is not induced by ischemic injury. Circulation 1996;94:2373-80.

21. Biasucci LM, Ciliberto G, Liuzzo G et al. Elevated levels of Interleukin-6 in unstable angina. Circulation 1996;94:874-7.

22. Ceriello A, Pirisi M, Giacomello R et al. Fibrinogen plasma levels as a marker of thrombin activation: new insights on the role of fibrinogen as a cardiovascular risk factor. Thromb Haemost 1994;17:593-5.

23. Becker RC, Cannon CP, Bovill EG et al., for the TIMI III Investigators. Prognostic value of plasma fibrinogen concentration in patients with unstable angina and non-Q-wave myocardial infarction. Am J Cardiol 1996;78:142-7.

EFFECTS OF CORONARY ENDOTHELIUM ON SYSTOLIC MYOCARDIAL FUNCTION

Jan Baan, Paul Steendijk, Jan Baan Jr.

Summary

Homeometric autoregulation (HAR) of the heart describes the effect of a change in arterial pressure on ventricular performance. When afterload is increased, the ventricle maintains its output (stroke volume) while end-diastolic volume remains unaltered. In other terms, this effect comes down to an increased end-systolic pressure generated at identical end-systolic volume, a clear mark of increased inotropic state of the ventricle. When realizing that increased aortic pressure is accompanied by increased coronary perfusion pressure and flow it is plausible that the mechanism for the phenomenon resides in the coronary vasculature. A paracrine effect of not only endocardial but also vascular endothelial factors on myocardial cells has been shown to exist recently. Studies sofar were performed mainly in isolated cardiac muscle and isolated perfused heart preparations. This study represents an initial attempt to demonstrate the involvement of the coronary vascular endothelium in HAR in the intact animal. This was done by disabling the vascular endothelium by intra coronary injection of Triton X-100 in anaesthetized sheep in which left ventricular pressure and volume (conductance catheter) were measured during different afterload conditions. The limited set of experiments indicate that disabling the vascular endothelium indeed tends to obliterate the HAR effect, which leads to the preliminary conclusion that endothelial cell factors have a positive inotropic effect in the heart in situ.

E.E. van der Wall et al. (eds.), Vascular Medicine, 33-43.
© 1997 *Kluwer Academic Publishers.*

Introduction

Our interest in the effects of loading conditions on left ventricular (LV) performance in situ dates back to 1985. The development of the conductance catheter enables one to study ventricular pressure-volume relationships in the intact animal and patients.[1] Earlier, these relationships had been measured primarily in the isolated canine heart, in which Suga and Sagawa, using an intraventricular balloon to measure and control volume, had shown the remarkable ability of the end-systolic pressure-volume relation (ESPVR) to reflect the contractile performance of the ventricle, hardly influenced by loading conditions. A steeper ESPVR (increased elastance, Ees) reflected enhanced inotropy and the reverse was true for a decreased inotropy.[2] Later, Lew showed in the in-situ canine heart that a leftward shift of the ESPVR without much change in its slope was equally characteristic for an increased inotropic state.[3] In our studies of the behaviour of the ESPVR under different loading conditions we showed that increasing afterload by gradual (partial) aortic occlusion led to a much steeper relationship than increased preload by volume loading.[4,5] Later, we showed that this effect was similar when afterload was modified in a steady-state fashion[6] and that the effect remained present after surgical denervation of the heart.[7] An important clue for the mechanism of this phenomenon was thought to lie in the mechanism of shortening deactivation: when the heart produces increased stroke volume (i.e. increased muscle shortening) with volume loading, the pressure (i.e. muscle force) decreases in comparison to the situation in which the heart produces decreasing stroke volume with aortic occlusion. To a certain extent, this phenomenon, originally described by Brady for cardiac muscle,[8] was also present in the isolated heart as found by Suga et al.[9], but in the intact heart the observed difference in ESPVR for preload versus afterload changes was much larger. In our group, Van der Linden et al. succeeded in quantifying the difference in slopes almost completely by a stroke volume (i.e. shortening-related) effect, but effects of changes in intrinsic myocardial contractile performance were characterized only in terms of the early-systolic parameter dP/dtmax, corrected for its dependence on pre- and afterload.[10]

To rule out the effects of shortening deactivation on the behaviour of the ESPVR, we performed a study in newborn lambs in which the relationships were measured under different steady-state afterload conditions using partial to total occlusion of the descending aorta, and varying preload by vena caval occlusion. Like before in the canine experiments,[6] the ESPVR shifted leftward to a smaller volume intercept as afterload was higher. However, by comparing heartbeats with equal end-diastolic volume (EDV) from different afterload conditions, we found that on these beats stroke volume (SV) was nearly equal (differences were statistically nonsignificant) while, by design, systolic LV pressure was higher.[11] (Figure 1.) This is considered a classical example of the phenomenon of homeometric autoregulation (HAR). The left part, however, also shows that each step of increased afterload, a higher end-systolic pressure (ESP) is generated at identical end-systolic volume (ESV). In other words, the same ESP is generated at increasingly smaller ESV values. A similar behaviour was shown for the related variables stroke work and dP/dtmax (both matched for identical EDV), which increased for higher afterloads.[11]

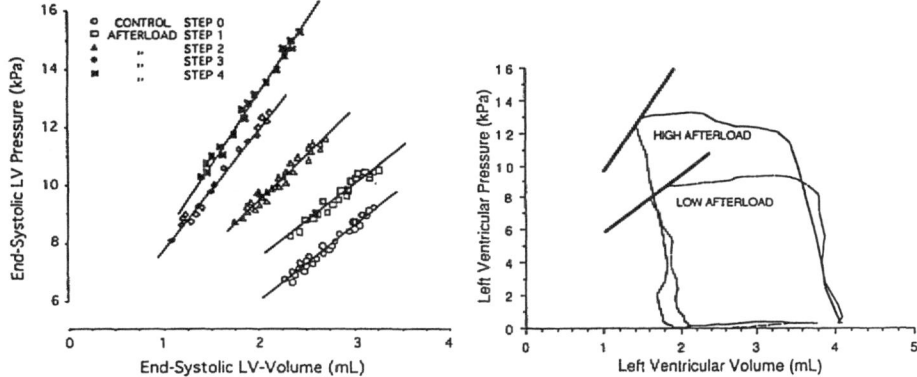

Figure 1. *Left: End-Systolic Pressure-Volume relations (ESPVR) in a lamb at 5 different levels of afterload differing at least 1 kPa between steps. At each afterload step, ESPVR were obtained by vena caval occlusion. With each step, relations became somewhat steeper and shifted to the left, indicating increased inotropic state. Right: Effect of increase in afterload on the P-V loop at matched preload conditions. The increased afterload caused beats ejecting from the same preload to reach a higher systolic pressure and stroke work, while end-systolic volume and stroke volume remained constant. The heavy lines indicate the ESPVR's in both conditions (Reproduced by permission from Klautz et al.[11])*

Homeometric autoregulation

The phenomenon was originally described by Von Anrep who found evidence for increased cardiac performance after increasing arterial pressure.[12] It was later confirmed by the work of Sarnoff et al. who studied LV pressure and volume in the isolated canine heart-lung preparation in which stroke volume was controlled by a pump.[13] After increasing aortic pressure they found that SV was maintained at equal EDV after this had undergone a small and transient increase. They coined the term homeometric autoregulation (HAR), discerning the effect from the well-known Starling effect or heterometric regulation, by which performance is increased by increased filling.[13] The existence of the HAR effect in the normally contracting heart in situ has been doubted until recently.[14] Causes for the effect have been attributed alternatively to (a), ischemia-caused poor performance of the isolated heart preparation, which presumably suffers from insufficient endocardial perfusion, improved by the increase in coronary perfusion concomitant with the increased afterload,[15] or (b) the so-called erectile effect of increased coronary pressure which would tend to stretch the myocardium in such a way as to enhance its performance through the Starling mechanism.[16] Neither of these effects probably play an important role, because in case of (a), the effect would not be observed in the normally working, healthy heart as found in our experiments, and in case of (b), the effect should have been accompanied by an observed increase in EDV.

There is probably a close resemblance of the HAR effect with the well-known Gregg effect, which describes the increase in myocardial performance and oxygen consumption upon an increase in coronary perfusion pressure or flow.[17] The effect was recently shown to be unequivocally present in isolated papillary and trabecular muscle,[18] the isolated canine heart studied by ESPVR and Suga's concept of pressure-volume area (PVA)-related myocardial oxygen consumption,[19] as well as in the intact dog preparation.[20] All of these studies show a marked positive inotropic effect of increased perfusion, although its existence is still doubted in more recent studies.[21] An important difference in comparison to the HAR phenomenon, however, lies in the experimental setup in which the Gregg phenomenon is demonstrated. Invariably this employs a separate perfusion of the left coronary artery, thus uncoupling coronary perfusion pressure from aortic pressure, while the HAR effect deals with the more normal physiological situation of coupled coronary and aortic pressure. Moreover, while it is a standard and classical question in studying the Gregg effect, myocardial oxygen consumption is generally no issue in studies of the HAR effect, because the ventricular performance increase by raising afterload invariably is accompanied by increased stroke work which by necessity entails increased oxygen demand.

In spite of these differences, it is very likely that the effects of changes in afterload and coronary perfusion pressure or flow on ventricular performance have a common mechanism which, by straightforward reasoning, may lie in a messenger transmitted to the myocardium via the coronary vessel wall. In this connection, it seems logical to suppose that the coronary vascular endothelium should play an important role.

The role of the endothelium

The group of Brutsaert was the first to hypothesize and prove a role for the *endocardial* endothelium in influencing myocardial performance. Using isolated trabecular muscle strips, Brutsaert and his colleagues showed that damage or removal of endocardial endothelium diminished force development in late systole and earlier relaxation of isotonically contracting muscle fibres.[22] A similar effect on LV pressure was observed later in the intact heart after damaging the endocardium by ultrasound.[23] These effects are probably caused by increased myofibrillar calcium sensitivity.[24,25] Subsequently, studies have been published in which the effects of coronary endothelial products on myocardial mechanics were measured, mostly in isolated muscle strips or isolated hearts.[26-28] In the putative role of coronary perfusion pressure and flow we must realize that, especially in a preparation in which (diastolic and systolic) muscle length is unaltered, the only components of the ventricle undergoing appreciable mechanical changes during a change in perfusion pressure are the cells in the coronary vascular wall. Especially the endothelium is affected by changes in radial stress induced by pressure and in shear stress induced by flow. These mechanical disturbances have been shown in numerous studies to induce metacrine and paracrine effects. Mechanical stimulation of isolated endothelial cells leads to increased intracellular calcium spreading to adjacent cells, most likely through stretch-activated ion channels,[29] while flow-induced shear stress was shown to elevate endothelial cGMP.[30] Cyclic strain was shown to increase endothelial nitric oxide synthase (NOS) activity.[31]

Products of the endothelial cell include EDRF, presently identified as nitric oxide (NO), endothelin (ET-1), prostanoids, PGE2, natriuretic products, but the list is not complete as other factors presently unidentified yet, such as 'myofilament desensitizing agent', may also be present.[32] NO has different effects on myocardial contractile performance, positive or negative depending on its concentration, while endothelin-1 is one of the most potent vasoconstrictors through its positive inotropic action, which it exerts its effects not only on vascular smooth muscle, but also on myocardium.[33] Interestingly, sodium nitroprusside, as exogenous donor of NO, has negative effects on systolic pressure and speeds up relaxation when injected into the coronary arterial tree in human subjects, and the same phenomenon was observed when substance P, which releases NO from the coronary endothelium, was injected.[34] Strikingly, no effects of these drugs were seen on the early-systolic contractility parameter dP/dtmax, while, in addition, they have important effects on diastolic chamber compliance.

Pilot experiment with disabling endothelial function

In a pilot study with young sheep (25-35 kg), we aimed at constructing

ESPVR's at different afterloads with and without a functional vascular endothelium to determine its effects on the HAR phenomenon. The sheep were anaesthetized with ketamine (4-10 mg/kg/hr i.v.) and xylazine (1 mg/kg i.m.), and instrumented with a Millar 5F catheter-tip micro manometer for LV pressure measurement, and a 6F, 12-pole conductance catheter (Sentron, Roden, NL) to measure LV volume, using a LEYCOM Sigma-5DF signal conditioner-processor (CardioDynamics, Zoetermeer, NL). A balloon catheter was placed in the inferior vena cava for volume reduction for the purpose of obtaining ESPVR. A second balloon catheter was placed in the descending thoracic aorta which, by different degrees of inflation, enabled us to obtain 4 steady-state levels of pressure in the ascending aorta i.e. step 1) no occlusion, step 2) slight occlusion, step 3) severe occlusion, and step 4) total occlusion.

A fluid-filled catheter was placed in the ascending aorta to measure aortic and coronary perfusion pressure. After opening the chest through the 5th intercostal space, the pericardial sac was opened and a flow probe (Transonic Systems, Inc, Ithaca, NY) was fitted around the left circumflex coronary artery for measurement of coronary flow. Coronary vascular resistance in this bed was measured by dividing perfusion pressure by flow. Next, a 4F catheter was placed in the same coronary artery for infusion of drugs (see below) and Triton X-100, a substance which has been shown to obliterate the function of the endothelium, probably without actually destroying the cells.[27] The initial dosage used was the same as used by the above investigators, but it was increased as required to obtain the desired effect of dysfunctional endothelium (repeated injections of 0.5 ml, 0.25% Triton X-100).

The latter effect was tested by the method introduced by Furchgott through intracoronary infusion of acetylcholine (target blood concentration 10^{-5} to 10^{-6} M) which gives vasodilation when the endothelium is intact.[35] After an effective dosage of Triton X-100, the vasodilatory action of acetylcholine was reversed to a vasoconstrictive one, while the endothelium-independent vasodilatory action of papaverine was maintained. Vasoconstriction as well as dilation was tested by calculating the coronary vascular resistance of the left circumflex arterial bed.

Before and after effective dysfunction of the endothelium, tested as indicated above, P-V loops of the left ventricle were obtained by vena caval balloon occlusion at each of the 4 levels of afterload.

So far, two experiments were carried out successfully. The results, however, were almost identical. In spite of the circumstance that, in this preliminary study, Triton X-100 was injected only into the circumflex coronary artery, thus leaving the left anterior descending coronary artery unaffected, there was a clear difference in the behaviour of the ESPVR. With intact endothelium, the ESPVR of the afterloaded runs in steps 2-4, i.e. increased with respect to step 1 (normal afterload), were remarkably steeper and displaced to the left, thus reflecting an intact HAR phenomenon, similar to the effect observed previously in the newborn lamb (Figure 1, left). In contrast, after successful Triton X-100 treatment all ESPVR lines were much closer together or even coincided for the 4 afterload steps.

Discussion

Our preliminary conclusion from these findings is that indeed the coronary vascular endothelium plays an important role in the phenomenon of homeometric autoregulation, possibly by no longer being able to produce an (as yet unknown) substance which enables the myocardium to respond to the increased afterload conditions with increased contractile performance. Endothelin-1 may play an important role in this effect, in the light of its known positive inotropic effects[28,33,36] and the fact that ET_A receptors are present on myocytes.[37] On the other hand, endothelium mediated release of NO in proper concentrations cannot be excluded either.

The only study known to us at this moment to have investigated the effect of dysfunctioning endothelium (also using Triton X-100) on effects of increased perfusion is the recently published work by Westerhof's group.[38] These investigators studied the isovolumically contracting, Langendorff, crystalloid perfused rat heart specifically to investigate the Gregg effect. They found no influence of the coronary arterial endothelium on this phenomenon. However, the fact that these hearts were perfused with a crystalloid instead of by whole blood might explain their findings which seem to deviate from our results. Effective dysfunction of the endothelium, namely, may be obtained by brief perfusion with Krebs solution at high pressure[39] or hypotonic Tyrode solution.[40] Thus, the possibility exists that the procedure of preparing the Langendorff setup and the perfusion with a blood substitute has in fact modified the response of the endothelium to the Triton X-100 treatment. Besides, the difference in species (rat versus sheep) may have been of influence. However, it should be noted that, generally, the load depndence observed by us in vivo, also in dogs, was much larger than in those instances when it was observed in the isolated canine heart preparation.[9]

It is interesting that Van der Linden's sophisticated statistical analysis of our previous data obtained in the dog indicated no appreciable role for modification of contractile performance by increased afterload conditions insofar as indicated by the (load corrected) pre-ejection parameter dP/dtmax. Using this approach Van der Linden et al. were not able to analyze an end-systolic parameter.[10] Similarly, practically no effects on dP/dtmax were observed by dysfunction of either endocardial[22] or vascular endothelium,[33] while the effects in late systole were always considerable. Together with the finding that the calcium transient in myocytes is hardly affected by the presence of endothelial products,[33,36] this points again to a modified sensitivity of the myofibrils for calcium during shortening, while the positive dF/dt of the fibre (i.e. positive dP/dt in the ventricle) reflects the actual value of the calcium transient.[41] A similar dissociation between the pre-ejection parameter dP/dtmax and the (end-systolic) ESPVR in response to the sarcoplasmic reticulum blocker ryanodine was recently found in our group.[42] Finally, in terms of clinical relevance of our findings, a few remarks are appropriate. The identity of cardioregulatory substances produced by endothelial cells or the secondary messenger effects of the same in myocytes may have great clinical importance as stressed in recent review and editorial papers.[33,43] According to Shah,[33] endothelial control of cardiac function may be of the same importance as the control exerted by the neurohumoral system. The above substances seem to have a direct relationship with one of the most important functions of the heart, namely to maintain cardiac output under normal physiological conditions as well as during stress whether related to exercise, hypertension or heart disease. Quite possibly, the normal heart of a young person has a well-functioning HAR effect, allowing it to maintain or increase stroke volume (and cardiac output) primarily through reduction in end-systolic volume, i.e. without having to rely appreciably on the Frank-Starling mechanism, thus keeping cardiac volume within normal limits. In the aging person as well as those suffering from ischemic or valvular heart disease, this autoregulatory mechanism may deteriorate or even disappear, causing the heart to adapt to increased circulatory demands by increasing its diastolic volume as shown by Lakatta's group.[44] This phenomenon might eventually lead to a process of chronic dilation, remodelling and cardiac failure.

References

1. Baan J, van der Velde ET, de Bruin HG et al. Continuous measurement of left ventricular volume in animals and humans by conductance catheter. Circulation 1984;70:812-23.
2. Suga H, Sagawa K. Instantaneous pressure-volume relationships and their ratio in the excised, supported canine left ventricle. Circ Res 1974;35:117-26.
3. Lew WYW. Time-dependent increase in left ventricular contractility following acute volume loading in the dog. Circ Res 1988;63:635-47.
4. Baan J, de Bruin HG, van der Velde ET. Emax for the left ventricle in situ is influenced by muscle shortening. J Physiol 1985;366:66P.
5. Baan J, van der Velde ET. Sensitivity of left ventricular end-systolic pressure-volume

relation to the type of loading intervention in dogs. Circ Res 1988;62:1247-58.

6. van der Velde ET, Burkhoff D, Steendijk P, Karsdon J, Sagawa K, Baan J. Nonlinearity and afterload sensitivity of the end-systolic pressure-volume relation of the canine left ventricle in vivo. Circulation 1991;83:315-27.

7. Schipper IB, Steendijk P, Klautz RJM, van der Velde ET, Baan J. Cardiac sympathetic denervation does not change the load dependence of the left ventricular end-systolic pressure/volume relationship in dogs. Eur J Physiol (Pflugers Arch) 1993;425:426-33.

8. Brady AJ. Length-tension relations in cardiac muscle. Am Zoologist 1967;7:603-10.

9. Suga H, Sagawa K, Demer L. Determinants of instantaneous pressure in canine left ventricle: time and volume specification. Circ Res 1980;46:256-63.

10. van der Linden LP, van der Velde ET, van Houwelingen HC, Bruschke AVG, Baan J. Determinants of end-systolic pressure during different load alterations in the in-situ left ventricle. Am J Physiol (Heart Circ Physiol 36) 1994;267:H1895-H1906.

11. Klautz RJM, Teitel DF, Steendijk P, van Bel F, Baan J. Interaction between afterload and contractility in the newborn heart. Evidence of homeometric autoregulation in the intact circulation. J Am Coll Cardiol 1995;25:1428-35.

12. Von Anrep G. On the part played by the suprarenals in the normal vascular reactions of the body. J Physiol (London) 1912;45:307-17.

13. Sarnoff SJ, Mitchell JH, Gilmore JP, Remensnyder JP. Homeometric autoregulation in the heart. Circ Res 1960;8:1077-91.

14. Elzinga G, Noble MIM, Stubbs J. The effect of an increase in aortic pressure upon the inotropic state of cat and dog left ventricles. J Physiol (London) 1977;273:597-615.

15. Downey JM. Myocardial contractile force as a function of coronary blood flow. Am J Physiol 1976;230:1-6.

16. Arnold G, Kosche F, Miessner E, Neitzert A, Lochner W. The importance of the perfusion pressure in the coronary arteries for the contractility and the oxygen consumption of the heart. Pflugers Arch 1968;299:339-56.

17. Gregg DE. Effect of coronary perfusion pressure or coronary flow on oxygen usage of the myocardium. Circ Res 1963;13:497-500.

18. Schouten VJA, Allaart CP, Westerhof N. Effect of perfusion pressure on force of contraction in thin pappillary muscles and trabeculae from rat heart. J Physiol 1992;451:585-604.

19. Goto Y, Slinker BK, LeWinter MM. Effect of coronary hyperemia on Emax and oxygen consumption in blood-perfused rabbit hearts. Energetic consequences of Gregg's phenomenon. Circ Res 1991;68:482-92.

20. Iwamoto T, Bai X-J, Downey HF. Coronary perfusion related changes in myocardial contractile force and systolic ventricular stiffness. Cardiovasc Res 1994;28:1331-6.

21. Dankelman J, van der Ploeg CPB, Spaan JAE. Transients in myocardial O2 consumption after abrupt changes in perfusion pressure in goats. Am J Physiol (Heart Circ Physiol 39) 1996;270:H492-H499.

22. Brutsaert DL, Meulemans AL, Sipido KR, Sys SU. Effects of damaging the endocardial surface on the mechanical performance of isolated cardiac muscle. Circ Res 1988;62:358-66.

23. De Hert S, Gillebert TC, Brutsaert DL. Alteration of left ventricular endocardial function of intracavitary high-power ultrasound interacts with volume, inotropic state, and alpha1-adrenergic stimulation. Circulation 1993;87:1275-85.

24. Brutsaert DL, Andries LJ. The endocardial endothelium. Am J Physiol (Heart Circ

Physiol 32) 1992;263:H985-H1002.

25. Wang J, Morgan JP. Endocardial endothelium modulates myofilament Ca2 + responsiveness in aequorin-loaded ferret myocardium. Circ Res 1992;70:754-60.

26. Ramaciotti C, McClellan G, Sharkey A, Rose D, Weisberg A, Winegrad S. Cardiac endothelial cells modulate contractility of rat heart in response to oxygen tension and coronary flow. Circ Res 1993;72:1044-64.

27. Li K, Rouleau JL, Andries LJ, Brutsaert DL. Effect of dysfunctional vascular endothelium on myocardial performance in isolated papillary muscles. Circ Res 1993;72:768-77.

28. McClellan G, Weisberg A, Winegrad S. Effect of endothelin-1 on actomyoasin ATPase activity. Implications for the efficiency of contraction. Circ res 1996;78:1044-50.

29. Demer LL, Wortham CM, Dirksen ER, Sanderson MJ. Mechanical stimulation induces intercellular calcium signalling in bovine aortic endothelial cells. Am J Physiol (Heart Circ Physiol 33) 1993;264:H2094-H2102.

30. Ohno M, Gibbons GH, Dzau VJ, Cooke JP. Shear stress elevates endothelial cGMP. Circulation 1993;88:193-7.

31. Awolesi MA, Widmann MD, Sessa WC, Sumpio BE. Cyclic strain increases endothelial nitric oxide synthase activity. Surgery 1994;116:439-45.

32. Shah AM, Mebazaa A, Wetzel RC, Lakatta EG. Novel cardiac myofilament desensitizing factor released by endocardial and vascular endothelial cells. Circulation 1994;89:2492-7.

33. Shah AM. Paracrine modulation of heart cell function by endothelial cells. Cardiovasc Res 1996;31:847-67.

34. Paulus WJ, Vantrimpoint PJ, Shah AM. Acute effects of nitric oxide on left ventricular relaxation and disatolic distensibility in man. Circulation 1994;89:2070-8.

35. Furchgott RF, Zawadski JV. The obligatory role of endothelial cells in the relaxation of arterial smooth muscle by acetylcholine. Nature 1980;288:373-6.

36. Mebazaa A, Mayoux E, Maeda K et al. Paracrine effects of endocardial endothelial cells on myocyte contraction mediated via endothelin. Am J Physiol (Heart Circ Physiol 34) 1993;265):H1841-H1846.

37. Moody CJ, Dashwood MR, Sykes RM et al. Functional and autoradiographic evidence for endothelin 1 receptors on human and rat cardiac myocytes. Comparison with single smooth muscle cells. Circ Res 1990;67:764-9.

38. Dijkman MA, Heslinga JW, Sipkema P, Westerhof N. Perfusion-induced changes in cardiac contractility and oxygen consumption are not endothelium-dependent. Cardiovasc Res 1997;33:593-600.

39. McClellan G, Weisberg A, Rose D, Winegrad S. Endothelial cell storage and release of endothelin as a cardioregulatory mechanism. Circ Res 1994;75:85-96.

40. Pelissier T, Miranda HF, Bustamente D, Paeile C, Pinardi G. Removal of endothelial layer in perfused mesenteric vascular bed of the rat. J Pharmacol Meth 1992;27:41-4.

41. Yue DT. Intracellular [Ca2 +] related to rate of force development in twitch contraction of heart. Am J Physiol (Heart Circ Physiol 21) 1987;252:H760-H770.

42. Klautz RJM. Myocardial Contractility in the Immature Heart and in Experimental Congenital Heart Disease. Doctoral thesie. Leiden, 1995: Chapter 3.

43. Colucci WS. Myocardial endothelin. Does it play a role in myocardial failure? Circulation 1996;93:1069-72.

44. Rodeheffer RJ, Gerstenblith G, Becker LC, Fleg JL, Weisfeldt ML, Lakatta EG.

Exercise cardiac output is maintained with advancing age in healthy human subjects: cardiac dilatation and increased stroke volume compensate for a diminished heart rate. Circulation 1984;69:203-13.

ENDOTHELIAL FUNCTION AND CALCIUM METABOLISM

Hubert W. Vliegen, J. Wouter Jukema, Arnoud van der Laarse,
Hermann Haller

Summary

The endothelium plays a crucial role in the regulation of the vessel wall
under physiological and pathological conditions.[1] The endothelium lines all
vessels of the body and is the most important structure for communication
between the blood stream and the vessel wall.[2] One function is to act as a
barrier that prevents noxious agents from entering the vessel wall. Other
functions of healthy endothelium include antithrombotic properties that
inhibit the adhesion of blood cells (thrombocytes, erythrocytes, and
leukocytes) to the vessel wall. Hence, endothelial cells are crucial for
maintaining laminar blood flow. A third function of the endothelium is a
secretory function. Endothelial cells can release their secretory products into
the vessel wall as well as into the blood stream. Of particular importance for
the physiological function of the vessel wall is the vasorelaxing function of
endothelial cells[1] due to secretion of endothelium-derived relaxing factor
(EDRF).[3] Under physiological conditions, EDRF is released permanently and
ensures the patency of normal vessels.[4] In addition, endothelial cells can
release vasoconstrictive factors such as endothelin into the vessel wall.[5,6]
Furthermore, studies over recent years have identified growth factors and
chemotactic substances which are produced by damaged or overstimulated
endothelial cells and which play a crucial part in structural changes of the
vessel wall.[7,8]
The most important vasorelaxing factor secreted by endothelial cells is nitric

E.E. van der Wall et al. (eds.), Vascular Medicine, 45-53.
© 1997 *Kluwer Academic Publishers.*

oxide (NO) or EDRF. NO is synthesized in endothelial cells from the amino acid L-arginine by NO-synthase.[9] The latter enzyme is continuously active and thus ensures the permanent release of NO. Disturbances of endothelial cell function lower the release of NO and thus reduce vasorelaxation.[10,11] In addition to NO, endothelial cells also release prostaglandins with vasodilatory action such as prostacyclin. Prostacyclin induces vasorelaxation and inhibits platelet aggregation.[12] It is possible that the endothelium secretes additional vasorelaxing substances that have not yet been identified.

The influence of calcium antagonists on endothelial function

Calcium antagonists may influence endothelial cell function and its interactions with blood cells by different modes of action. However, up to now only little is known about the direct effects of calcium antagonists on endothelial cell function.[13] In contrast to their effects in vascular smooth muscle, calcium antagonists do not influence calcium homeostasis in endothelial cells.[14] Intracellular calcium release and transmembranous calcium influx upon stimulation of endothelial cells by agonists are not affected by calcium antagonists.[15] This is due to the fact that endothelial cells apparently do not possess voltage-operated, L-type calcium channels.[14] Therefore, calcium antagonists do not appear to have any adverse effects on the calcium-dependent formation of NO. However, contradictory reports have appeared in the literature that describe an increased NO release by calcium antagonists,[15] but the exact mechanism of how calcium antagonists may interfere with NO production and release has not yet been elucidated. One possibility is that calcium antagonists interfere with the hypoxia-induced alterations of damaged endothelium.[16]

Recently it has been shown that calcium antagonists interfere with the interaction between endothelial and vascular smooth muscle cells.[17] Activated endothelial cells release endothelin which is a strong activator of vascular smooth muscle contraction. Presumably, this effect of endothelin on vascular smooth muscle contractility is mostly mediated via the L-type calcium channel.[18] This effect of endothelin on the contractility of vascular smooth muscle can be almost abolished by the concomitant administration of calcium antagonists.[19] Kiowski et al. have demonstrated in patients that calcium antagonists are very effective in preventing the endothelin-induced contraction.[20] These findings indicate that calcium antagonists may be effective drugs under conditions of endothelial dysfunction with increased release of endothelin in the vessel wall.

In addition to the effects on vascular smooth muscle, Haller et al. recently showed that calcium antagonists also inhibit the endothelin-induced activation of macrophages. It was observed that endothelin induces release of oxygen free radicals in human macrophages. When these macrophages are incubated with nitrendipine, the endothelin-induced superoxide radical release is markedly diminished.[21] A comparable effect of calcium antagonists on leukocytes has also been shown by other investigators.[22,23]

The increased binding of blood cells to the vessel wall with subsequent cell activation can also be influenced by calcium antagonists. Firstly, calcium antagonists lead to relaxation of the blood vessel and thereby improve the flow conditions. Laminar flow in relaxed blood vessels diminishes cell-cell interaction. Furthermore, calcium antagonists specifically interact with the different cell types, i.e., platelets, leukocytes, and endothelial cells, which play a role in the pathogenesis of atherosclerosis.

It has been demonstrated in patients that the administration of calcium antagonists results in a slightly decreased aggregation of platelets in vivo.[24] One of the mechanisms contributing to this effect is a lowered release of thromboxane from thrombocytes during treatment with calcium antagonists.[25]

Antiatherosclerotic effect of calcium antagonists

It has been speculated since the early 1970's that calcium antagonists might stop the sclerotic process and calcification of the vessel wall. Recently, new concepts of this antiatherosclerotic effect have been proposed.[26] Fleckenstein and coworkers performed many animal studies that provided the basic data for an antiatherosclerotic action of calcium antagonists.[27] Most of the investigations by Fleckenstein's group were done in rats. Others examined the antiatherosclerotic effects of calcium antagonists in rabbits on a high-cholesterol diet or in genetic models of hypercholesterolemia. Many but not all of these studies have shown that calcium antagonists (at high doses) can prevent or reduce the deposition of cholesterol or calcium in the vessel wall.

The results of these animal studies and the cellular mechanisms of calcium antagonist action in the pathogenesis of atherosclerosis described above served as a basis for designing several clinical trials to investigate the possible antiatherosclerotic effects of calcium antagonists in patients. Such clinical studies face a number of serious problems. Since atherosclerotic changes develop over many years or even decades, it is of course difficult to evaluate the effects of treatment during a relatively short period of time (maximally 1-3 years). Therapeutic benefits of the administered agents might not become apparent during the study period. Another question that arises relates to the vascular region to be used for evaluating the antiatherosclerotic effect. Atherosclerosis does not affect all vascular regions simultaneously, and it is also possible that calcium antagonists act differently in the various vascular regions in accordance with different pathogenic mechanisms of atherosclerosis in these regions.

Clinical trials on coronary atherosclerosis in humans with calcium antagonists

Therapy with lipid lowering drugs and therapy with calcium antagonists have been tested as pharmacological approaches for prevention of atherosclerosis progression. Lipid lowering therapy now has undoubtedly proven to be an effective therapeutic modality to retard progression of coronary atherosclerosis. Evidence indicating that calcium antagonists inhibit atherosclerosis is less unequivocal. Many investigations lend support to the view that a number of key processes in atherosclerosis may be influenced by calcium antagonists. From the "negative" and "positive" studies with calcium antagonists performed in animals and man we must conclude that apparently some but not all types or stages of the atherosclerotic process are inhibited by calcium antagonists.

In humans, Loaldi et al.[28] demonstrated a reduction in progression of preexisting stenoses and reduction of new lesion formation in patients treated with nifedipine as compared to patients treated with propranolol or isosorbide dinitrate. However, in two placebo controlled randomized clinical trials, the International Nifedipine Trial on Antiatherosclerotic Therapy (INTACT) study[29] and the Montreal Heart study,[30] calcium antagonists did not influence the overall rate of progression and regression of coronary atherosclerosis, although these trials also showed significantly less progression of minimal lesions or less new lesion formation in the patients treated with calcium antagonists.

Schroeder et al.[31] investigated the effect of diltiazem on coronary artery disease in heart transplant recipients. These patients are prone to accelerated coronary artery disease which is the major cause of late morbidity and mortality. Treatment with diltiazem resulted in prevention of the usual reduction in coronary artery diameter.

To assess whether lipid lowering therapy and treatment with calcium antagonists may have an additive or synergistic beneficial effect on human atherosclerosis, which is conceivable since their anti-atherosclerotic properties differ, data of the angiographic lipid lowering trial "REGRESS" (pravastatin versus placebo)[32] were reviewed in this regard.[33] In REGRESS, patients in the pravastatin group, had significantly less progression if co-treated with calcium antagonists as compared to those who received no co-treatment, whereas in the placebo group (no pravastatin) no effect of calcium antagonist treatment was observed (Figure 1).

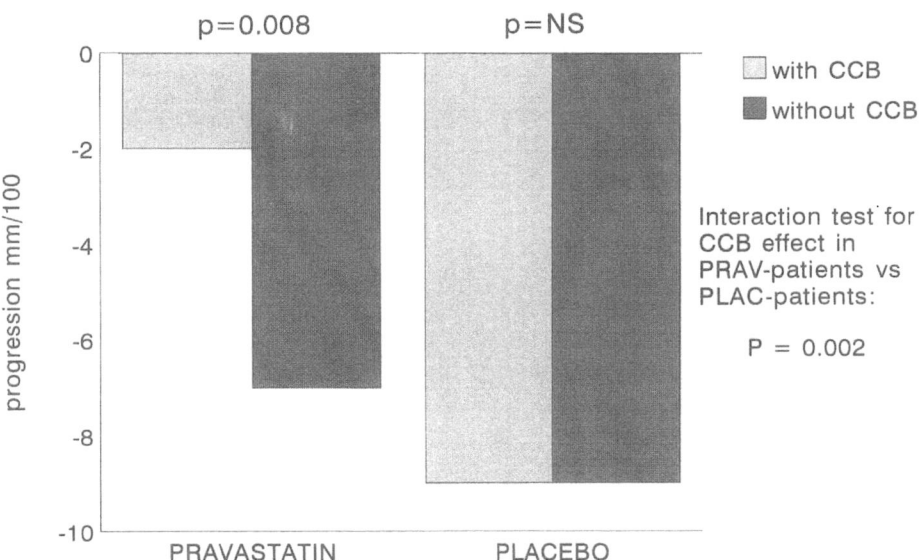

Figure 1. *Angiographic progression (change of minimum obstruction diameter (MOD)) for patients with and without calcium channel blocker (CCB) co-treatment in the pravastatin group as well as in the placebo group in the REGRESS study (32,33).*
Patients in the pravastatin group have significantly less progression if co-treated with CCBs as compared to no CCB co-treatment (p = 0.008), whereas in the placebo (no pravastatin) group no effect of CCB treatment is observed.

With respect to angiographic new lesion formation, in the pravastatin group there were 50% less patients with new angiographic lesions if co-treated with calcium antagonists as compared to the group receiving no co-treatment, whereas in the placebo (no pravastatin) group again no significant effect of treatment with calcium antagonists was observed (Figure 2). No beneficial effects of treatment with calcium antagonists on clinical events were observed during the 2 year study follow-up. In view of the correlation between angiographic progression and subsequent clinical events as demonstrated in several large trials, it is not unrealistic to anticipate in this population also a beneficial effect on clinical events with longer follow-up.[34-36]
We can only speculate about the mechanism by which calcium

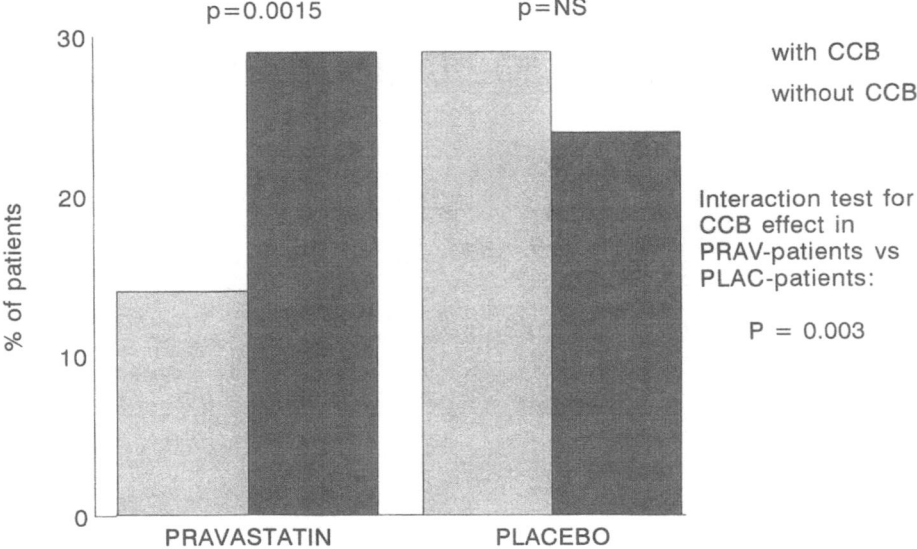

Percentage of patients with new lesions

with CCB

without CCB

Interaction test for
CCB effect in
PRAV-patients vs
PLAC-patients:

P = 0.003

Figure 2. *Angiographic new lesion formation for patients with and without calcium channel blocker (CCB) co-treatment in the pravastatin group as well as in the placebo group in the REGRESS study (32,33).*
In the pravastatin group there are significantly less patients with new lesions if co-treated with CCBs as compared to no CCB co-treatment (p = 0.0015), whereas in the placebo (no pravastatin) group no significant effect of CCB treatment is observed.

antagonists may augment the beneficial effects of lipid lowering by pravastatin. The mechanisms which may contribute to this effect include stimulation of cholesteryl ester hydrolase activity in vascular smooth muscle cells,[38] improvement of hypercholesterolemia-induced endothelial dysfunction, and inhibition of vascular smooth muscle cell proliferation and migration.[37,38] Furthermore, an increased resistance to oxidation of LDL cholesterol is associated with diminished atherogenicity.[39] Antioxidants are considered to protect LDL cholesterol from oxidation. Several investigators have demonstrated that certain calcium antagonists have antioxidant properties.[40] Lower concentrations of LDL in plasma and an improved protection against its oxidation may act synergistically in preventing progression of atherosclerosis.

Although the REGRESS trial was not designed to evaluate combination therapy, the results suggest strongly that addition of calcium antagonists to HMG-CoA reductase inhibitor therapy (pravastatin) acts synergistically in

51

retarding the progression of established coronary atherosclerosis. These results appear to warrant prospective randomized trials to determine in a more definitive manner the merits of this combination in the prevention of progression of coronary atherosclerosis. A number of studies in this field are currently being designed or already underway.

References

1. Luscher TF, Vanhoutte PM. The endothelium: modulator of cardiovascular function. CRC Press, Boca Raton 1990.
2. Dzau VJ, Gibbons GH. Cell biology of vascular hypertrophy in systemic hypertension. Am J Cardiol l988;62:30G-35G.
3. Vallance P, Collier J, Moncada S. Effects of endothelium-derived nitric oxide on peripheral arteriolar tone in man. Lancet 1989;1:997-1000.
4. Luscher TF. Imbalance of endothelium-derived relaxing and contracting factors: a new concept in hypertension? Am J Hypertens 1990;3:317-30.
5. Yanagisawa X, Kurihara H, Kimura S, Mitsiu Y, Kobayashi M, Watanabe TX, Masaki T. A novel potent vasoconstrictor peptide produced by vascular endothelial cells. Nature 1988;388:411-5.
6. Panza JA, Quyyumi AA, Brush JE Jr, Epstein SE. Endothelium-dependent vascular relaxation in patients with essential hypertension. N Engl J Med 1990;323:22-7.
7. DiCorleto PE, Fox PL. Growth factor production by endothelial cells. In: Una R (ed) Endothelial cells, vol 2. CRC Press, Boca Raton 1988:51-62.
8. Egleme C, Creesier F, Wood JM. Local formation of angiotensin II in the rat aorta. Effect of endothelium. Br J Pharmacol 1990;100:237-40.
9. Palmer RJM, Ashtor DS, Moncada S. Vascular endothelial cells synthesize nitroxide from L-arginine. Nature 1988;333:664-6.
10. Lorenzi M, Cagliero E. Pathobiology of endothelial and other vascular cells in diabetes mellitus; call for data. Diabetes 1991;40:653-9.
11. Jensen T, Bjerre-Knudsen J, Feldt-Rasmussen B, Deckert. Features of endothelial dysfunction in early diabetic nephropathy. Lancet 1989;1:461-3.
12. Guerra R, Brotherton AFA, Goodwin PJ, Clark CR, Armstrong ML, Harrison DG. Mechanisms of abnormal endothelium-dependent vascular relaxation in atherosclerosis: implications for altered autocrine and paracrine functions of DRF. Blood Vessels 1989;26:300-14.
13. Ciriaco E, Abbate F, Ferrante F, Laura R, Amenta F. Structural changes in the endothelium of the femoral artery of spontaneously hypertensive rats: sensitivity to isradipine treatment. J Hypertens 1993;11:515-22.
14. Himmel HM, Whorton AR, Strauss HC. Intracellular calcium, currents, and stimulus - response coupling in endothelial cells. Hypertension 1993;21:112-27.
15. Gunther J, Dhein S, Rosen R, Klaus W, Fricke U. Nitric oxide (EDRF) enhances the vasorelaxing effect of nitrendipine in various isolated arteries. Basic Res Cardiol 1992;87:452-60.
16. Wilkie ME, Stevens CR, Cunningham J, Blake D. Hypoxia-induced von Willebrand factor release is blocked by verapamil. Miner Electrolyte Metab 1992;18:141-4.
17. Luscher TF, Espinosa E, Dubey RK, Yang Z. Vascular biology of human coronary artery and bypass graft disease. Curr Opin Cardiol 1993;8:963-74.

18. Yang Z, Bauer E, von Segesser L, Stulz P, Turina M, Luscher TF. Different mobilization of calcium in endothelin-i-induced contractions in human arteries and veins: effects of calcium antagonists. J Cardiovasc Pharmacol 1990;16:654-60.
19. Goto K, Kasuya Y, Matsuki N, Takuwa Y, Kurihara H, Kimura S, Yanagisawa M, Masaki T. Endothelin activates the dihydropyridine - sensitive, voltage-dependent calcium channel in vascular smooth muscle. Proc Natl Acad Sci USA 1989;86:3915-8.
20. Kiowski W, Luscher TF, Linder L, Buhler FR. Endothelin-1 induced vasoconstriction in Man: reveral by calcium channel blockade but not by nitrovasodilators or EDRF. Circulation 1991;83:469-75.
21. Haller H, Schaberg T, Lindschau C, Quass P, Lode H, Distler A. Endothelin increases intracellular free calcium, protein phosphorylation and O2-production in human alveolar macrophages. Am J Physiol 1991;261:L713-L723.
22. Wright B, Zeitman I, Greig R, Poste G. Inhibition of macrophage function by calcium channel blockers and calmodulin antagonists. Cell Immunol 1985;95:46-53.
23. Jouvin-Marche E, Cerrina J, Coeffier E, Duroux P, Benviste J. Effect of the calcium antagonist nifedipine on the relase of PAF, slow-reacting substance and beta-glucuronidase from human neutrophils. Eur J Pharmacol 1983;89:19-26.
24. Haller H, Lenz T, Ludersdorf M, Distler A, Philipp T. Changes in sensitivity to angiotensin II in platelets. J Cardiovasc Pharmacol l987;l0 [Suppl l0]:S44-S46.
25. Tschöpe D, Kaufmann L, Roesen P, Ohlrogge R, Gries FA. Influence of a single dose of nitrendipine on whole platelet activity in healthy subjects. J Cardiovasc Pharmacol 1988;12:SI67-S169.
26. Collins P, Rosano GM, Jiang C, Lindsay D, Sarrel PM, Poole-Wilson PA. Cardiovascular protection by oestrogen - a calcium antagonist effect? Lancet 1993;341:1264-5.
27. Fleckenstein-Grun G, Frey M, Thimm F, Hofgartner W, Fleckenstein A. Calcium overload an important cellular mechanism in hypertension and arteriosclerosis. Drugs 1992;1:23-30.
28. Loaldi A, Polese A, Montorsi P et al. Comparison of nifedipine, propranolol and isosorbide dinitrate on angiographic progression and regression of coronary arterial narrowings in angina pectoris. Am J Cardiol 1989;64:433-9.
29. Lichtlen PR, Hugenholtz PG, Rafflenbeul W, Hecker H, Jost S, Deckers JW, on behalf on the INTACT group investigators. Retardation of angiographic progression of coronary artery disease by nifedipine. Lancet 1990;335:1109-13.
30. Waters D, Lespérance J, Francetich M et al. A controlled clinical trial to assess the effect of calcium channel blocker on the progression of coronary atherosclerosis. Circulation 1990;82:1940-53.
31. Schroeder JS, Gao SZ, Alderman EL, Hunt SA, Johnstone I, Boothroyd DB, Wiederhold V, Stinson EB. A preliminary study of diltiazem in the prevention of coronary artery disease in heart transplant recipients. N Engl J Med 1993;328:164-70.
32. Jukema JW, Bruschke AVG, van Boven AJ et al. on behalf of the REGRESS study group. Effects of lipid lowering by pravastatin on progression and regression of coronary artery disease in symptomatic men with normal to moderately elevated serum cholesterol levels. Circulation 1995;91:2528-40.
33. Jukema JW, Zwinderman AH, van Boven AJ, Reiber JHC, van der Laarse A, Lie KI, Bruschke AVG. Evidence for a synergistic effect of calcium channel blockers with lipid-lowering therapy in retarding progression of coronary atherosclerosis in

symptomatic patients with normal to moderately raised cholesterol levels. Arterioscler Thromb Vasc Biol 1996;16:425-30.

34. Buchwald H, Matts JP, Fitch LL et al. for the Program on the Surgical Control of the Hyperlipidemias (POSCH) Group. Changes in sequential coronary arteriograms and subsequent coronary events. JAMA 1992;268:1429-33.

35. Waters D, Craven TE, Lespérance J. Prognostic significance of progression of coronary atherosclerosis. Circulation 1993;87:1067-75.

36. Azen SP, Mack WJ, Cashin-Hemphill L, LaBree L, Shircore AM, Selzer RH, Blankenhorn DH, Hodis HN. Progression of coronary artery disease predicts clinical coronary events. Long-term follow-up from the Cholesterol Lowering Atherosclerosis Study. Circulation 1996;93:34-41.

37. Waters D, Lespérance J. Calcium channel blockers and coronary atherosclerosis: From the rabbit to the real world. Am Heart J 1994;128:1309-16.

38. Etingin OR, Hajjar DP. Calcium channel blockers enhance cholesteryl ester hydrolysis and decrease total accumulation in human aortic tissue. Circulation Research 1990;66:185-90.

39. Witztum JL. The oxidation hypothesis of atherosclerosis. Lancet 1994;344:793-5.

40. Mak IT, Weglicki WB. Comparative antioxidant activities of propranolol, nifedipine, verapamil, and diltiazem against sarcolemmal membrane lipid peroxidation. Circ Res 1990;66:1449-52.

ENDOTHELIAL (DYS)FUNCTION, LIPID REDUCTION AND BALLOON ANGIOPLASTY

Han J.G.H. Mulder, Martin J. Schalij

Summary

The endothelium is an important anatomical structure which is present throughout the whole vascular system. This review will focus on the endothelial function of the coronary artery system, especially in relation to cholesterol reduction and percutaneous transluminal coronary angioplasty (PTCA). The review is divided into four parts; 1) endothelial function; 2) endothelial dysfunction; 3) restoring endothelial function by cholesterol reduction; and 4) endothelial (dys)function and PTCA.

Endothelial function

The endothelium

The coronary arteries are composed of three layers (Figure 1). The intima, the media and the adventitia, separated from another by the *internal elastic lamina* and the *external elastic lamina*. The innermost layer, or *intima*, consists of the *endothelium* and a thin layer of loose connective tissue, the *sub-endothelial space*. The *media* is built up of spiraling layers of smooth muscle cells lying in a stromal meshwork of elastic and collagen fibers. The *adventitia*, finally, consists of a layer of loosely arranged collagen and elastic fibers, rich in lymphatics and nerves.

The endothelium is a flattened, monolayer cell structure throughout the body

E.E. van der Wall et al. (eds.), Vascular Medicine, 55-82.
© 1997 *Kluwer Academic Publishers.*

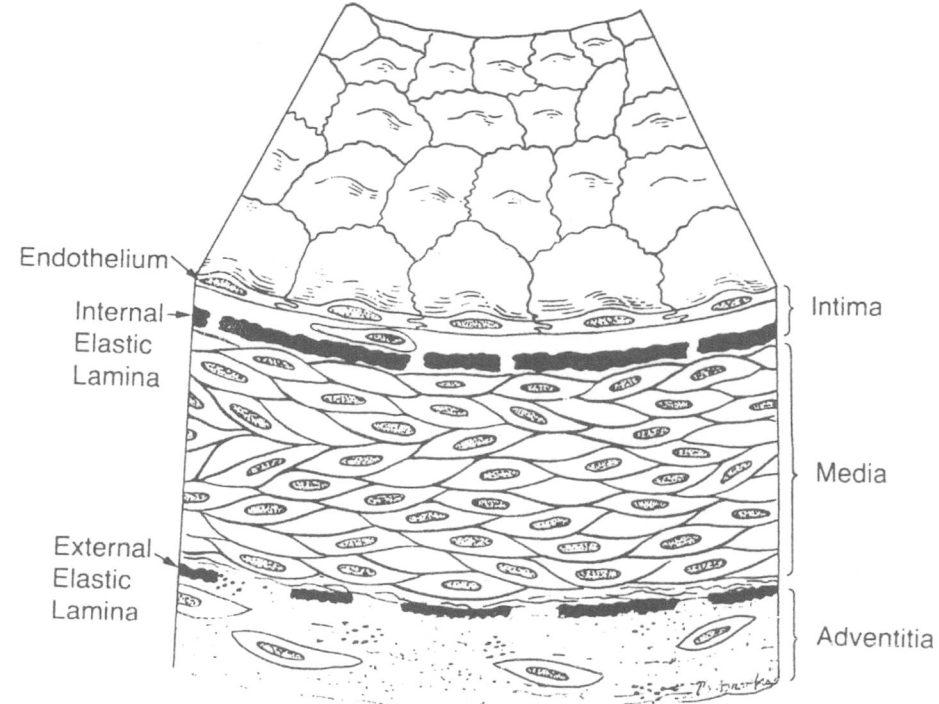

Figure 1. Cross-section of a coronary artery. (Reprinted by permission from Ross et al., 1976)

at the inner surface of all vessels. In man, it is equivalent in mass to five normal hearts and in area to half a dozen tennis courts. Originally the endothelium was considered to be only a selective barrier for macromolecules. The experiments by Furchgott et al.[1] in 1980 changed this perspective dramatically.

Endothelial (dys)function
The experiments of Furchgott et al.[1] and others demonstrated that endothelial cells are pivotal to blood vessel physiology. They appeared to be small regulating units, essential to many functions. Several functions of importance to the vascular system can be recognized:[2]
(1) *Semi selective physical barrier.* The endothelium is a physical barrier between the blood and the surrounding structures.
(2) *Promotion and inhibition of vascular growth.* Endothelium can promote or inhibit cell growth. For example, nitric oxide, released by the endothelium, inhibits cell growth and endothelin, also released by endothelial cells, promotes cell growth.

(3) *Local hemo-coagulation regulation.* The endothelial cell surface can express pro- and anti-thrombotic qualities. Anti-thrombotic compounds produced by endothelial cells are, for example, nitric oxide and prostacyclin (inhibition of platelet aggregation). Pro-thrombotic compounds produced by endothelial cells are, for example, the Von Willebrand factor and the plasminogen activator inhibitor (PAI-1).

(4) *Synthesis of cell adhesion molecules.* The expression of adhesion molecules is an important step in the process of atherosclerosis.[3] Examples of adhesion molecules, expressed by the endothelium, are VCAM (vascular cell adhesion molecule) and ICAM (intercellular adhesion molecule).

(5) *Processing of lipid-rich particles.* The endothelial surface harbors lipoprotein lipase (LPL). This enzyme plays an important role in the metabolism of triglyceride-rich particles.

(6) *Regulation of vasomotor tone.* The endothelial cells are important regulators of the vascular smooth muscle tone.

Endothelial dysfunction occurs when the endothelial cells are affected by, for example, atherosclerosis. This results in impaired regulatory properties.

Endothelium-dependent vasomotion
The vascular smooth muscle tone is regulated, among other factors, by endothelial cell derived substances. The endothelial cells can be regarded as local sensors, adapting the smooth muscle tone to different impulses such as blood flow velocity and vasoactive compounds. Vasorelaxation, controlled by the endothelium is referred to as "endothelium-dependent vasorelaxation" (EDV). This is in contrast to "endothelium independent vasomotion" (EIDV), which is the result of substances acting directly on the smooth muscle cells The execution of endothelium dependent vasomotion involves a complex biochemical pathway. This is a multi-step pathway, interacting with many parts of the endothelial cell's metabolism. This is why disturbance of the endothelium-dependent vasomotion is seen as a sign of general decline of the endothelial cell and the functions it exhibits. In this perspective, endothelium-dependent vasomotion can be regarded as a "thermometer" of endothelial health.

The endothelium dependent vasomotion pathway
Though the endothelial cells are capable of producing vaso-constrictive substances, the ability to produce vasodilating substances seems to be more important.[4] In 1980 Furchgott[1] postulated the existence of a vasodilating substance released by the endothelium, calling it EDRF (endothelium derived relaxant factor). Since then it has become clear that EDRF is more than one substance. Nitric oxide is considered to be the most important of them.[4] Nitric oxide (NO) as relaxing factor was discovered in 1987 by Palmer et al.[5]

58

Myers et al.[6] refined this discovery in 1990 by adding that NO is part of a compound, probably a nitrosothiol. The NO itself is a soluble gas and has a very short life time. After being synthesized it is quickly oxidated and converted to nitrite and nitrate.[7] The rapid breakdown ensures that there is little downstream activity within the vascular compartment and that each millimeter of endothelium controls no more than a small part of vascular wall. The exogenous counterparts of NO producing cells are the nitro-donating drugs, for example nitroglycerin, which deliver NO directly to the smooth muscle cells.

Nitric oxide is synthesized through a biochemical pathway, known as the "*L-arginine/NO pathway*".[8] This pathway can be simplified to the following summary (Figure 2); an endothelium dependent vasodilator arrives at the cell membrane and activates a specific receptor (muscarinic, etc.). Receptor activation leads to initiation of a second messenger pathway, resulting in increased activity of nitric oxide synthetase (NOS). NOS aids the transform l-arginine (l-arg) into nitric oxide and l-citrulline (l-cit). The molecule NO diffuses out of the endothelial cell and a portion of it will arrive at the smooth muscle cell layer beneath the endothelium. Here the NO will activate the soluble enzyme guanylate cyclase which up-regulates c-GMP (cyclic-guanosine monophosphate), resulting in smooth muscle cell relaxation. Also depicted in the figure is the action of nitro-donating drugs, delivering NO directly to the smooth muscle cells.

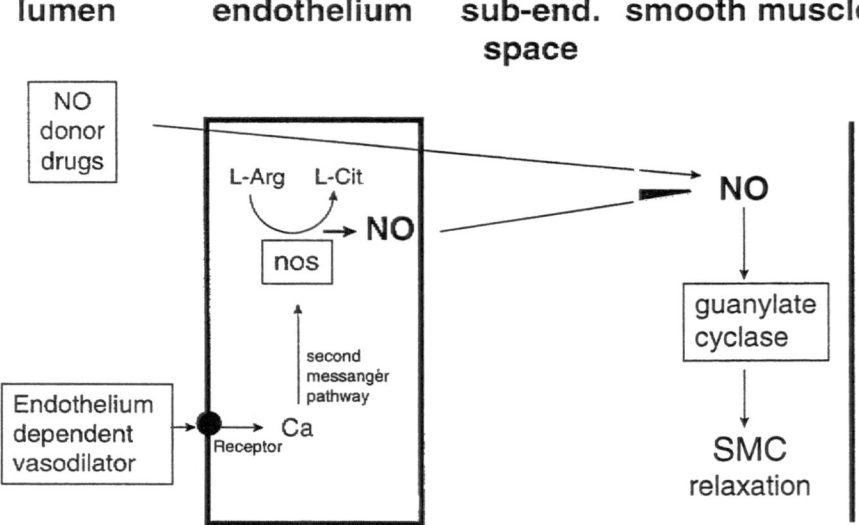

Figure 2. *The l-arginine/NO pathway in context of the vasomotion. L-arg, l-arginine; L-cit, l-citrulline; NOS, nitric oxide synthetase; Ca, calcium; SMC, smooth muscle cells; sub-end. Space, sub-endothelial space*

Nitric oxide synthetase (NOS) is the key enzyme in the pathway of NO synthesis.[8] Several isoforms of the NOS-enzyme exist in different tissues and with different names.[9] These isoforms were originally named on the basis of the tissue archetype, for example, neuronal-derived NOS (nNOS) and endothelial-derived NOS (eNOS). Recently, however, eNOS has been discovered in several other cell types like cardiac myocytes and platelets.[9] This has led to a numerical name designation in the order of discovery of the known three isoforms (NOS1, NOS2, NOS3). Because of the ubiquitous presence of NO-synthesizing systems, the acronym EDNO (endothelium-derived nitric oxide) has been introduced to prevent confusion.

Besides its importance to the vasomotion, EDNO is also important to other regulatory functions of the endothelium. For example, EDNO inhibits platelet aggregation,[10] and vascular smooth muscle cell proliferation.[11] It also prevents expression of adhesion molecules for instance neutrophils[12] and it has a role in the radical scavenging process.[13]

Other endothelium derived vasoactive substances
Soon after its discovery it became apparent that EDNO could not act by itself. Although it is probably the most important vasoactive substance released by the endothelium, subsequent investigations indicated that there had to be other endothelium derived vasoactive substances. The endothelium-derived hyperpolarizing factor (EDHF) is one of them.[14] EDHF seems to relax smooth muscle cells independently of guanylate cyclase in contrast to EDNO.[15] The exact identity of EDHF still remains uncertain, though research is pointing at a cytochrome P-450 derived, arachidonic acid metabolite.[16] Prostacyclin (PGI_2) is another vaso-relaxant produced by the endothelium.[17] It increases the c-AMP (cyclic-adenosine monophosphate) in smooth muscle cells. Like the raise of c-GMP in case of EDNO, this results in smooth muscle cell relaxation.

In addition to vasodilating factors, endothelium-derived vaso-constricting factors have been identified. Endothelin-1(ET-1) is one of them. This peptide, discovered in 1988 by Yanagisawa et al.,[18] exhibits strong vasoconstrictor activity. Until now, not much is known about circumstances of activation and release. Other endothelium-derived vaso-constricting factors are angiotensin-II,[19] a well-known product of the renin-angiotensin system, and the vaso-constrictive prostanoids.[20]

Induction of vasomotion
Acetylcholine (a muscarinic receptor activator), is a vasodilator *in-vivo* and a vasoconstrictor *in-vitro*. This apparent paradox was unraveled in 1980,[1] when the importance of intact (healthy, vivid) endothelium was recognized for turning the acetylcholine-effect from vasoconstrictive into vasodilating.

Now we know that acetylcholine causes vasoconstriction through its direct action on muscarinic receptors of the vascular smooth muscle cells. The degree of constriction is blunted by the concomitant release of NO through activation of the muscarinic receptors on endothelial cells. Thus, activation of muscarinic receptors on endothelial cells cause induction of the l-arginine/NO pathway resulting in vasodilatation, while activation of muscarinic receptors on smooth muscle cells cause vasoconstriction (Figure 3). These antagonizing forces give a resulting tone of the smooth muscle.

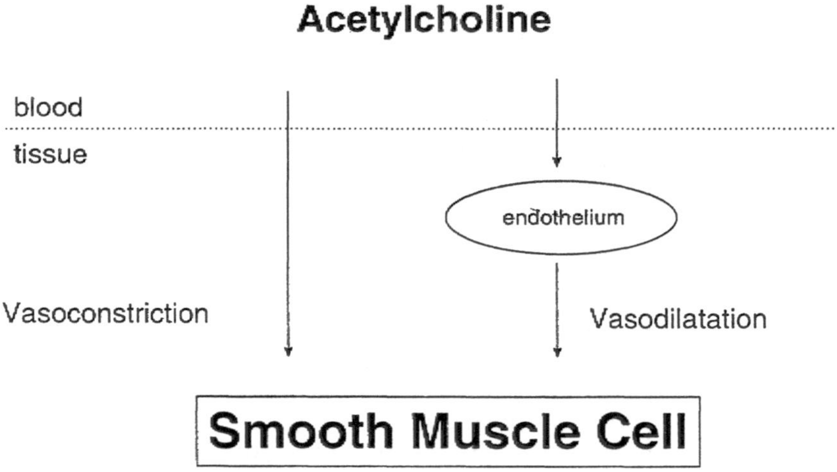

Acetylcholine

Figure 3. The *"double agent"* acetylcholine. See text.

There are other endothelium receptor agonists, in addition to acetylcholine, which also have this effect. Examples of these so called *"double agents"* are serotonin and norepinephrine. Examples of single agents (only induction of the l-arginine/NO pathway) are bradykinin, substance-P and thrombin. Single and double agents are widely utilized in the vascular system. Platelet aggregation, for example, triggers EDNO release in the healthy endothelium.[21] This effect is due to serotonin (5-HT) and adenosine diphosphate (ADP), released by aggregating platelets. As described above, serotonin is a double agent, causing vasodilation, inhibition of platelet aggregation, and inhibition of platelet adhesion to the endothelial cells. This results in elimination of the microaggregate and thereby the prevention of vascular occlusion. The opposite is true in the case of endothelial dysfunction where the synthesis of opposing EDNO is compromised.

Physical stimuli are another group of important stimuli for endothelium dependent vaso-relaxation. The most important among them is "shear stress" or viscous drag. This is the longitudinal force exerted by the blood flow velocity upon the endothelial cell layer. Increase of shear stress causes an increase of EDNO production. This results in vasodilation and causes a fall in blood flow velocity and related shear stress[22] which can be considered as a feedback, regulatory mechanism. The induction of the l-arginine/NO pathway by shear stress is the consequence of conductance changes of potassium channels in the endothelial membrane.[23] This leads to an increase of cytosolic calcium, resulting in activation of endothelial NOS.

The EDNO production is directly related to blood flow velocity under normal physiologic conditions. Besides receptor-agonist initiated EDNO release, however, there is also a continuous basal release.[24] Next to the importance for basal vessel tone, this is also important for regulatory functions such as smooth muscle cell inhibition and prevention of expression of adhesion-molecules.

The assessment of endothelial function
Endothelium-dependent vasorelaxation (EDV) may be regarded as a thermometer of endothelial health. To use this effectively and comparably, it is necessary to quantify the "degree" of EDV. This is established by giving EDV impulses [chemical (acetylcholine) or physical (flow increase)] to the endothelium after which the reaction is compared to a reference standard. As reference standard, the physiologically, maximal, achievable vasodilation is used, comparable to the situation in which the endothelial cells would produce an abundance of EDNO. This situation can be simulated by endothelium independent vasodilators (EIDV) like nitroglycerin.

Invasive assessment of endothelial function of epicardial conductance vessels
Ludmer et al.[25] introduced the technique of intracoronary, endothelial function assessment in humans. The technique at present still resembles the original technique. After acquiring baseline coronary angiograms of the coronary artery of interest, graded concentrations of acetylcholine is infused. After each intra-coronary acetylcholine infusion an angiogram is taken, which will be analyzed afterwards using quantitative coronary analysis techniques. The quantified endothelium-dependent vascular response to acetylcholine can then be compared to the quantified endothelium-independent vascular response to nitroglycerin.

Noninvasive assessment of endothelial function
Two noninvasive methods have been developed for assessment of endothelial function. In principle they measure flow or diameter changes in a limb without invading the body. For drug administration, however, artery cannulation may be required.

First, the mercury strain-gauge plethysmography technique[26] is performed on the forearm. By inflating upperarm cuffs to supra-diastolic pressure values, venous return is stopped. This will result in a time related, volume increase of the forearm, directly related to the (unimpaired) arterial forearm blood flow. The change in circumference of the forearm alters the electrical resistance of a strain-gauge applied around it. These resistance changes can be reduced to changes in blood flow, which in turn are regarded as a measure of endothelial function.

Second, fore-arm B-mode ultrasonography as a method for endothelial function assessment was introduced in 1992 by Celermajer et al.[27] The brachial artery diameter change in response to increased blood flow is measured. After a 5 minute period of ischemia (upper arm occlusion) as provocation for increased blood flow, the normal brachial artery diameter will increase up to 20%, with good individual reproducibility. Blood flow related shear stress is one of the main modulators of EDNO release. This explains why blood flow-induced vasodilatation (reactive hyperemia) of the brachial artery is a measure of endothelial function. When endothelial dysfunction aggravates, the diameter augmentation will be depressed or even vasoconstriction may occur. The advantages of noninvasive measurements are obvious, although not always sufficient. When the interest is focused on systemic endothelial function an estimate of the general state of endothelial health is enough. However, when local endothelial function has to be assessed (coronary artery segments), invasive methods are inevitable.

Endothelial (dys)function

Endothelial dysfunction, as expressed earlier, is the impairment of various regulating functions expressed by the endothelium. Clinical relevant sources of endothelial dysfunction are hypercholesterolemia and atherosclerosis. Endothelial dysfunction is next to being caused by atherosclerosis, also an amplifier of the atherosclerotic process and a major causal factor in the occurrence of ischemic symptoms and associated events.

Atherogenesis
In the early days, atherosclerosis was thought to be a degenerative process, an inevitable consequence of aging. Virchow[28] believed that atherosclerosis developed as a form of low-grade injury to the artery wall. This would result in a type of inflammatory insudate, which in turn caused the passage and accumulation of plasma constituents in the intima of the arterial wall. Among other concepts, this hypothesis led to the "response to injury" hypothesis;[29] "injury" to the endothelium would initiate the atherosclerotic lesion development. Atherosclerosis today is seen as a chronic inflammatory

condition which is converted into an acute clinical event by plaque rupture or plaque instability.[30] The basic mechanisms inducing this sequence are thought to involve low density lipoproteins (LDL) and oxidative processes. When atherogenesis is looked upon in a contemporary perspective the following aspects of atherogenesis, relevant to endothelial (dys)function, can be singled out;[3] (Figure 4)

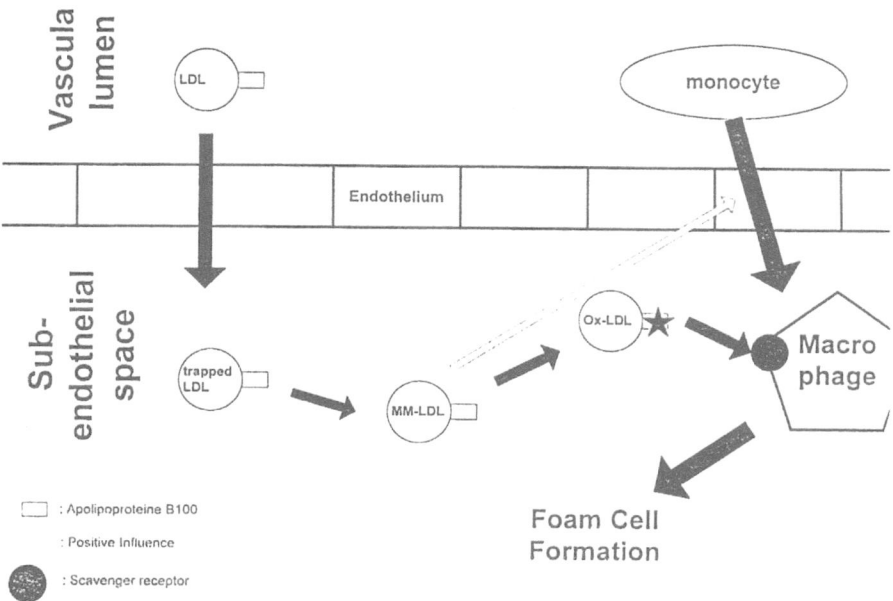

Figure 4. *Outline of the initiation of atherosclerosis. LDL, low density lipoprotein; MM-LDL, mildly modified LDL; Ox-LDL, oxidated LDL. See text.*

The first step in development of atherosclerotic lesions is the concentration dependent process of lipoproteins (mainly LDL) into the subendothelial space. The LDL becomes entrapped in the subendothelial, three-dimensional cagework of fibers, after which it is oxidized by endothelial, smooth muscle and inflammatory cell released substances. This oxidative modification is thought to occur in two stages. The first oxidation stage happens before monocytes are recruited into the arterial wall. Initially, the LDL particle is protected against this mild oxidative modification by lipophilic antioxidants (like vitamin E). However, after depletion, the polyunsaturated fatty acids of the phospholipids will be modified. Also conversion of phosphatidylcholine (lecithin) into lysophosphatidylcholine (Lyso PC or lysolecithin) takes place. At the early stage of oxidation, the apo-B100 (apolipoprotein B100, the protein by which LDL is recognized) is still unmodified, so the LDL particle can still be recognized by the "normal" B/E receptors (receptors at the surface of hepatic cells, intended to recognize, among others, the apo-B100 molecules) as native LDL. In this initial stage of oxidation, the LDL is referred to as minimal modified LDL (MM-LDL). MM-LDL attracts plasma monocytes directly through chemotaxis and indirectly through its ability to stimulate the endothelial cell to express adhesion molecules. These monocytes are converted into macrophages in the sub-endothelial space and with their enormous oxidative capacity, convert MM-LDL into Ox-LDL(Oxidated LDL). At this stage of LDL oxidation the amino acid residues on the apo-B100 protein become oxidized which is accompanied by the loss of recognition of the LDL particle by the normal B/E-receptor and a concomitant shift to recognition by the scavenger/ox-LDL receptors. These scavenger receptors are present on macrophages and smooth muscle cells which leads to the uptake of LDL by receptors the expression of which is not regulated by the intracellular lipid concentration. The result is the formation of "foam cells"; the hallmark of atherosclerosis. The lesion grows through the imbedding of new mononuclear cells, proliferation of macrophages and smooth muscle cells and the accumulation of extracellular lipid in a necrotic core. Finally thrombosis may be initiated by intimal plaque rupture or "activated" endothelium.

For more than 20 years an increase of serum LDL level has been associated with the development of atherosclerosis.[31] More recent is the premise that the oxidative modification of LDL (and possibly other lipoproteins) is pivotal in the initiation and progression of atherosclerosis. This "oxidation hypothesis"[32] of atherosclerosis has been confirmed now by an impressive body of evidence.[33]

Oxidated LDL has many atherogenic properties which can not be duplicated by native LDL,[34] for example, chemotaxis of monocytes, inhibition of macrophage mobility, foam cell formation, up-regulation of endothelial adhesion molecules, proliferative effects on smooth muscle cells, cytotoxicity to endothelial cells and inhibition of endothelium dependent-vasomotion. Lysophosphatidylcholine (Lyso PC), one of the lipid components unique to oxidating LDL, mimics many of the pro-atherogenic effects of ox-LDL. This component of ox-LDL might be the most important in the context of endothelial dysfunction.

Endothelial dysfunction and atherosclerosis
In 1983, Shimokawa et al.,[35] among others, demonstrated that infusion of vasoactive agents like histamine caused vasoconstriction in atherosclerotic arteries. Apart from this kind of observations was the discovery of Furchgott et al.[1] that several vasoactive substances cause release of a potent vasodilator only in the presence of intact endothelium. These observations

together have led to the speculation that atherosclerosis might be related to endothelial dysfunction.

The relations between the morphological aspects of atherosclerosis and endothelial dysfunction were the first to be recognized and Ludmer et al.[25] (Figure 5) were the first to demonstrate, in 1986, the correlation between endothelial dysfunction and the severity of atheroma. In their experiments the dose response to the double agent acetylcholine showed a shift from dilatation towards increasing degrees of constriction in relation to the graded, morphologic, severity of underlying atheroma, while the response to nitroglycerin was unaffected. The latter would suggest an unimpaired function of the vascular smooth muscle. During the following years, endothelial dysfunction was also demonstrated in smooth coronary arteries with visible atherosclerosis elsewhere in the coronary system.[36]

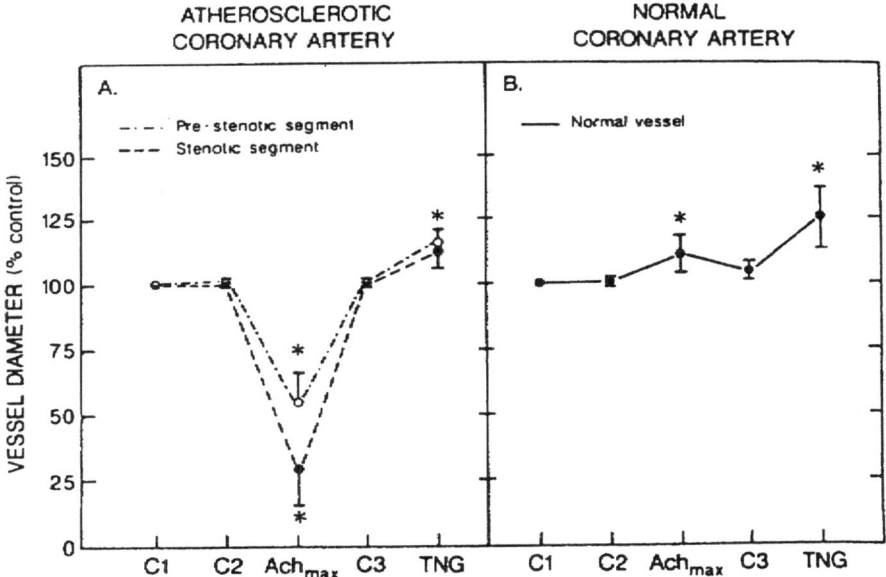

Figure 5. *Responses of coronary arteries to the endothelium-dependent vasodilator acetylcholine and the endothelium-independent vasodilator nitroglycerin, in 8 atherosclerotic coronary arteries and 4 (angiographic) normal coronary arteries. C1/C2/C3, control infusions; Ach_{max}, response to maximal dose of acetylcholine; TNG, response to nitroglycerin. (Reprinted by permission from Ludmer et al.[25])*

Today, there is an advancing body of evidence that endothelial dysfunction is more related to enhanced cholesterol levels (and more specific ox-LDL levels) than to the formation and progression of atherosclerotic lesions. Experiments in humans have shown that there is a direct link between endothelial function and cholesterol serum levels.[37] Furthermore, it is demonstrated that hypercholesterolemia impairs endothelium-dependent relaxation of the microcirculation, where overt atherosclerosis does not develop.[38] This, together with the fact that selective LDL removal, directly improves endothelial function,[39] leads to the hypothesis that atherogenic plasma itself can induce disorders of endothelial function.

Possible explanations for disturbance of endothelial function
Central to the concept of the genesis of endothelial dysfunction is endothelial stress. This is the burden put upon endothelial cells by their environment. Although the endothelial cells have their own maintenance systems, the prolongation or intensification of stress will result in endothelial dysfunction. The causes of endothelial stress can be divided into metabolic (hypercholesterolemia, diabetes, smoking, infection, ischemia), physical (PTCA, hypertension) and degenerative (age) causes.

Among the metabolic stress causes, hypercholesterolemia-related "oxidative stress" seems to be very important. Oxidative stress is the total burden of potentially harmful reactive biochemical species that are present in tissues as a consequence of the routine cellular oxidative metabolism. Increased oxidative stress refers to a state in which the production of these species is enhanced.[13] One source of oxidative stress for the endothelium is formed by the oxygen-derived radicals like superoxides, which can be generated by injury, ischemia, ox-LDL, activated leukocytes, smooth muscle cells and the endothelium itself.[13] Superoxides are produced as a byproduct of many cellular reactions and are normally maintained at very low levels by the activity of radical scavenging systems. The dysfunctional state of the endothelium might be due to increased production of reactive species or by a relative shortage of scavengers.

It has been shown that hypercholesterolemic rabbits have increased levels of superoxide radicals, which can be brought to normal levels upon dieting.[40] The most important source of these superoxides appears to consist of endothelial and smooth muscle cells. Membrane-bound oxidases,[41] activated by ox-LDL,[42] seem to be the cause. Cholesterol reduction reduces the amount of available LDL for oxidation and can, in this fashion, diminish oxidative stress.

The effects of hypercholesterolemic related oxidative stress and related side effects on endothelial cells are multiple. Oxygen radicals such as hydrogen peroxide and hydroxide participate in lipid peroxidation and damage of the cellular membranes. Also impaired signal transduction is demonstrated, caused by alterations of the G-protein (an important protein, associated with the membrane receptors).[43] Furthermore, decreased activity of eNOS[44] and changed bioactivity of EDNO are demonstrated.[45]

Next to hypercholesterolemia and atherosclerosis there are other factors related to endothelial dysfunction. They overlap with the known risk factors for ischemic heart diseases such as hypertension, aging, and diabetes.

Endothelial dysfunction and ischemic events
Endothelial dysfunction is probably a very important step in the generation of the clinical symptoms, generally associated with the atherosclerotic process. The endothelium in a healthy person maintains a balance in the circulatory system, aptly reacting to changing circumstances such as sympathetic activation, shear stress, etc. When endothelial dysfunction occurs, the reactions to environmental stimuli become inadequate. The endothelium gets "activated".
In stable angina, important triggers of chest pain are sympathetic activation, mental stress and cold exposure. Endothelial dysfunction is probably an important factor in the cause of angina, in the presence of stenosis.[46] Dysfunction may just override the critical level of luminal narrowing, compromising the oxygen supply.
The pathological substrate of unstable angina is seen as plaque rupture or plaque activation with subsequent platelet activation and thrombus formation.[30] There are several mechanisms by which dysfunctional endothelium interferes with the progression of unstable angina. For example, platelets release serotonin during the process of thrombosis. This is a double agent, so in case of endothelial dysfunction, the vasoconstrictive impulse will be unopposed. Thrombin, a substance produced after initiation of the coagulation cascade, is a single agent for vasodilation. Also this effect is compromised in case of endothelial dysfunction. In patients with atherosclerosis, indeed vasoconstriction is demonstrated distal to the site of the thrombus formation.[47]

Restoring endothelial function by cholesterol reduction

Modes of cholesterol reduction
Until 1987, lipid reduction therapy was limited to diet, bile sequestrants, nicotinic acid and fibrates. Unfortunately, these therapies had limited efficacy and tolerability. Next to diet, fibrates were the therapy of choice. They were relatively well tolerated and produced a moderate reduction of LDL cholesterol, a moderate increase of high density lipid-cholesterol and a substantial reduction of triglycerides. The introduction of lovastatin (a 3-hydroxy-3-methyl-glutaryl-coenzyme A (HMG-CoA) reductase inhibitor) in 1987 changed this preference in treatment completely.
In the 1960s it was discovered that the feedback suppression of cholesterol

synthesis in the liver, by dietary cholesterol, is mediated through changes in the activity of HMG-CoA reductase enzyme. This microsomal enzyme catalyzes the conversion of HMG-CoA to mevalonate and is the rate-limiting enzyme in cholesterol synthesis. These findings started the search for a HMG-CoA reductase inhibitor. The first result of this search was the fungal metabolite mevastatin (formerly ML-236B), which was isolated from the micro-organism *Penicillium Citrinum* in 1973.[48] Related compounds were isolated in the following years and by 1980 it had been shown that mevastatin reduced LDL-cholesterol levels in humans.[49] These findings gave rise to more research which resulted in four approved HMG-CoA reductase inhibitor drugs by 1996. The currently used statins reduce total serum cholesterol levels by 15-30% and LDL-cholesterol levels by 20-40%. They also cause a modest increase in high density lipid-cholesterol (5-10%), and a reduction of triglycerides by up to 20%.[50] In general they are tolerated well. Studies have shown that HMG-CoA reductase inhibitors upregulate the hepatic B/E-receptors by decreasing the intra-cellular cholesterol contents of the liver cell. This is a feedback mechanism. The increased receptor density causes more apo B/E containing particles (among which LDL) to be withdrawn from the circulation.

New developments concern the introduction of a new generation of potent HMG-CoA reductase inhibitors. They not only have increased reduction capabilities with respect to serum cholesterol (up to 60% of the LDL-cholesterol) in primary hypercholesterolemia but they also reduce triglyceride concentrations in patients with primary hypertriglyceridemia by more than 40%.[51]

Cholesterol lowering trials and cardiovascular events
Many clinical trials have convincingly demonstrated the beneficial effect of cholesterol-lowering therapy on both cardiovascular mortality and morbidity.[52-54] Besides these impressive clinical effects, it was demonstrated that cholesterol-lowering caused reduced progression and in some instances, regression, of atherosclerotic coronary lesions.[55-57] The average small change in diameter stenosis (1 to 2 %), resulting from cholesterol reduction, appears not to be sufficient to explain the observed decrease of the event rate. Also in other studies it seems that angiographic severity of stenosis is poorly correlated to physiological parameters and clinical events.[58] For example, Ambrose et al.[59] found an average stenosis diameter reduction of 48% at infarct-related lesions and that only 22% of the infarct related lesions had a stenosis diameter reduction of more than 70%. Similar results have been reported by others.[60]

All of this together leads to the conclusion that lesion diameter improvement is not the only factor causing the event rate to drop with cholesterol reduction therapy. Evidence is accumulating that improvement of endothelial function and plaque stability by cholesterol reduction are more responsible for this.[58]

Endothelial function and cholesterol reduction
Reduction in cholesterol levels results in improved endothelial function. This was first demonstrated in vessels of hypercholesterolemic monkeys in whom endothelial function was completely restored after dieting.[61] The first of endothelial function improvement in human coronary arteries *in-vivo* was given by Leung et al.[62] in 1993. For cholesterol reduction they used diet and bile sequestrants. Recent studies, using statins to lower cholesterol resulted in even more endothelial function improvement.[63] (Figure 6) Since then several trials have been conducted to prove that reduction of LDL-related endothelial stress factors, like oxidative resistance of LDL, also result in improvement of endothelial function.[64]

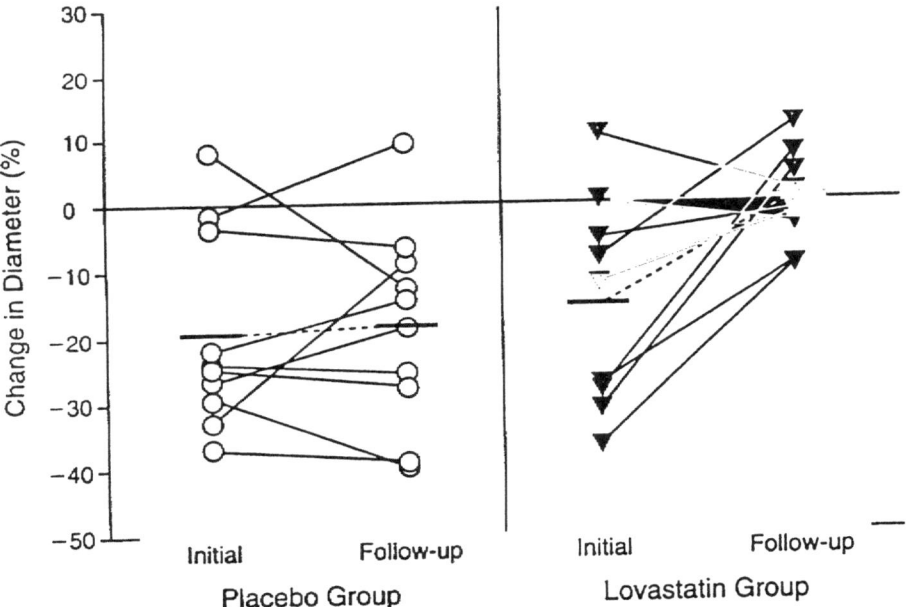

Figure 6. Individual responses to peak-dose acetylcholine among those in the placebo group (10 patients) and the lovastatin group (9 patients), who were studied initially(IN) and at follow-up(FU) (5,5 months). (Reprinted by permission from Treasure et al.[63])

Improvement of endothelial function with cholesterol reduction therapy becomes apparent within weeks[65] in case of statin therapy and almost immediately in case of LDL-apheresis.[39] It is even possible to prevent deterioration of endothelial function when a cholesterol rich diet is administered parallel with statins in mice.[66] All these effects are probably related to LDL and oxidative stress levels.[13,58] Both of them are effectively counteracted with cholesterol lowering strategies.

The mechanism by which serum cholesterol reduction decreases the frequency of ischemic events, in the absence of a substantial change in lesions, is not completely clear, but improvement of endothelial dysfunction seems to be an important one. Endothelial dysfunction related to hypercholesterolemia and atherosclerosis can exacerbate unstable coronary syndromes by virtue of the pathological responses to substances associated with plaque rupture (i.e. serotonin, thrombin, catecholamines). The dysfunction reflects an underlying pathologic state in which the endothelium supports thrombosis and inhibits fibrinolysis. These pro-thrombotic and antifibrinolytic abnormalities have a clear implication for (un)stable ischemic syndromes.

The hypolipidemic effect is probably not the only effect of HMG-CoA reductase inhibitors on the course of cardiac events. Mevalonic acid, the product of the enzyme reaction inhibited by HMG-CoA reductase inhibitors, is not only the precursor of cholesterol but also of numerous other isoprenoid metabolites such as dolichol, ubiquinone and isopentenyladenosine.[67] All of these metabolites are essential to normal cell function, for example, in the control of cell proliferation. So beyond their effects on plasma lipids, the statins also appear to have direct, anti-atherosclerotic effects on the vessel wall.[68] Until now, however, the underlying mechanism is not fully clear.

Endothelial (dys)function and percutaneous transluminal coronary angioplasty

Percutaneous transluminal coronary angioplasty
Since the introduction by Andreas Gruentzig in 1977,[69] PTCA procedures have become the first choice treatment for coronary artery stenosis in single and two vessel disease. The initial success rate is over 90%, however restenosis, occurring in 30% to 40% of the patients within the first six months, is still a major problem.[70]

The events happening after angioplasty can be divided into three, partially overlapping, phases.[71] (Figures 7 and 8) Phase 1, the elastic recoil, happens within the first 24 hours. This acute lumen loss is caused by the elastic properties of the stenotic wall. Phase 2, is the mural thrombus formation. During the first 2 to 3 weeks, platelet depositions take place, forming a adhesive thrombus with all its accompanying paracrine effects. Phase 3 is the phase of smooth muscle cell activation with subsequent migration and

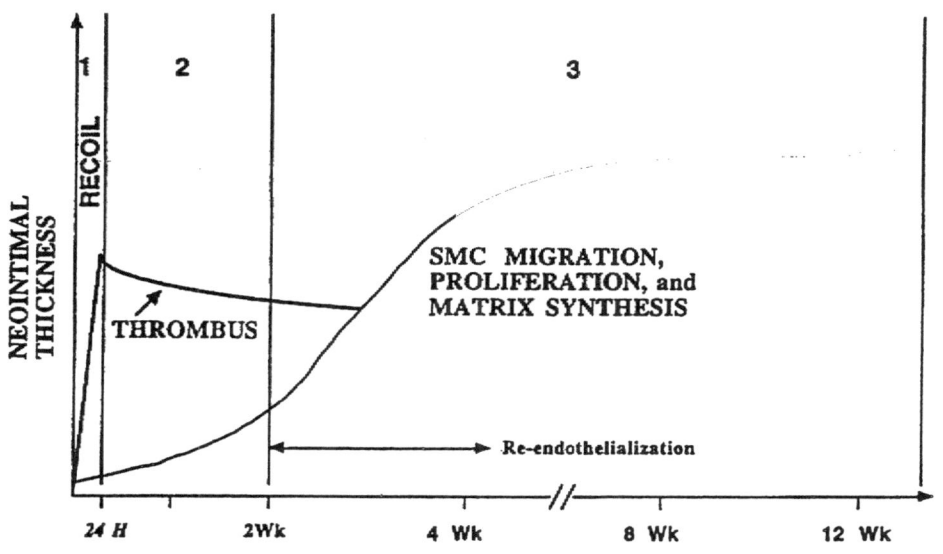

Figure 7. *The three sequential phases of vascular response to balloon angioplasty, in normal pig coronary arteries. SMC, smooth muscle cell; H, hour; Wk, week. (Reprinted by permission from Gallo et al.[71])*

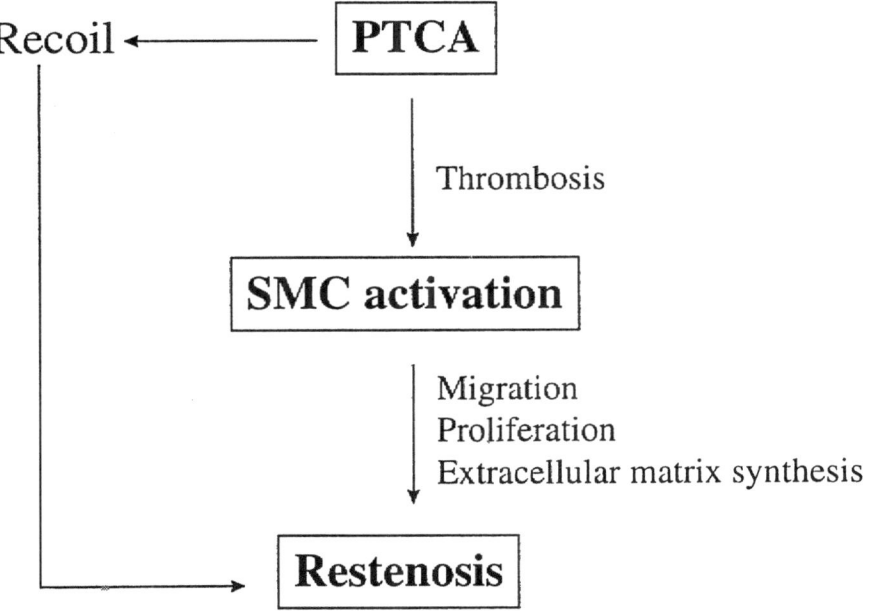

Figure 8. *The process of restenosis genesis. PTCA, percutaneous transluminal coronary angioplasty; SMS, smooth muscle cell.*

proliferation of smooth muscle cells. This is accompanied by extracellular matrix formation (intimal hyperplasia). This phase commences in the first week and tends to cease within 3 months. About 40% of the activated medial smooth muscle cells actually migrates to the intima region through breaks in the internal elastic membrane. This is were the proliferation·and synthesis of extracellular matrix takes place.

Following PTCA, elastic recoil is the most important, acute event with respect to restenosis. Within the first minute after final balloon deflation there is a significant reduction in luminal cross sectional area. The chronic processes like cell growth and proliferation are also initiated by the dilation of smooth muscle. Early markers for smooth muscle activation, the proto-oncogenes, are visible within 30 minutes after injury.[72] The proliferation in smooth muscle cells last up to 4 weeks, during which a different kind of smooth muscle cell is generated: the synthetic smooth muscle cells. These cells have lower contractile abilities and seem to be totally focused on extracellular matrix production. The added wall volume, 4 weeks after PTCA, mainly reflects the synthesis of extracellular matrix by the synthetic smooth muscle cells.[73] In the perspective of smooth muscle cell proliferation also re-endothelialization is important. It seems that the intimal thickening response to injury depends on the rate and pattern of endothelial regeneration. Areas that are quickly covered by endothelium are protected from accumulation of smooth muscle cells.[74]

Next to the above-described intimal hyperplasia there is the factor of arterial remodeling in the restenosis process. Arterial remodeling is well described in *de-novo* atherosclerosis as an adaptive enlargement response to plaque extension, maintaining the lumen area until the plaque occupies 40% of the area circumscribed by the internal elastic lamina.[75] Recently it has been shown in animal experiments that there is an important role for failure in compensatory enlargement (vascular remodeling) in the restenosis process.[76] Whatever the actual underlying mechanism may be, until now, in spite of encouraging animal experiments, no systemic pharmacologic agent has been proven to produce a clinical, valid reduction of restenosis.

Endothelium and PTCA
Studies have demonstrated that balloon dilation results in the disruption of both atherosclerotic plaque and arterial wall, with rupture of intima and media.[77] Animal studies have also shown that the intima of coronary arteries is completely denuded after PTCA, exposing a thrombogenic and adhesive subendothelial layer.[78] This results in platelet and leucocyte adhesion with formation of local thrombus and concomitant release of growth factors.

The degree of injury is important. If the internal elastic lamina remains intact, platelet adherence to the lesion is transient and there is no formation of a fibrin-rich thrombus. Re-endothelialization will be completed within a week and the signs of injury will be gone. On the surface of deeply injured arteries, however, mural thrombi are present for over a week. This will lead to delayed or even incomplete re-endothelialization. The process of re-endothelialization itself starts from the edge of the injury and from the orifice of collateral arteries. The intact endothelial cells at these injury borders enter the replication cycle within hours after angioplasty. The replication process is initiated by loss of contact, stretch and growth factors,[79] and will cease within 6 to 10 weeks, depending on the extent of injury.[80]

In the perspective of vascular remodeling, it has been shown that an increase of lumen area occurs in response to long-term increase in flow velocity. This shear stress induced remodeling response is dependent upon intact endothelium.[81] The presence of dysfunctional endothelium may contribute, in this fashion, to the restenosis process.[82]

Endothelial function and PTCA
The lifespan of the endothelial cell is about 30 years. Unfortunately, regenerated cells (neo-endothelium), apart from having different anatomic features, like the polygonal shapes and misalignment with the blood flow, also possess a diminished functional capability. The dysfunctional neo-endothelium, which is less able to produce EDNO, may contribute to the development of intimal thickening indirectly through the loss of platelet inhibition (which in turn results in the release of growth factors) and directly through the loss of inhibition of smooth muscle cell growth.[83] In particular the responses to serotonin and α2-adrenergic agonists, both patho-physiologically important substances, seem to be impaired.[84] The reasons for the dysfunction are not clear. Receptor pathway impairment[85] and dysfunctional eNOS have been proposed.[86]

In conclusion it seems that the endothelium has the ability for quick anatomical regeneration, though functional regeneration lags behind.

In-vivo studies of PTCA and endothelial function
Several research projects have been undertaken to assess endothelial function after PTCA, however, there are only a few *in-vivo* studies, reporting the intra-coronary assessment of endothelial function with acetylcholine. El-Tamimi et al.[87] were the first to apply quantitative coronary analysis and graded acetylcholine-dose infusion technique for endothelial function assessment. They demonstrated a dose-dependent constriction of the dilated segment and together with the results of other subsequent studies it was concluded that the dilated segment had a dose-dependent reaction to acetylcholine although it was more constrictive than other segments. Furthermore, it appeared that the segment distal to the PTCA lesion reacted

less well than other segments.[88] Unfortunately, the studies consisted of small groups of patients or they were not homogeneous with respect to risk factors. The latter is very important. Sakai et al.,[89] for example, demonstrated a clear relationship between the endothelial function of the dilated segment and the cholesterol level 3 to 6 months after PTCA.

An important conclusion drawn from these studies appears to be that the dilated segment does react in an acetylcholine dose-dependent fashion. Thus, regenerated endothelium has the capacity to produce vasomotion which is contrary to earlier beliefs and although endothelial function is worse than in not-dilated segments, it has been shown that the function is related to cholesterol plasma levels (Figures 9-12).

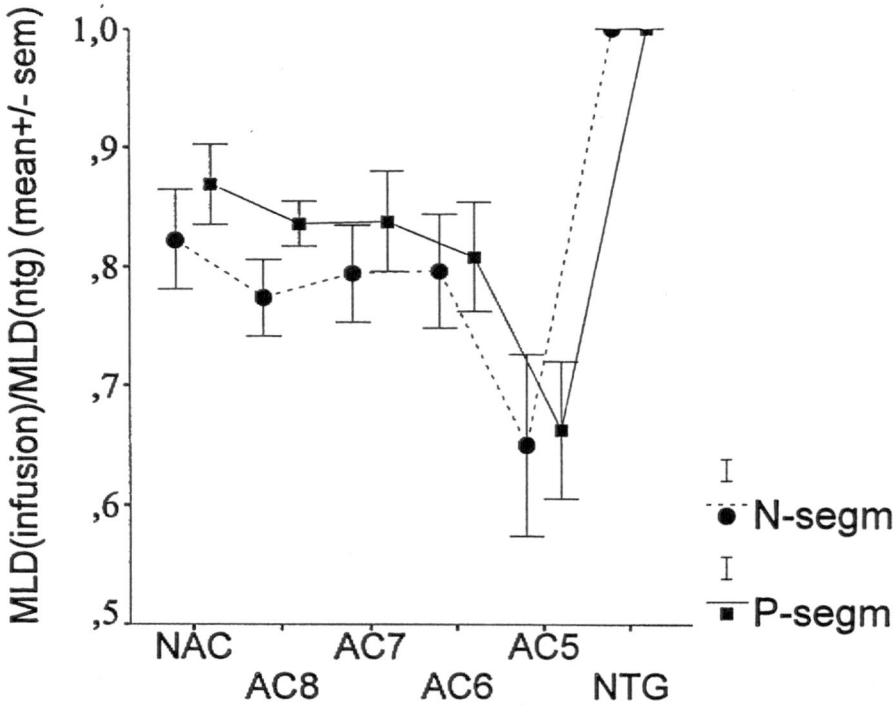

Figure 9. Vasomotion of the dilated segment compared to the angiographically normal segment, 2 months after PTCA. SE, standard error; MLD(infusion)/MLD(ntg), this is the ratio of the minimum lumen diameter at a certain infusion, divided by the minimum lumen diameter at nitroglycerin infusion; P-seg, dilated segment; N-segm, angiographically normal segment; Ac-8/5, acetylcholine infusions expressed as locally estimated concentrations, ranging from 10^{-8} to 10^{-5} mol/liter; NTG, nitroglycerin. PREFACE study, preliminary results in 10 patients.

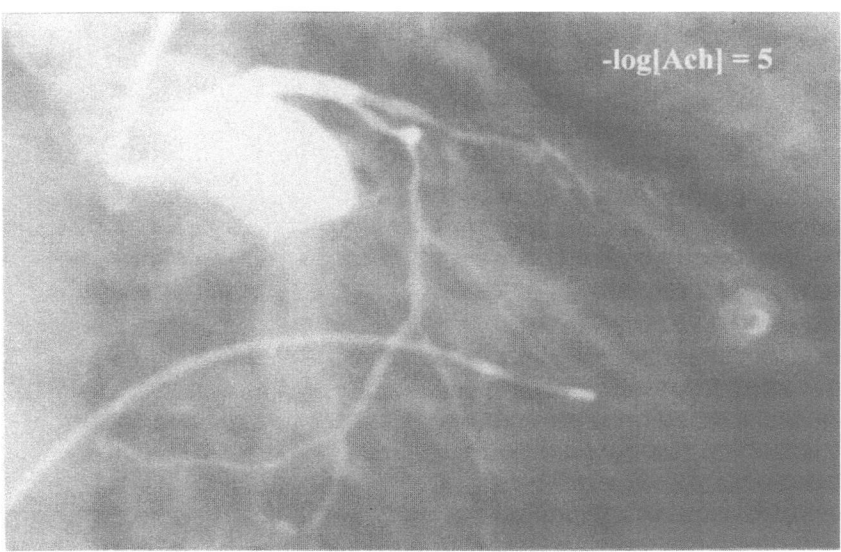

Figure 10. Angiograms made at peak-acetylcholine infusions. A major response is seen in this patient. PREFACE study, preliminary results.

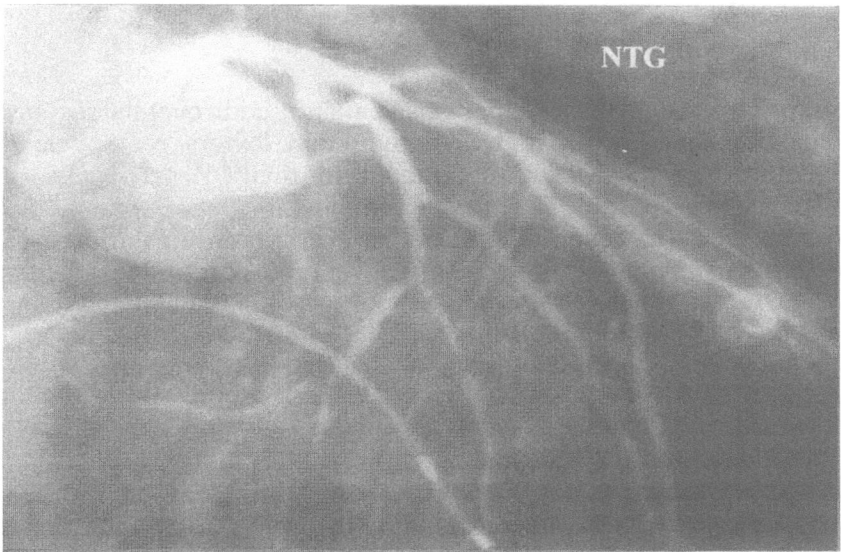

Figure 11. Angiograms made during nitroglycerin infusion just after the angiogram shown in figure 10 was made. Complete normalization is seen. PREFACE study, preliminary results.

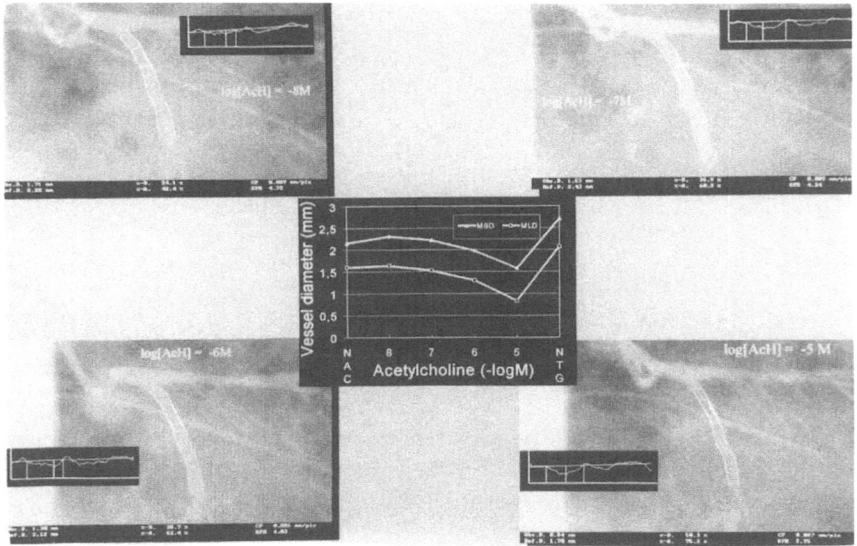

Figure 12. Compilation of the infusions sequence angiograms made in one patient and the quantitative coronary angiography results. MSD, mean segment diameter; MLD, minimum luminal diameter; NAC, saline; NTG, nitroglycerin. PREFACE study, preliminary results.

Cholesterol reduction and PTCA

Cholesterol reduction and restenosis remain a controversial issue. Several studies have suggested that lipid reduction lowers restenosis rate.[90-93] However, others have failed to demonstrate this.[94-96]

The results of REGRESS,[56] a cholesterol-lowering, two-year angiographic follow-up study to assess the effect of pravastatin on the progression of coronary atherosclerosis, show a lower restenosis rate. In patients treated with PTCA, the pravastatin group had 47% fewer clinical events and 61% fewer re-PTCAs, compared to the placebo group. Since REGRESS was not designed to evaluate these problems, this difference can not be explained definitively.

Reducing restenosis rate and other cardiovascular events by improving endothelial function

Research has been undertaken to prove that direct improvement of endothelial function is beneficial to the event rate after PTCA. Drugs like angiopeptin and angiotensinogen converting enzyme inhibitors, which proved to be effective in animals, did not have the desired effect in recent clinical trials.[97,98] Also bypassing the endothelial cell employing novel, NO donating drugs didn't seem effective.[99] It has been shown that deterioration in endothelial function leads to ischemic cardiovascular events (chronic and acute) and that improvement of endothelial dysfunction is observed with cholesterol lowering medication. It is well-known that following PTCA the neo-endothelium is partially dysfunctional and has to regenerate functionally over a period of time. Consequently, a reduction in lipid related "stress" could improve and accelerate functional regeneration, with beneficial effects on cardiovascular event rates. This is why the PREFACE study (Pravastatin Related Effects Following Angioplasty on Coronary Endothelium) was initiated. This randomized, placebo controlled, clinical trial is designed to evaluate the effect of pravastatin therapy on the endothelial function of dilated segments in 80 patients. The results of this study will be known within several years.

References

1. Furchgott RF, Zawadzki JV. The obligatory role of endothelial cells in the relaxation of arterial smooth muscle by acetylcholine. Nature 1980;288:373-6.
2. Vanhoutte PM. Endothelium and control of vascular function. State of the Art lecture. Hypertension 1989;13:658-67.
3. Berliner JA, Navab M, Fogelman AM ET AL. Atherosclerosis: basic mechanisms. Oxidation, inflammation, and genetics. Circulation 1995;91:2488-96.
4. Moncada S, Higgs A. The l-arginine-nitric oxide pathway. N Engl J Med 1993;329:2002-12.
5. Palmer RMJ, Ferrige AG, Moncada S. Nitric oxide release accounts for the biological activity of endothelium-derived relaxing factor. Nature 1987;327:524-6.
6. Myers PR, Minor R Jr., Guerra R Jr., Bates JN, Harrison DG. Vasorelaxant properties of the endothelium-derived relaxing factor more closely resemble S-nitrosocysteine than nitric oxide. Nature 1990;345:161-3.
7. Kelm M, Schrader J. Control of coronary vascular tone by nitric oxide. Circ Res 1990;66:1561-75.
8. Moncada S. The first Robert Furchgott lecture: from endothelium-dependent relaxation to the L-arginine: NO pathway. Blood Vessels 1990;27:208-17.
9. Sase K, Michel T. Expression and regulation of endothelial nitric oxide synthase. Trends Cardiovasc Med 1997;7:28-37.
10. Radomski MW, Palmer RMJ, Moncada S. The role of nitric oxide and cGMP in platelet adhesion to vascular endothelium. Biochem Biophys Res Commun 1987;148:1482-91.
11. Scott-Burden T, Vanhoutte PM. The endothelium as a regulator of vascular smooth muscle proliferation. Circulation 1993;87:V-51-V-55.
12. Provost P, Lam JY, Lacoste L, Merhi Y, Waters D. Endothelium-derived nitric oxide attenuates neutrophil adhesion to endothelium under arterial flow conditions. Arteriosclér Thromb 1994;14:331-5.
13. Keaney JF Jr., Vita JA. Atherosclerosis, oxidative stress, and antioxidant protection in endothelium-derived relaxing factor action. Prog Cardiovasc Dis 1995;38:129-54.
14. Chen G, Suzuki H, Weston AH. Acetylcholine releases endothelium-derived hyperpolarizing factor and EDRF from rat blood vessels. Br J Pharmacol

1988;95:1165-74.

15. Bolotina VM, Najibi S, Palacino JJ, Pagano PJ, Cohen RA. Nitric oxide directly activates calcium-dependent potassium channels in vascular smooth muscle. Nature 1994;368:850-3.

16. Hecker M, Bara AT, Bauersachs J, Busse R. Characterization of endothelium-derived hyperpolarizing factor as a cytochrome P450-derived arachidonic acid metabolite in mammals. J Physiol Lond 1994;481:407-14.

17. Siegel G, Schnalke F, Stock G, Grote J. Prostacyclin, endothelium-derived relaxing factor and vasodilatation. Adv Prostaglandin Thromboxane Leukot Res 1989;19:267-70.

18. Yanagisawa M, Kurihara H, Kimura S. A novel potent vasoconstrictor peptide produced by vascular endothelial cells. Nature 1988;332:411-5.

19. Lincoln J, Loesch A, Burnstock G. Localization of vasopressin, serotonin and angiotensin II in endothelial cells of the renal and mesenteric arteries of the rat. Cell Tissue Res 1990;259:341-4.

20. Lin L, Nasjletti A. Role of endothelium-derived prostanoid in angiotensin-induced vasoconstriction. Hypertension 1991;18:158-64.

21. Cohen RA, Shepherd JT, Vanhoutte PM. Vasodilatation mediated by the coronary endothelium in response to aggregating platelets. Bibl Cardiol 1984;35-42.

22. Pohl U, Holtz J, Busse R, Bassenge E. Crucial role of endothelium in the vasodilator response to increased flow in vivo. Hypertension 1986;8:37-44.

23. Olesen SP, Clapham DE, Davies PF. Haemodynamic shear stress activates a K+ current in vascular endothelial cells. Nature 1988;331:168-70.

24. Kelm M, Feelisch M, Spahr R, Piper HM, Noack E, Schrader J. Quantitative and kinetic characterization of nitric oxide and EDRF released from cultured endothelial cells. Biochem Biophys Res Commun 1988;154:236-44.

25. Ludmer PL, Selwyn AP, Shook TL et al. Paradoxical vasoconstriction induced by acetylcholine in atherosclerotic coronary arteries. N Engl J Med 1986;315:1046-51.

26. Fitchett DH. Forearm arterial compliance: a new measure of arterial compliance? Cardiovasc Res 1984;18:651-6.

27. Celermajer DS, Sorensen KE, Gooch VM et al. Non-invasive detection of endothelial dysfunction in children and adults at risk of atherosclerosis. Lancet 1992;340:1111-5.

28. Virchow R (ed): Phlogose und thrombose in gefassytem, gesammelte abhandlungen zur wissenschaftlichen medicin. Frankfurt am main, Meidinger Sohn and Co. 1856

29. Ross R. The pathogenesis of atherosclerosis; an update. N Engl J Med 1986;314:488-500.

30. Fuster V, Badimon L, Badimon JJ, Chesebro JH. The pathogenesis of coronary artery disease and the acute coronary syndromes. N Engl J Med 1992;326:242-50 and 310-8.

31. Kannel WB, Castelli WP, Gordon T, McNamara PM. Serum cholesterol, lipoproteins, and the risk of coronary heart disease. The Framingham study. Ann Intern Med 1971;74:1-12.

32. Steinberg D, Parthasarathy S, Carew TE, Khoo JC, Witztum JL. Beyond cholesterol. Modifications of low-density lipoprotein that increase its atherogenicity. N Engl J Med 1989;320:915-23.

33. Witztum JL. The oxidation hypothesis of atherosclerosis. Lancet 1994;344:793-5.

34. Holvoet P, Collen D. Oxidized lipoproteins in atherosclerosis and thrombosis. FASEB J 1994;8:1279-84.

35. Shimokawa H, Tomoike H, Nabeyama S et al. Coronary artery spasm induced in atherosclerotic miniature swine. Science 1983;221:560-2.
36. Werns SW, Walton JA, Hsia HH, Nabel EG, Sanz ML, Pitt B. Evidence of endothelial dysfunction in angiographically normal coronary arteries of patients with coronary artery disease. Circulation 1989;79:287-91.
37. Cox DA, Cohen ML. Effects of oxidized low-density lipoprotein on vascular contraction and relaxation: clinical and pharmacological implications in atherosclerosis. Pharmacol Rev 1996;48:3-19.
38. Sellke FW, Armstrong ML, Harrison DG. Endothelium-dependent vascular relaxation is abnormal in the coronary microcirculation of atherosclerotic primates. Circulation 1990;81:1586-93.
39. Tamai O, Matsuoka H, Itabe H, Wada Y, Kohno K,.Imaizumi T. Single LDL apheresis improves endothelium-dependent vasodilatation in hypercholesterolemic humans. Circulation 1997;95:76-82.
40. Ohara Y, Peterson TE, Sayegh HS, Subramanian RR, Wilcox JN, Harrison DG. Dietary correction of hypercholesterolemia in the rabbit normalizes endothelial superoxide anion production. Circulation 1995;92:898-903.
41. Mohazzab KM, Kaminski PM, Wolin MS. NADH oxidoreductase is a major source of superoxide anion in bovine coronary artery endothelium. Am J Physiol 1994;266:H2568-72.
42. Ohara Y, Peterson TE, Zheng B, Kuo JF, Harrison DG. Lysophosphatidylcholine increases vascular superoxide anion production via protein kinase C activation. Arterioscler Thromb 1994;14:1007-13.
43. Shimokawa H, Flavahan NA, Vanhoutte PM. Loss of endothelial pertussis toxin-sensitive G protein function in atherosclerotic porcine coronary arteries. Circulation 1991;83:652-60.
44. Liao JK, Shin WS, Lee WY, Clark SL. Oxidized low-density lipoprotein decreases the expression of endothelial nitric oxide synthase. J Biol Chem 1995;270:319-24.
45. Myers PR, Wright TF, Tanner MA, Ostlund RE Jr. The effects of native LDL and oxidized LDL on EDRF bioactivity and nitric oxide production in vascular endothelium. J Lab Clin Med 1994;124:672-83.
46. Bogaty P, Hackett D, Davies G, Maseri A. Vasoreactivity of the culprit lesion in unstable angina. Circulation 1994;90:5-11.
47. Zeiher AM, Schachinger V, Weitzel SH, Wollschlager H, Just H. Intracoronary thrombus formation causes focal vasoconstriction of epicardial arteries in patients with coronary artery disease. Circulation 1991;83:1519-25.
48. Endo A, Kuroda M, Tsujita Y. ML-236A, ML-236B, and ML-236C, new inhibitors of cholesterogenesis produced by Penicillium citrinium. J Antibiot Tokyo 1976;29:1346-8.
49. Yamamoto A, Sudo H, Endo A. Therapeutic effects of ML-236B in primary hypercholesterolemia. Atherosclerosis 1980;35:259-66.
50. Hunninghake D. HMG-CoA reductase inhibitors. Curr Opin Lipidol 1992;3:22-8.
51. Bakker-Arkema RG, Davidson MH, Goldstein RJ et al. Efficacy and safety of a new HMG-CoA reductase inhibitor, atorvastatin, in patients with hypertriglyceridemia. JAMA 1996;275:128-33.
52. Scandinavian Simvastatin Survival Study Group. Randomised trial of cholesterol lowering in 4444 patients with coronary heart disease: the Scandinavian Simvastatin Survival Study (4S). Lancet 1994;344:1383-9.
53. Shepherd J, Cobbe SM, Ford I et al. Prevention of coronary heart disease with

pravastatin in men with hypercholesterolemia. West of Scotland Coronary Prevention Study Group. N Engl J Med 1995;333:1301-7.

54. Sacks FM, Pfeffer MA, Moye LA et al. The effect of pravastatin on coronary events after myocardial infarction in patients with average cholesterol levels. N Engl J Med 1996;335:1001-9.

55. Waters D, Higginson L, Gladstone P et al. Effects of monotherapy with an HMG-CoA reductase inhibitor on the progression of coronary atherosclerosis as assessed by serial quantitative arteriography: The Canadian coronary atherosclerosis intervention trial. Circulation 1994;89:959-68.

56. Jukema JW, Bruschke AV, van-Boven AJ et al. Effects of lipid lowering by pravastatin on progression and regression of coronary artery disease in symptomatic men with normal to moderately elevated serum cholesterol levels. The Regression Growth Evaluation Statin Study (REGRESS). Circulation 1995;91:2528-40.

57. Tamura A, Mikuriya Y, Nasu M et al. Effect of pravastatin (10 mg/day) on progression of coronary atherosclerosis in patients with serum total cholesterol levels from 160 to 220 mg/dl and angiographically documented coronary artery disease. Am J Cardiol 1997;79:893-6.

58. Levine GN, Keaney JF Jr., Vita JA. Cholesterol reduction in cardiovascular disease. Clinical benefits and possible mechanisms. N Engl J Med 1995;332:512-21.

59. Ambrose JA, Tannenbaum MA, Alexopoulos D et al. Angiographic progression of coronary artery disease and the development of myocardial infarction. J Am Coll Cardiol 1988;12:56-62.

60. Little WC, Constantinescu M, Applegate RJ et al. Can coronary angiography predict the site of a subsequent myocardial infarction in patients with mild-to-moderate coronary artery disease? Circulation 1988;78:1157-66.

61. Harrison DG, Armstrong ML, Freiman PC, Heistad DD. Restoration of endothelium-dependent relaxation by dietary treatment of atherosclerosis. J Clin Invest 1987;80:1808-11.

62. Leung WH, Lau CP, Wong CK. Beneficial effect of cholesterol-lowering therapy on coronary endothelium-dependent relaxation in hypercholesterolaemic patients. Lancet 1993;341:1496-500.

63. Treasure CB, Klein JL, Weintraub WS et al. Beneficial effects of cholesterol-lowering therapy on the coronary endothelium in patients with coronary artery disease. N Engl J Med 1995;332:481-7.

64. Anderson TJ, Meredith IT, Yeung AC, Frei B, Selwyn AP, Ganz P. The effect of cholesterol-lowering and antioxidant therapy on endothelium-dependent coronary vasomotion. N Engl J Med 1995;332:488-93.

65. O'Driscoll G, Green D, Taylor RR. Simvastatin, an HMG-Coenzyme A reductase inhibitor, improves endothelial function within 1 month. Circulation 1997;95:1126-31.

66. Kamata K, Kojima S, Sugiura M, Kasuya Y. Preservation of endothelium-dependent vascular relaxation in cholesterol-fed mice by the chronic administration of prazosin or pravastatin. Jpn J Pharmacol 1996;70:149-56.

67. Grunler J, Ericsson J, Dallner G. Branch-point reactions in the biosynthesis of cholesterol, dolichol, ubiquinone and prenylated proteins. Biochim Biophys Acta 1994;1212:259-77.

68. Corsini A, Mazzotti M, Raiteri M et al. Relationship between mevalonate pathway and arterial myocyte proliferation: in vitro studies with inhibitors of HMG-CoA reductase. Atherosclerosis 1993;101:117-25.

69. Gruentzig AR. Transluminal dilatation of coronary-artery stenosis. Lancet 1978;1:263.
70. McBride W, Lange RA, Hillis LD. Restenosis after successful coronary angioplasty. Pathophysiology and prevention. N Engl J Med 1988;318:1734-7.
71. Gallo R, Chesebro JH, Badimon L, Fuster V, Bedimon JJ. Restenosis after coronary angioplasty Cardiol Rev 1996;4:146-52.
72. Bauters C, de-Groote P, Adamantidis M et al. Proto-oncogene expression in rabbit aorta after wall injury. First marker of the cellular process leading to restenosis after angioplasty? Eur Heart J 1992;13:556-9.
73. Thyberg J, Hedin U, Sjolund M, Palmberg L, Bottger BA. Regulation of differentiated properties and proliferation of arterial smooth muscle cells. Arteriosclerosis 1990;10:966-90.
74. Stemerman MB, Spaet TH, Pitlick F, Cintron J, Lejnieks I, Tiell ML. Intimal healing. The pattern of reendothelialization and intimal thickening. Am J Pathol 1977;87:125-42.
75. Glagov S, Weisenberg E, Zarins CK, Stankunavicius R, Kolettis GJ. Compensatory enlargement of human atherosclerotic coronary arteries. N Engl J Med 1987;316:1371-5.
76. Post MJ, Borst C, Kuntz RE. The relative importance of arterial remodeling compared with intimal hyperplasia in lumen renarrowing after balloon angioplasty. A study in the normal rabbit and the hypercholesterolemic Yucatan micropig. Circulation 1994;89:2816-21.
77. Block PC, Myler RK, Stertzer S, Fallon JT. Morphology after transluminal angioplasty in human beings. N Engl J Med 1981;305:382-5.
78. Steele PM, Chesebro JH, Stanson AW et al. Balloon angioplasty. Natural history of the pathophysiological response to injury in a pig model. Circ Res 1985;57:105-12.
79. Casscells W. Migration of smooth muscle and endothelial cells. Critical events in restenosis. Circulation 1992;86:723-9.
80. Reidy MA, Clowes AW, Schwartz SM. Endothelial regeneration. V. Inhibition of endothelial regrowth in arteries of rat and rabbit. Lab Invest 1983;49:569-75.
81. Langille BL, O'Donnell F. Reductions in arterial diameter produced by chronic decreases in blood flow are endothelium-dependent. Science 1986;231:405-7.
82. Gibbons GH, Dzau VJ. The emerging concept of vascular remodeling. N Engl J Med 1994;330:1431-8.
83. Cornwell TL, Arnold E, Boerth NJ, Lincoln TM. Inhibition of smooth muscle cell growth by nitric oxide and activation of cAMP-dependent protein kinase by cGMP. Am J Physiol 1994;36:C1405-C1413.
84. Shimokawa H, Aarhus LL, Vanhoutte PM. Porcine coronary arteries with regenerated endothelium have a reduced endothelium-dependent responsiveness to aggregating platelets and serotonin. Circ Res 1987;61:256-70.
85. Baykal D, Schmedtje JF, Runge MS. Role of the thrombin receptor in restenosis and atherosclerosis. Am J Cardiol 1995;75:82B-87B.
86. Myers PR, Webel R, Thondapu V et al. Restenosis is associated with decreased coronary artery nitric oxide synthase. Int J Cardiol 1996;55:183-91.
87. el-Tamimi H, Davies GJ, Crea F, Maseri A. Response of human coronary arteries to acetylcholine after injury by coronary angioplasty. J Am Coll Cardiol 1993;21:1152-7.
88. Vassanelli C, Menegatti G, Zanolla L, Molinari J, Zanotto G, Zardini P. Coronary vasoconstriction in response to acetylcholine after balloon angioplasty: possible role

of endothelial dysfunction. Coron Artery Dis 1994;5:979-86.

89. Sakai A, Hirayama A, Adachi T et al. Is the presence of hyperlipidemia associated with impairment of endothelium-dependent neointimal relaxation after percutaneous transluminal coronary angioplasty? Heart Vessels 1996;11:255-61.

90. Gellman J, Ezekowitz MD, Sarembock IJ et al. Effect of lovastatin on intimal hyperplasia after balloon angioplasty: a study in an atherosclerotic hypercholesterolemic rabbit. J Am Coll Cardiol 1991;17:251-9.

91. Reis GJ, Kuntz RE, Silverman DI, Pasternak RC. Effects of serum lipid levels on restenosis after coronary angioplasty. Am J Cardiol 1991;68:1431-5.

92. Sahni R, Maniet AR, Voci G, Banka VS. Prevention of restenosis by lovastatin after successful coronary angioplasty. Am Heart J 1991;121:1600-8.

93. Adachi H, Niwa A, Shinoda T. Prevention of restenosis after coronary angioplasty with low-density lipoprotein apheresis. Artif Organs 1995;19:1243-7.

94. Weintraub WS, Boccuzzi SJ, Klein JL et al. Lack of effect of lovastatin on restenosis after coronary angioplasty. Lovastatin Restenosis Trial Study Group. N Engl J Med 1994;331:1331-7.

95. Onaka H, Hirota Y, Kita Y et al. The effect of pravastatin on prevention of restenosis after successful percutaneous transluminal coronary angioplasty. Jpn Circ J 1994;58:100-6.

96. O'Keefe JH Jr., Stone GW, McCallister BD Jr. et al. Lovastatin plus probucol for prevention of restenosis after percutaneous transluminal coronary angioplasty. Am J Cardiol 1996;77:649-52.

97. Emanuelsson H, Beatt KJ, Bagger JP et al. Long-term effects of angiopeptin treatment in coronary angioplasty. Reduction of clinical events but not angiographic restenosis. European Angiopeptin Study Group. Circulation 1995;91:1689-96.

98. Faxon DP. Effect of high dose angiotensin-converting enzyme inhibition on restenosis: final results of the MARCATOR Study, a multicenter, double-blind, placebo-controlled trial of cilazapril. The Multicenter American Research Trial With Cilazapril After Angioplasty to Prevent Transluminal Coronary Obstruction and Restenosis (MARCATOR) Study Group. J Am Coll Cardiol 1995;25:362-9.

99. Lablanche JM, Grollier G, Lusson JR et al. Effect of the direct nitric oxide donors linsidomine and molsidomine on angiographic restenosis after coronary balloon angioplasty. The ACCORD Study. Angioplastic Coronaire Corvasal Diltiazem. Circulation 1997;95:83-9.

Abbreviations:
ApoB100 = apolipoprotein B100
c-AMP = cyclic adenosine monophosphate
c-GMP = cyclic guanosine monophosphate
EDHF = endothelium derived hyperpolarizing factor
EDNO = endothelium derived nitric oxide
EDR = endothelium dependent reaction
EDV = endothelium dependent vasorelaxation
HMG-CoA = 3-hydroxy-3-methyl-glutaryl-coenzyme A
LDL = low density lipoprotein
Lyso PC = lysophosphatidylcholine
MM-LDL = minimal modified LDL
NO = nitric oxide
NOS = nitric oxide synthetase
Ox-LDL = oxidated LDL
PTCA = percutaneous transluminal coronary angioplasty
QCA = quantitative coronary analyzes

STATE-OF-THE-ART
DIAGNOSIS IN MYOCARDIAL ISCHEMIA

Jeroen J. Bax, Ernst E. van der Wall

Summary

In the last decade substantial improvements have been made in the diagnostic capabilities to detect myocardial ischemia. Particularly, the development and advancement of noninvasive imaging modalities have resulted in increased understanding of the functional sequelae of coronary artery stenosis. Imaging techniques such as stress perfusion scintigraphy and dobutamine echocardiography have found a niche in the diagnostic armamentarium of the clinical cardiologist in search of adequate methods to delineate or to exclude myocardial ischemia. One of the latest developments in this field is magnetic resonance imaging by virtue of its capability to evaluate myocardial perfusion and function. As the main subject of this chapter is dedicated to the state-of-the-art diagnosis of myocardial ischemia, the topic of the chapter is confined to stress myocardial perfusion scintigraphy as most of the experience world-wide has been obtained in this field of imaging. Especially the relative merits of single photon emission computed tomography (SPECT) and positron emission tomography (PET) will be addressed.

Evaluation of coronary artery disease by SPECT

Over the past 25 years, much progress has been made in the detection and evaluation of coronary artery disease (CAD) by radionuclide imaging. Sofar,

E.E. van der Wall et al. (eds.), Vascular Medicine, 83-101.
© 1997 *Kluwer Academic Publishers.*

PET has mainly been used in the research setting and can provide adequate information on myocardial perfusion, particularly in terms of absolute quantification of myocardial perfusion. However, PET imaging has been used for the evaluation of myocardial viability which relies on the combined evaluation of perfusion (not necessarily a PET tracer) and metabolism (generally a PET tracer). The role of PET in the assessment of myocardial viability will be discussed below.

In the clinical setting however, mainly single photon emitting agents are used for the evaluation of CAD. In the 1970s already, many studies demonstrated the use of thallium-201 (TI-201) to evaluate myocardial perfusion. Initially, these studies were performed using conventional planar scintigraphy, while nowadays most centers use SPECT imaging. SPECT has the advantage of offering a three-dimensional presentation of the heart, resulting in reduced overlap of the myocardium and other structures. Furthermore, a better assessment of location and extent of perfusion defects is possible with SPECT, due to improved lesion contrast.

Other developments include the shift from using TI-201 to the application of technetium-99m (Tc-99m) based agents. These agents have several advantages over TI-201, related to the different physical properties of the Tc-99m tracers. The shorter half-life (6 hours) of Tc-99m allows the administration of up to 10 times higher doses as compared to TI-201, resulting in improved count statistics. Also, the higher photon energy (140 keV) of the Tc-99m tracers reduces attenuation and scatter.

Much effort has also been invested in the development of alternative stress protocols using pharmacologic stress agents, including dipyridamole, adenosine and dobutamine.

Finally, SPECT imaging has also been shown to have prognostic value in patients with known or suspected CAD. Several parameters (lung uptake of TI-201 immediately after stress, the presence and extent of reversible defects) are associated with high risk for future cardiac events. In the next few paragraphs these issues will be addressed.

The different tracers in the detection of CAD

Thallium-201

After intravenous injection of TI-201, the extraction rate by the myocardium is 85-90% of the injected dose. TI-201 distributes proportionally to regional myocardial perfusion, although at high flow rates extraction may become rate limiting.[1,2] In addition, Pohost et al.[3] showed that at low flow rates TI-201 may overestimate actual flow.

TI-201 is a potassium analog and its uptake in the myocardium is partly dependent on active transport mediated by the sodium-potassium ATP-ase pump, whereas the remainder enters the myocyte passively.[1,2]

Its application in combination with physical exercise has been validated in many studies, showing accurate detection, localization and quantification of CAD. In a meta-analysis by Detrano et al.[4] 56 reports (published between 1977 and 1986) were reviewed. The sensitivity and specificity of stress-redistribution TI-201 scintigraphy for the detection of CAD were based on the presence of any perfusion defect on the stress image (either reversible or irreversible on the delayed image). In all studies coronary angiography was used as the gold standard for the diagnosis of CAD (50 to 70% narrowing in luminal diameter of at least 1 vessel). A total of 6038 patients were studied; 4240 patients had CAD on angiography, whereas 1798 did not. TI-201 scintigraphy correctly identified 3609 patients, yielding a sensitivity of 85%. Similarly, a specificity of 85% was found. Comparable results were described by Gerson[5] (30 studies) and Kotler et al.[6] (33 stress-redistribution studies): the average sensitivity and specificity were 84% and 88% respectively.

The majority of the studies included in these meta-analyses were performed with conventional planar scintigraphy. More recent studies have employed SPECT. Fintel et al.[7] compared planar TI-201 imaging with SPECT in 112 patients undergoing cardiac catheterization. The authors showed that SPECT showed a higher sensitivity than planar imaging. Also, SPECT had a significantly higher sensitivity in the detection of single vessel disease; for the detection of multi-vessel disease both modalities were comparable. It also appeared that SPECT was superior over planar imaging in identifying lesions in the left anterior descending and circumflex coronary arteries.

Analysis of combined data of 6 TI-201 SPECT studies[8] (with a total of 1042 patients) has demonstrated a sensitivity for the detection of CAD of 90% (ranging from 82% to 98%) and a specificity of 70% (ranging from 43% to 91%) (Figure 1). Virtually all patients (99%) with a previous myocardial infarction had an abnormal TI-201 study, whereas 85% of the patients without a previous infarction had an abnormal scintigram.[8] The somewhat lower specificity of TI-201 SPECT may partially be ascribed to referral bias,[9] since patients with an abnormal TI-201 study may be more often referred for cardiac catheterization. In this context, the term "normalcy rate", which is defined as the frequency of a normal TI-201 test in patients with a low likelihood of CAD, may be more appropriate than specificity. Combined data of 3 TI-201 SPECT studies showed a normalcy rate of 89%.[9-11]

The sensitivities for the detection of single vessel, double vessel and triple vessel disease were respectively 83%, 93% and 95%.[8] Moreover, the sensitivity and specificity for the detection of involvement of individual vessels were also high (Figure 1). SPECT identified significantly more stenoses in the left anterior descending and right coronary arteries as compared to stenoses in the left circumflex coronary artery (Figure 1).

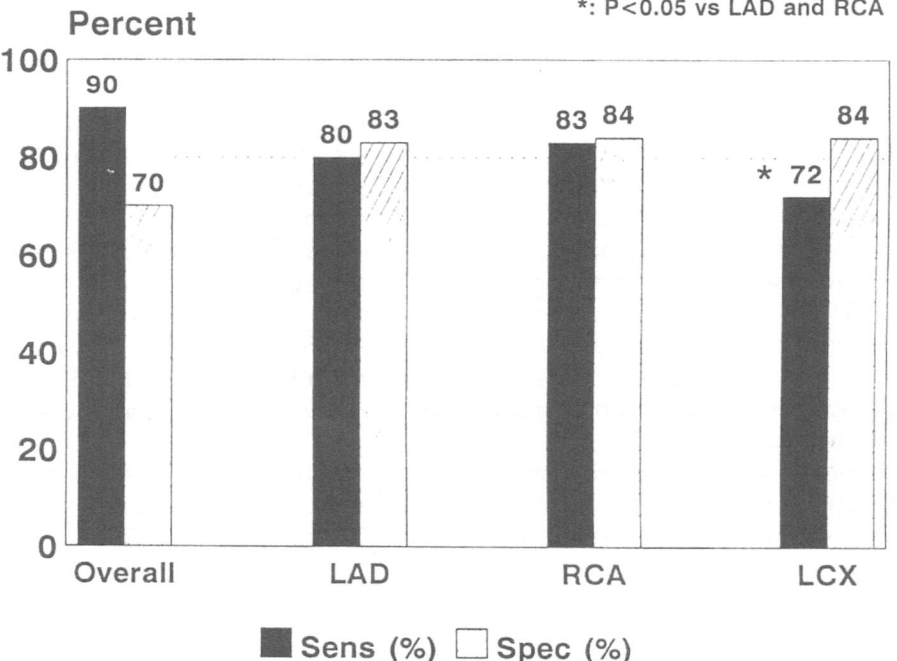

Figure 1. Sensitivity and specificity of TI-201 SPECT to assess coronary artery disease; the sensitivities and specificities for the different vessels are also shown (data based on reference #94).

Technetium-99m labeled agents

Recently, Tc-99m based agents have been introduced for the assessment of myocardial perfusion, including Tc-99m sestamibi, Tc-99m teboroxime and Tc-99m tetrofosmin.

The most experience has been gained with Tc-99m sestamibi. Although the extraction fraction of Tc-99m sestamibi is relatively low (65%),[12] still a good relation between the initial myocardial uptake of Tc-99m sestamibi and regional myocardial blood flow was demonstrated.[12] Like TI-201, Tc-99m sestamibi also underestimates flow at high flow rates and tends to overestimate flow at low flow rates.[13]

Unlike TI-201, the myocardial clearance time is prolonged (5 hours) and the redistribution is minimal.[12,14] These properties allow for the use of Tc-99m sestamibi imaging in acute ischemic syndromes and for gated SPECT imaging.[15,16] Gated SPECT imaging enables simultaneous assessment of ventricular function and perfusion, which is currently being evaluated.[16] Since Tc-99m sestamibi does not redistribute, separate injections are necessary to assess defect reversibility. Two imaging protocols have been proposed.[17] The conventional two-day protocol employs separate stress (day 1) and rest acquisitions (day 2). This protocol provides optimal defect contrast since it avoids contamination from the previous acquisition. Moreover, if the stress study is normal, the rest study is not necessary. The one-day protocol (either stress/rest or rest/stress) is less time-consuming, but the defect contrast is inferior as compared to the two-day protocol, due to the activity from the first study.[18]

Several studies have compared the use of Tc-99m sestamibi versus Tl-201 in the detection of CAD[19-23] (Table 1), showing a good agreement between the two tracers in the assessment of CAD.

Table 1. Comparative studies evaluating Tl-201 and Tc-99m sestamibi imaging for the identification of patients with coronary artery disease ("gold standard": angiography) (based on reference #94).

Author, ref	n	sens (%)		spec (%)	
		Tl-201	MIBI	Tl-201	MIBI
Taillefer[19]	65	74	70	-	-
Iskandrian[20]	40	82	82	82	100
Maddahi[21]	153	90	89	41	49
Kahn[22]	38	84	95	-	-
Kiat[23]	19	80	93	75	75

MIBI: technetium-99m sestamibi; Tl-201: thallium-201 chloride

Cramer et al.[24] compared planar Tc-99m sestamibi imaging with SPECT; the authors concluded that (similar as to Tl-201[7]) SPECT was superior in the detection of lesions in the left anterior descending and circumflex coronary arteries.

The other novel Tc-99m labeled tracers include Tc-99m teboroxime and Tc-99m tetrofosmin. Tc-99m teboroxime has a myocardial extraction rate of approximately 90% over a wide range of flow-rates,[25] both under ischemic and nonischemic conditions,[26] making this tracer most suitable for the detection of CAD. The rapid wash-out after the initial accumulation in the myocardium however, makes imaging with Tc-99m teboroxime technically difficult. Imaging should be completed within 2 to 8 minutes from the time of injection, requiring the use of multi-headed SPECT systems to reduce acquisition time, and the administration of pharmacological stress with the patient already in position for imaging. At this moment the precise value of this tracer in the detection of CAD has not been established.

Tc-99m tetrofosmin has more or less the same physical properties as compared to Tc-99m sestamibi.[27] Sinusas et al.[27] showed that myocardial Tc-99m tetrofosmin uptake correlated well with myocardial blood flow, comparable to the other tracers; similarly, at high flow rates, Tc-99m tetrofosmin also tended to underestimate myocardial flow. Tamaki et al.[28] described a head-to-head comparison of stress/rest Tc-99m tetrofosmin SPECT and stress/redistribution Tl-201 SPECT in 25 patients who underwent angiography; the sensitivities for the detection of CAD were comparable for Tc-99m tetrofosmin and Tl-201 (95% versus 100%). Van Eck-Smit et al.[29] compared the one-day and two-day protocols, showing comparable diagnostic accuracy for the detection of CAD for both protocols.

Thus, despite the preferable physical properties of the Tc-99m tracers, the available evidence indicates that their diagnostic accuracy (to detect CAD) is comparable to that of Tl-201.

The alternative pharmacologic stress protocols in the detection of CAD

Dipyridamole

Dipyridamole produces vasodilation of the coronary arteries, while the peripheral arterioles are less affected. The mechanism of this dilation of the coronary arteries is an increased level of adenosine caused by inhibition of cellular uptake of adenosine and also by inhibition of breakdown of adenosine.[30] Dipyridamole is usually administered intravenously employing a dose of 0.56 mg/kg (0.14 mg/min for 4 minutes).

Ranhosky et al.[31] evaluated the safety and side-effects of dipyridamole Tl-201 scintigraphy in 3911 patients. Four patients had a myocardial infarction within 24 hours of administration, leading to death in 2 patients, and 6 patients had acute bronchospasm. Minor side-effects were relatively common (46.5%) and included chest pain, dizziness, nausea, flushing, hypotension and headaches (Table 2). Aminophylline, which is an adenosine antagonist, was used to reverse the side-effects, and brought relief in 96.7% of the patients.

The most important contraindication for dipyridamole imaging is the presence or history of asthma, since dipyridamole may also act on bronchial smooth muscle and induce bronchospasm. The sensitivity and the specificity for the detection of CAD with dipyridamole Tl-201 scintigraphy are comparable to exercise Tl-201 scintigraphy. In a pooled analysis of 11 studies Beller showed a sensitivity of 85% and a specificity of 91%.[32]

Table 2. Prevalence of frequent side-effects with dipyridamole, adenosine and dobutamine Tl-201 imaging (based on reference #95).

	Dipyridamole Rahonsky, 1990 (3911 pts)	Adenosine Verani, 1990 (89 pts)	Dobutamine Hays, 1993 (144 pts)
Chest pain	19.7%	57%	31%
Headache	12.2%	35%	14%
Dizziness	11.8%	-	4%
ST-T changes on ECG	7.5%	12%	50%
Nausea	4.6%	-	9%
Hypotension	4.6%	-	-
Flushing	3.4%	29%	14%
Dyspnea	2.6%	15%	14%
Palpitation	-	-	29%

Adenosine

Adenosine acts directly on the coronary arteries, and has the advantage over dipyridamole of a more rapid onset of vasodilation and a shorter half-life (< 2 seconds),[33] which leads to a reduction in the duration of side-effects; the dose can be titrated if desired in the individual patient.

Since the mechanism is comparable to that for dipyridamole, asthma is a contraindication to adenosine Tl-201 as well.

The use of adenosine in combination with Tl-201 scintigraphy was introduced by Verani et al.[34] The authors used a stepwise infusion protocol of adenosine in 89 patients, beginning with a dose of 50µg/kg/min, increasing in 1-minute increments to 75, 100 and 140µg/kg/min. Mild side-effects (chest pain, flushing, headache, dyspnea) were noted frequently (Table 2); more severe side-effects included first-degree atrioventicular block (10% of patients), and ischemic ST-T depression (12% of patients). All side-effects disappeared within 1 to 2 minutes after discontinuing administration of adenosine without the use of aminophyllin or other agents. Using this technique, they found a sensitivity of 83% versus a specificity of 94% for detecting CAD. In a more recent report, Verani and Mahmarian described their experiences in almost 1000 patients using a dose of adenosine of 140 µg/kg/min, showing a sensitivity of 87% and a specificity of 94%.[35]

Dobutamine

Dobutamine is a ß1-specific agonist and increases myocardial oxygen demand by increasing heart rate, contractility and arterial blood pressure. Dobutamine is extremely useful in patients unable to exercise who have a history of reactive airway disease. Dobutamine is infused intravenously at incremental doses of 5, 10, 20, 30 and 40 µg/kg/min at 3-5 min intervals. Atropine (0.25-1.0 mg) can be added if the heart rate response to dobutamine is inadequate. Hays and colleagues[36] described a series of 144 patients studied with dobutamine Tl-201 scintigraphy. Minor side-effects were experienced in 75% of patients (Table 2). All side-effects disappeared within a few minutes after discontinuation of dobutamine infusion. Side-effects can be antagonized by beta-blocking agents. These investigators found a sensitivity of 86% versus a specificity of 90% for detecting CAD. Hence all three pharmacological stress agents are useful alternatives for detecting CAD in patients unable to exercise. Each test has a high sensitivity and specificity for the detection of CAD, comparable to physical exercise. All substances have a relatively good safety profile although side-effects are common in all tests. In patients with asthma, dipyridamole and adenosine are contraindicated, whereas dobutamine Tl-201 scintigraphy provides a good alternative.

Prognostic value of Tl-201 imaging

Although stress-redistribution Tl-201 scintigraphy was initially used as a diagnostic tool for detecting CAD, the prognostic value has been shown in many subsets of patients with CAD, including those with recent myocardial infarction.[37]

Brown et al.[38] were the first to describe a direct relation between the risk of future cardiac events and the amount of ischemically jeopardized myocardium. Their study population existed of 100 patients referred for evaluation of chest pain; all underwent stress-redistribution Tl-201 scintigraphy. Determining the number of myocardial segments with transient Tl-201 defects was superior in predicting cardiac events (cardiac death or infarction) as compared to clinical; exercise ECG and angiographic data. In 1926 patients with stable angina undergoing stress-redistribution Tl-201 SPECT Machecourt et al.[39] showed that the extent of reversible Tl-201 defects was the best predictor for long-term outcome.

Pollock and colleagues[40] investigated the incremental prognostic value of stress-redistribution Tl-201 imaging as compared to clinical and catheterization data. It was demonstrated that stress-redistribution Tl-201 imaging added significant prognostic information compared with clinical and exercise ECG data in both groups.

On the other hand, patients with (proven) coronary artery disease may also show a normal scintigram. In sharp contrast with the predictive value of abnormal stress-redistribution TI-201 studies is the prognostic value of a normal TI-201 scintigram. It has been shown in several studies[38,41-47] that patients with a normal TI-201 study have an excellent prognosis. In a recent review the mean cardiac event rate (death and infarction) in 3573 patients with normal scintigrams was 0.9% per year.[37]

Not only extent and severity of perfusion defects can be determined by TI-201 stress-redistribution scintigraphy but also the presence of increased lung uptake of TI-201. This increased lung TI-201 activity represents the sequestration of TI-201 in pulmonary edema due to exercise-induced left ventricular dysfunction. This is primarily present in patients with extensive CAD and left ventricular dysfunction.[48] Gill and coworkers[43] showed that increased lung uptake of TI-201 is a powerful predictor of adverse outcome in patients with known or suspected CAD.

Evaluation of myocardial viability by PET and SPECT

Clinical relevance of viability

It is generally accepted that impaired left ventricular function is not necessarily an irreversible process. Many studies have shown that revascularization may improve regional and global ventricular function.[49-51] Reversal of myocardial dysfunction is particularly relevant in patients with depressed ventricular function, since this is an important prognostic factor.[52] Pigott et al.[53] showed that in patients with a left ventricular ejection fraction ≤35%, the 7-year survival was 63% after surgical revascularization as compared to 34% when patients were treated medically.

Further insight into the mechanisms which determine the presence or absence of functional recovery after revascularization, has been derived from the characterization of dysfunctional myocardium. Many studies have shown that dysfunctional but viable myocardium can improve in contractile function after revascularization.[54-61] In contrast, contractile function failed to improve when viability could not be demonstrated.[54-61] Therefore, a careful selection of those patients who may benefit from a revascularization procedure is needed, especially since surgical revascularization in patients with depressed ventricular function is associated with a high mortality, varying from 5-37%.[62]

Dysfunctional but viable myocardium has been demonstrated to have several characteristics: 1. cell membrane integrity, 2. preserved glucose metabolism and 3. inotropic reserve.[63] These characteristics form the basis for the various techniques that are currently available for the assessment of myocardial viability in patients with chronic coronary artery disease. The assessment of contractile reserve is possible with stress echocardiography using dobutamine. Since this chapter only focuses on radionuclide imaging, the reader is referred to recent review articles by various experts.[63,64]

Assessment of cell membrane integrity
Thallium-201 imaging relies on the principle that integrity of cell membrane is the hallmark of viable myocardium.[65] Many protocols have been proposed; the clinically most accurate protocols are stress-redistribution-reinjection[57] and rest-redistribution.[58]
Bonow et al.[66] compared the value of Tl-201 stress-redistribution-reinjection imaging with FDG PET and showed concordance between the 2 techniques in 88% of segments regarding the presence or absence of viable myocardium. It also appeared that quantitation of Tl-201 activity is important, as the majority of mild-to-moderate (Tl-201 activity $\geq$50% of normal) fixed defects on the redistribution images[66] and reinjection images[67] were viable on FDG PET. Reanalysis of the available reports in the literature[57,60,61,68-72] revealed that Tl-201 reinjection imaging has a high sensitivity (average 86%) but a relatively low specificity (average 47%) to detect improvement of contractility after revascularization (Table 3).
Gewirtz et al.[73] initially reported that resting Tl-201 perfusion defects on the initial images (obtained 15 minutes after tracer injection) may show redistribution over the next 2-4-hours.
Several studies evaluated the use of Tl-201 rest-redistribution imaging to predict improvement of regional contractility after revascularization.[58,74-80] In these studies the average sensitivity and specificity were 90% and 54% (Table 3).
More recently, the use of an immediate reinjection protocol has been investigated: reinjection is performed after obtaining the stress image and 1 hour later a second scintigram is obtained.[81,82] This procedure may eliminate the need for the additional 3-4-hour redistribution imaging and offers reduced imaging time and may increase patient throughput.[81,82] These data need to be confirmed by studies showing improvement of ventricular function in viable segments as assessed by this protocol.

Assessment of preserved glucose metabolism
Since the early 1980s the fluorine-18 labeled radionuclide F18-fluoro-deoxyglucose (FDG) has been used to detect myocardial glucose uptake.[83] The initial trans-sarcolemmal uptake of FDG is closely related with glucose

Table 3. Sensitivities and specificities for the different techniques, based on weighted means from the available studies, presented with their 95% CI (data based on reference #72).

Technique	sens (%)	95% CI	spec (%)	95% CI
FDG PET	88	84-91	73	69-77
TI-201 Reinj	86	83-89	47	43-51
TI-201 RR	90	87-93	54	49-60

95% CI:95% confidence intervals; FDG:F18-fluorodeoxyglucose; TI-201:thallium-201;RR: rest-redistribution

uptake. The clinical applicability of FDG is based on the effective intracellular trapping after phosphorylation to FDG-6-phosphate. In contrast to glucose-6-phosphate, FDG-6-phosphate is no substrate for further metabolism.[84]
In the last years, a lot of evidence has accumulated showing that FDG in combination with PET can detect viable myocardium. Tillisch et al.[54] showed that contractility improved after revascularization in 85% of the dysfunctional regions that were viable on FDG PET. In contrast, regional contractile dysfunction did not improve in 92% of the segments that were nonviable on FDG PET. In the last years, many studies that evaluated functional outcome after revascularization have confirmed these findings[56,70,85-93]; the 12 available FDG-perfusion studies reported high sensitivies (average 88%) and somewhat lower specificities (average 73%) to predict functional outcome (Table 3).[72]
It appeared that dysfunctional segments with either normal perfusion and normal FDG uptake or decreased perfusion but preserved FDG uptake (perfusion-metabolism mismatch pattern) showed improvement in contraction, whereas segments with decreased perfusion and concordantly reduced FDG uptake (perfusion-metabolism match) did not show improvement of function. The match pattern represents scarred tissue, whereas the mismatch pattern is thought to represent jeopardized yet viable myocardium.[83] Even more important in the clinical setting, is improvement of global ventricular function. In the study by Tillisch et al.[54], the left ventricular ejection fraction (LVEF) improved from $30 \pm 11\%$ to $45 \pm 14\%$ in patients with dysfunctional segments of which 2 or more were viable on FDG PET, whereas the LVEF did not improve in patients with dysfunctional segments of which 1 or less were viable.

Noninvasive assessment of coronary endothelial function by PET

Using invasive methods, coronary endothelial function is generally studied by examining the response of epicardial coronary arteries to intracoronary administered acetylcholine or to cold pressor testing. As invasive methods have substantial inherent limitations, it should be attempted to evaluate coronary endothelial function noninvasively. In particular PET imaging may play an important role in assessing endothelial function by virtue of its capability to accurately quantify myocardial perfusion in absolute terms (ml/min/g). In Groningen (The Netherlands) a standardized method has been developed to acquire parametric polar maps of myocardial perfusion. These polar maps show three-dimensional imaging of myocardial perfusion of 480 segments in the human ventricle. Using this capability of PET, we compared PET perfusion imaging (labeled ammonia) with intracoronary Doppler-flow velocity measurements in non-stenotic arteries of 10 patients with single-vessel disease.[96] Endothelium-related stress testing was performed using cold pressor testing and intracoronary acetylcholine administration. Positive correlations were found between 1) cold pressor Doppler-flow velocity responses and acetylcholine Doppler-flow velocity responses, 2) cold pressor PET perfusion responses and cold pressor Doppler-flow velocity responses, and 3) cold pressor PET perfusion responses and acetylcholine Doppler-flow velocity responses. The results of this study suggested that in angiographically normal coronary arteries both the flow velocity and the perfusion responses during cold pressor testing may be related to the response to acetylcholine. A subsequent study in 10 'healthy' smokers showed 1) increased PET perfusion at rest in smokers compared to non-smokers, 2) impaired myocardial perfusion response to cold pressor testing in smokers, and 3) myocardial perfusion heterogeneity at rest and during cold pressor testing in smokers.[97] It was concluded that in healthy subjects the long-term effects of smoking are related to abnormal coronary artery vasoactivity, presumably induced by an interplay of regional endothelial dysfunction and autonomic dysregulation. A very recent study in 25 patients with syndrome X showed that -using ammonia PET perfusion studies at rest, during cold pressor stimulation and dipyridamole stress testing - endothelial dysfunction and impaired vasodilator reserve were of no major pathophysiologic relevance.[98] Rather other mechanisms, such as increased sympathetic tone and focal release of vasoactive substances may play a role in the pathogenesis of syndrome X. To summarize, PET perfusion imaging allows the examine coronary endothelial function in a noninvasive, accurate and quantitative way.

Conclusion

Myocardial perfusion scintigraphy has made essential advances in the detection of myocardial ischemia. Both SPECT and PET have widened our scope by their unique abilities to assess the functional consequences of coronary atherosclerosis accurately and quantitatively. In particular SPECT perfusion imaging has become a standard procedure in many centers to elicit myocardial ischemia in patients referred for undiagnosed chest pain. PET perfusion imaging is mostly used in combination with a metabolic marker to demonstrate myocardial viability. However, several recent studies have definitely shown the value of PET perfusion imaging to evaluate endothelial function using endothelium-related stress responses and parametric polar mapping. Endothelial function was not only assessed in patients with coronary artery disease but also in patients with syndrome X and in asymptomatic smokers. Excellent correlations were found between PET assessment of endothelial function and intracoronary Doppler-flow velocity measurements. By virtue of its restricted availability, PET offers only limited access to the patient and has therefore currently no major role in routine patient care. In the near future, this might be changed by the increasing number of PET centers, and by the definite proof that the use of PET technology may be one of the most cost-effective approaches in patients in whom the question of myocardial perfusion, endothelial function, ischemia and viability is of paramount importance.

References

1. Weich HF, Strauss HW, Pitt B. The extraction of thallium-201 by the myocardium. Circulation 1977;56:188-91.
2. Grunwald AM, Watson DD, Holzgrefe HH et al. Myocardial thallium-201 kinetics in normal and ischemic myocardium. Circulation 1981;64:610-8.
3. Pohost GM, Zir LM, Moore RH et al. Differentiation of transiently ischemic from infarcted myocardium by serial imaging after a single dose of thallium-201. Circulation 1977;55:294-302.
4. Detrano R, Janosi A, Lyons KP et al. Factors affecting sensitivity and specificity of a diagnostic test: The exercise thallium scintigram. Am J Med 1988;84(4):699-710.
5. Gerson M. Test accuracy, test selection and test result interpretation in chronic coronary artery disease. In: Gerson MC, ed. Cardiac Nuclear Medicine. New York: McGraw-Hill, 1987:309-48.
6. Kotler TS, Diamond GA. Exercise thallium-201 scintigraphy in the diagnosis and prognosis of coronary artery disease. Ann Int Med 1990;113:684-702.
7. Fintel DJ, Links JM, Brinker JA et al. Improved diagnostic performance of exercise thallium-201 single photon emission-computed tomography over planar imaging in the diagnosis of coronary artery disease: A receiver-operating characteristic analysis. J Am Coll Cardiol 1989;13(3):600-12.

8. Mahmarian JJ, Verani MS. Exercise thallium-201 perfusion scintigraphy in the assessment of coronary artery disease. Am J Cardiol 1991;67:2D-11D.
9. Van Train K, Maddahi J, Berman DS et al. Quantitative analysis of tomographic stress thallium-201 myocardial scintigrams: A multicenter trial. J Nucl Med 1990;31:1168-79.
10. Iskandrian AS, Heo J, Kong B et al. Effect of exercise level on the ability of thallium-201-tomographic imaging in detecting coronary artery disease: Analysis of 461 patients. J Am Coll Cardiol 1989;14:1477-86.
11. Maddahi J, Van Train K, Prigent F et al. Quantitative single photon emission computed thallium-201 tomography for detection and localization of coronary artery disease: Optimization and prospective validation of a new technique. J Am Coll Cardiol 1989;14:1689-99.
12. Okada R, Glover D, Gaffney T et al. Myocardial kinetics of technetium-99m hexakis-2-methoxy-2-methylpropylisonitrile. Circulation 1988;77:491-8.
13. Melon PG, Beanlands RS, DeGrado TR, Nguyen N, Petry NA, Schwaiger M. Comparison of technetium-99m sestamibi and thallium-201 retention characteristics in canine myocardium. J Am Coll Cardiol 1992;20:1277-83.
14. Taillefer R, Primeau M, Costi P et al. Technetium-99m myocardial perfusion imaging in detection of coronary artery disease: Comparison between initial (1-hr) and delayed (3-hr) postexercise images. J Nucl Med 1991;32:2311-7.
15. Berman DS, Kiat H, Van Train KF et al. Technetium 99m sestamibi in the assessment of chronic coronary artery disease. Semin Nucl Med 1991;21:190-212.
16. Faber TL, Akers MS, Peshock RM et al. Three-dimensional motion and perfusion quantification in gated single-photon emission computed tomograms. J Nucl Med 1991;32:2311-7.
17. Berman DS, Kiat HS, Van Train KF et al. Myocardial perfusion imaging with technetium-99m-sestamibi: Comparative analysis of available imaging protocols. J Nucl Med 1994;35:681-8.
18. Verzijlbergen JF, Cramer MJM, Niemeyer et al. ^{99m}Tc sestamibi for planar myocardial perfusion imaging; Not as ideal as the physical properties. Nucl Med Comm 1991;12:381-91.
19. Taillefer R, Lambert R, Dupras G et al. Clinical comparison between thallium-201 and Tc-99m-methoxy isobutyl isonitrile (hexamibi) myocardial perfusion imaging for detection of coronary artery disease. Eur J Nucl Med 1989;15:280-6.
20. Iskandrian AS, Heo J, Kong B et al. Use of technetium-99m isonitrile (RP-30A) in assessing left ventricular perfusion and function at rest and during exercise in coronary artery disease, and comparison with coronary angiography and exercise thallium-201 SPECT imaging. Am J Cardiol 1989;64:270-5.
21. Maddahi J, Van Train KF, Prigent F et al. Myocardial perfusion imaging with technetium-99m sestamibi SPECT in the evaluation of coronary artery disease. Am J Cardiol 1990;66:55E-62E.
22. Kahn, JK, McGhie I, Akers MS et al. Quantitative rotational tomography with ^{201}Tl and ^{99m}Tc 2-methoxy-isobutyl-isonitrile. A direct comparison in normal individuals and patients with coronary artery disease. Circulation 1989;79:1282-93.
23. Kiat H, Maddahi J, Roy LT et al. Comparison of technetium-99m methoxyisobutyl isonitrille and thallium-201 for evaluation of coronary artery disease by planar and tomographic methods. Am Heart J 1989;117:1-11.
24. Cramer MJM, Van der Wall EE, Verzijlbergen et al. SPECT versus planar ^{99m}Tc-sestamibi myocardial scintigraphy: Comparison of accuracy and impact on patient

management in chronic ischemic heart disease. Q J Nucl Med 1997;41:1-9.

25. Leppo JA, Meerdink DJ. Comparative myocardial extraction of two technetium-labeled BATO derivatives (SQ30217, SQ32014) and thallium. J Nucl Med 1990;31:67-74.

26. Gray WA, Gewirtz H. Comparison of ^{99m}Tc-teboroxime with thallium for myocardial imaging in the presence of a coronary artery stenosis. Circulation 1991;84:1796-1807.

27. Sinusas AJ, Shi QX, Saltzberg MT et al. Technetium-99m tetrofosmin to assess myocardial blood flow; Experimental validation in an intact canine model of ischemia. J Nucl Med 1994;35:664-7

28. Tamaki N, Takahashi N, Kawamoto M et al. Myocardial tomography uusing technetium-99m-tetrofosmin to evaluate coronary artery disease. J Nucl Med 1994;35:594-600.

29. Van Eck-Smit BLF, Poots S, Zwinderman AH, Bruschke AVG, Pauwels EKJ, Van der Wall EE. Myocardial SPECT imaging with ^{99}Tc^{m}-tetrofosmin in clinical practice: Comparison of a 1 day and a 2 day imaging protocol. Nucl Med Comm 1997;18:24-30.

30. Knabb RM, Gidday JM, Ely SW, Rubio R, Berne RM. Effects of dipyridamole on myocardial adenosine and active hyperemia. Am J Physiol 1984;247:H804-H810

31. Rahonsky A, Kempthorne-Rawson J and the Intravenous Dipyridamole Thallium Myocardial Perfusion Imaging Study Group. Circulation 1990;81:1205-9.

32. Beller GA. Pharmacologic stress imaging. JAMA 1991;265;633-8.

33. Moser GH, Schrader J, Deursen A. Turnover of adenosine in plasma of human and dog blood. Am J Physiol 1989;256(Cell Physiol 25):C799-C806.

34. Verani MS, Mahmarian JJ, Hixson JB, Boyce TM, Staudacher RA. Diagnosis of coronary artery disease by controlled coronary vasodilation with adenosine and thallium-201 scintigraphy in patients unable to exercise. Circulation 1990;82:80-7.

35. Verani MS, Mahmarian JJ. Myocardial perfusion scintigraphy during maximal coronary artery vasodilation with adenosine. Am J Cardiol 1991;67:12D-17D.

36. Hays JT, Mahmarian JJ, Cochran A, Verani MS. Dobutamine thallium-201 tomography for evaluating patients with suspected coronary artery disease unable to undergo exercise or vasodilator pharmacologic stress testing. J Am Coll Cardiol 1993;21:1583-90.

37. Brown KA. Prognostic value of thallium-201 myocardial perfusion imaging. A diagnostic tool comes of age. Circulation 1991;83:363-81.

38. Brown KA, Boucher CA, Okada RD et al. Prognostic value of exercise thallium-201 imaging in patients presenting for evaluation of chest pain. J Am Coll Cardiol 1983;1:994-1001.

39. Machecourt J, Longere P, Fagret D et al. Prognostic value of thallium-201 single-photon emission computed tomographic myocardial perfusion imaging according to extent of myocardial defect. Study in 1926 patients with follow-up at 33 months. J Am Coll Cardiol 1994;23:1096-106.

40. Pollock SG, Abbott RD, Boucher CA, Beller GA, Kaul S. Independent and incremental prognostic value of tests performed in hierarchical order to evaluate patients with suspected coronary artery disease. Validation of models based on these tests. Circulation 1992;85:237-48.

41. Pamelia FX, Gibson RS, Watson DD, Craddock GB, Sirowatka J, Beller GA. Prognosis with chest pain and normal thallium-201 exercise scintigrams. Am J Cardiol 1985;55:920-6.

42. Wackers FJTh, Russo DJ, Russo D, Clements JP. Prognostic significance of normal quantitative planar thallium-201 stress scintigraphy in patients with chest pain. J Am Coll Cardiol 1985;6:27-30.

43. Gill JB, Ruddy TD, Newell JB, Finkelstein DM, Strauss HW, Boucher CA. Prognostic importance of thallium uptake by the lungs during exercise in coronary artery disease. N Engl J Med 1987;317:1485-9.

44. Koss JH, Kobren SM, Grunwald AM, Bodenheimer MM. Role of thallium-201 myocardial perfusion scintigraphy in predicting prognosis in suspected coronary artery disease. Am J Cardiol 1987;59:531-4.

45. Oosterhuis WP, Breeman A, Niemeyer MG et al. Patients with a normal exercise thallium-201 myocardial scintigram: always a good prognosis? Eur J Nucl Med 1993;20:151-8.

46. Brown KA, Rowen M. Prognostic value of a normal exercise myocardial perfusion imaging study in patients with angiographically significant coronary artery disease. Am J Cardiol 1993;71:865-7.

47. Abdel Fattah A, Kamal AM, Pancholy S et al. Prognostic implications of normal exercise tomographic thallium images in patients with angiographic evidence of significant coronary artery disease. Am J Cardiol 1994;74:769-71.

48. Boucher CA, Zir LM, Beller GA et al. Increased lung uptake of Tl-201 during exercise myocardial imaging: clinical, hemodynamic and angiographic implications in patients with coronary artery disease. Am J Cardiol 1980;46:189-96.

49. Brundage BH, Massie BM, Botvinick EH. Improved regional ventricular function after successful revascularization. J Am Coll Cardiol 1984;3:902-8.

50. Dilsizian V, Bonow RO, Cannon RO et al. The effect of coronary artery bypass grafting on left ventricular systolic function at rest: Evidence for preoperative subclinical myocardial ischemia. Am J Cardiol 1988;61:1248-54.

51. Elefteriades JA, Tolis Jr G, Levi E, Mills LK, Zaret BL. Coronary artery bypass grafting in severe left ventricular dysfunction: Excellent survival with improved ejection fraction and functional state. J Am Coll Cardiol 1993;22:1411-7.

52. The Multicenter Postinfarction Research Group. Risk stratification and survival after myocardial infarction. N Eng J Med 1983;309:331-6.

53. Pigott JD, Kouchoukos NT, Oberman A, Cutter GR. Late results of surgical and medical therapy for patients with coronary artery disease and depressed left ventricular function. J Am Coll Cardiol 1985;5:1036-45.

54. Tillisch J, Brunken R, Marshall R et al. Reversibility of cardiac wall-motion abnormalities predicted by positron tomography. N Engl J Med 1986;314:884-8.

55. Vom Dahl J, Eitzman DT, Al-Aouar ZR et al. Relation of regional function, perfusion and metabolism in patients with advanced coronary artery disease undergoing surgical revascularization. Circulation 1994;90:2356-66.

56. Knuuti MJ, Saraste M, Nuutila P et al. Myocardial viability: Fluorine-18-deoxyglucose positron emission tomography in prediction of wall motion recovery after revascularization. Am Heart J 1994;127:785-96.

57. Dilsizian V, Rocco TP, Freedman NM, Leon MB, Bonow RO. Enhanced detection of ischemic but viable myocardium by the reinjection of thallium after stress-redistribution imaging. N Engl J Med 1990;323:141-6.

58. Ragosta M, Beller GA, Watson DD, Kaul S, Gimple LW. Quantitative planar rest-redistribution Tl-201 imaging in detection of myocardial viability and prediction of improvement in left ventricular function after coronary artery bypass surgery in patients with severely depressed left ventricular function. Circulation 1993;87:1630-

41.

59. Arnese M, Cornel JH, Salustri A et al. Prediction of improvement of regional left ventricular function after surgical revascularization: A comparison of low-dose dobutamine echocardiography with 201-TL SPECT. Circulation 1995;91:2748-52.

60. Bax JJ, Cornel JH, Visser FC et al. Prediction of recovery of regional ventricular dysfunction following revascularization; Comparison of F18-fluorodeoxyglucose SPECT, thallium-201 stress-reinjection SPECT and dobutamine echocardiography. J Am Coll Cardiol 1996;28:558-64.

61. La Canna G, Alfieri O, Giubbini R, Gargano M, Ferrari R, Visioli O. Echocardiography during infusion of dobutamine for identification of reversible dysfunction in patients with chronic coronary artery disease. J Am Coll Cardiol 1994;23:617-26.

62. Maddahi J, Schelbert H, Brunken R, Di Carli M. Role of Tl-201 and PET imaging in evaluation of myocardial viability and management of patients with coronary artery disease and left ventricular dysfunction. J Nucl Med 1994;35:707-15.

63. Cornel JH, Bax JJ, Fioretti PM. Assessment of myocardial viability by dobutamine stress echocardiography. Curr Opin Cardiol 1996;11:621-6.

64. Marwick TH. Recent advances in stress echocardiography. Curr Opin Cardiol 1995;10:619-5.

65. Bonow RO, Dilsizian V. Assessing viable myocardium with thallium-201. Am J Cardiol 1992;70:10E-17E.

66. Bonow RO, Dilsizian V, Cuocolo A, Bacharach SL. Identification of viable myocardium in patients with chronic coronary artery disease and left ventricular dysfunction. Comparison of thallium scintigraphy with reinjection and PET imaging with 18-F-Fluorodeoxyglucose. Circulation 1991;83:26-37.

67. Dilsizian V, Freedman NMT, Bacharach SL, Perrone-Filardi P, Bonow RO. Regional Tl uptake in irreversible defects: Magnitude of change in Tl activity after reinjection distinguishes viable from nonviable myocardium. Circulation 1992;85:627-34.

68. Vanoverschelde J-LJ, D'Hondt A-M, Marwick T et al. Head-to-head comparison of exercise-redistribution-reinjection thallium single-photon emission computed tomography and low dose dobutamine echocardiography for prediction of reversibility of chronic left ventricular ischemic dysfunction. J Am Coll Cardiol 1996;28:432-42.

69. Ohtani H, Tamaki N, Yonekura Y et al. Value of thallium-201 reinjection after delayed SPECT imaging for predicting reversible ischemia after coronary artery bypass grafting. Am J Cardiol 1990;66:394-9.

70. Tamaki N, Ohtani H, Yamashita K et al. Metabolic activity in the areas of new fill-in after thallium-201 reinjection: Comparison with positron emission tomography using fluorine-18-deoxyglucose. J Nucl Med 1991;32:673-8.

71. Haque T, Furukawa T, Takahashi M, Kinoshita M. Identification of hibernating myocardium by dobutamine stress echocardiography: Comparison with thallium-201 reinjection imaging. AM Heart J 1995;130:553-63.

72. Bax JJ, Cornel JH, Visser FC, Fioretti PM, Wijns W. Which is the preferred technique to predict improvement of regional left ventricular dysfunction after coronary revascularization? Circulation 1996;94(Suppl.I):I-233 (Abstract).

73. Gewirtz H, Beller GA, Strauss HW, ,Dinsmore RE, Zir LM, McKusick KA, Pohost GM. Transient defect of resting thallium scans in patients with coronary artery disease. Circ 1979;53:707-13.

74. Mori T, Minamiji K, Kurogane H et al. Rest-injected thallium-201 imaging for assessing viability of severe asynergic regions. J Nucl Med 1991;32:1718-24.

75. Marzullo P, Parodi O, Reisenhofer B et al. Value of rest thallium-201/technetium-99m sestamibi and dobutamine echocardiography for detecting myocardial viability. Am J Cardiol 1993;71:166-72.

76. Udelson JE, Coleman PS, Metherall J et al. Predicting recovery of severe regional ventricular dysfunction; Comparison of resting scintigraphy with 201Tl and 99Tc-sestamibi. Circulation 1994;89:2552-61.

77. Qureshi U, Nagueh SF, Afridi I et al. Dobutamine echocardiography and quantitative rest-redistribution ^{201}Tl tomography in myocardial hibernation. Relation of contractile reserve to ^{201}Tl uptake and comparative prediction of recovery of function. Circulation 1997;95:626-35.

78. Alfieri O, La Canna G, Giubinni R, Pardini A, Zogno M, Fucci C. Recovery of myocardial function. Eur J Cardio-Thorac Surg 1993;7:325-30.

79. Charney R, Schwinger ME, Chun J et al. Dobutamine echocardiography and resting-redistribution thallium-201 scintigraphy predicts recovery of hibernating myocardium after coronary revascularization. Am Heart J 1994;128:864-9.

80. Perrone-Filardi P, Pace L, Prastaro M et al. Assessment of myocardial viability in patients with chronic coronary artery disease. Rest-4-hour-24-hour ^{201}Tl tomography versus dobutamine echocardiography. Circulation 1996;94:2712-9.

81. Van Eck-Smit BLF, van der Wall EE. Reinjection of thallium for detection of viable myocardium: Why not do it immediately? Br Heart J 1995;74:101-2.

82. Van Eck-Smit BLF, van der Wall EE, Kuijper AFM, Pauwels EKJ. Immediate thallium-201 reinjection following stress imaging: A novel timesaving approach for detection of myocardial viability. J Nucl Med 1993;34:737-43.

83. Schelbert HR. Metabolic imaging to assess myocardial viability. J Nucl Med 1994;35(Suppl):8S-14S.

84. Camici P, Ferrannini E, Opie LP. Myocardial metabolism in ischemic heart disease: Basic principles and application to imaging by positron emission tomography. Progr Cardiovasc Dis 1989;32:217-38.

85. Marwick TH, MacIntyre WJ, Lafont A, Nemec JJ, Salcedo EE. Metabolic responses of hibernating and infarcted myocardium to revascularization. Circulation 1992;85:1-347-53.

86. Gerber BL, Vanoverschelde J-LJ, Bol A et al. Myocardial blood flow, glucose uptake and recruitment of inotropic reserve in chronic left ventricular ischemic dysfunction. Implications for the pathophysiology of chronic hibernation. Circulation 1996;94:651-9.

87. Tamaki N, Yonekura Y, Yamashita K et al. PET using fluorine-18 deoxyglucose in evaluation of coronary artery bypass grafting. Am J Cardiol 1989;64:860-5.

88. Gropler RJ, Geltman EM, Sampathkumaran K et al. Comparison of carbon-11-acetate with fluorine-18-fluorodeoxyglucose for delineating viable myocardium by positron emission tomography. J Am Coll Cardiol 1993;22:1587-97.

89. Maes AF, Borgers M, Flameng W et al. Assessment of myocardial viability in chronic coronary artery disease using technetium-99m sestamibi SPECT. Correlation with histologic and positron emission tomographic studies and functional follow-up. J Am Coll Cardiol 1997;29:62-8.

90. Tamaki N, Kawamoto M, Tadamura E et al. Prediction of reversible ischemia after revascularization. Perfusion and metabolic studies with positron emission tomography. Circulation 1995;91:1697-705.

91. Baer FM, Voth E, Deutsch HJ, Schneider CA et al. Predictive value of low dose dobutamine transesophageal echocardiography and fluorine-18 fluorodeoxyglucose

positron emission tomography for recovery of regional left ventricular function after successful revascularization. J Am Coll Cardiol 1996;28:60-9.

92. Lucignani G, Paolini G, Landoni C et al. Presurgical identification of hibernating myocardium by combined use of technetium-99m hexakis 2-methoxyisobutylisonitrile SPECT and fluorine-18 fluoro-2-deoxy-D-glucose positron emission tomography in patients with coronary artery disease. Eur J Nucl Med 1992;19:874-81.

93. Carrel T, Jenni R, Haubold-Reuter S, Von Schulthess G, Pasic M, Turina M. Improvement of severely reduced left ventricular function after surgical revascularization in patients with preoperative myocardial infarction. Eur J Cardiothorac Surg 1992;6:479-84.

94. Keijer JT, Bax JJ, Van Rossum AC, Visser FC, Visser CA. Myocardial perfusion imaging: Clinical experience and recent progress in radionuclide scintigraphy and magnetic resonance imaging. Int J Card Imaging 1997;in press.

95. Bax JJ, Visser FC, Huitink JM, Visser CA. Exercise thallium-201 scintigraphy: Diagnostic and prognostic value in patients with known or suspected coronary artery disease. Cardiologie 1995;2:230-40.

96. Meeder JG, Peels JOJ, Blanksma PK et al. Comparison between PET-myocardial perfusion imaging and intracoronary Doppler-flow velocity measurements at rest and during cold pressor esting in angiographically normal coronary arteries in patients with single-vessel coronary artery disease. Am J Cardiol 1996;78:526-31.

97. Meeder JG, Blanksma PK, van der Wall EE et al. Long-term cigarette smoking is associated with increased myocardial perfusion heterogeneity assessed by positron emission tomography. Eur J Nucl Med 1996;23:1442-7.

98. Meeder JG, Blanksma PK, van der Wall EE et al. Coronary vasomotion in patients with syndrome X: evaluation with positron emission tomography and parametric myocardial perfusion imaging. Eur J Nucl Med 1997;24:530-7.

QUANTITATIVE CARDIOVASCULAR IMAGE ANALYSIS: CURRENT STATUS AND WHAT ARE REALISTIC EXPECTATIONS FOR THE FUTURE?

Johan H.C. Reiber, Bob Goedhart, Hans G. Bosch, Rob J. van der Geest, Jouke Dijkstra, Gerhard Koning, Mahmoud Ramze Rezaee, Boudewijn P.F. Lelieveldt, Albert de Roos, Ernst E. van der Wall, Albert V.G. Bruschke

Summary

Cardiology is typically an image oriented specialty. Single still images, but much more so dynamic and increasingly three-dimensional image sequences, play a major role in clinical decision making and clinical research trials. Of major interest is always the state of the coronary arteries and of the left ventricular function. In this chapter an overview is given of the various quantitative approaches using automated edge detection techniques which have been developed in our departments to: 1) assess the severity of disease of coronary obstructions from x-ray arteriography and intravascular ultrasound; and 2) assess the global and regional left ventricular function from x-ray angiography, echocardiography and magnetic resonance (MR) imaging. Also, the possibilities of MR flow velocity mapping are presented. In addition, for each modality and application a short description is given of the future developments and expectations. Finally, it is recognized that the automated combination of the data from the different imaging modalities (i.e. image fusion) will be a topic of major research in the future. As a current and practical example, the image fusion of biplane x-ray arteriography and 3D intravascular ultrasound is discussed.

103

E.E. van der Wall et al. (eds.), Vascular Medicine, 103-131.
© 1997 *Kluwer Academic Publishers.*

Introduction

Images and in particular dynamic sequences play a major role in clinical decision making and in clinical research trials in cardiology. Until today the anatomy of the coronary arteries can best be studied by the invasive cardiac catheterization procedure,[1,2] while the presence and amount of coronary calcium can be assessed by ultrafast computed tomography (CT).[3] Already for several years a significant amount of effort has been devoted to imaging the coronary arteries by noninvasive magnetic resonance (MR) imaging. Although significant progress has been made in the visualization of the proximal portions of the coronary vessels, expectations are that it will still take several years more before the entire coronary tree can be imaged with sufficient resolution.[4-6] Cross-sectional imaging of the individual coronary arteries and the assessment of the arterial wall sofar has been the exclusive domain of intravascular ultrasound (IVUS).[7] Developments are taking place to combine IVUS with Raman spectroscopy in an attempt to assess the chemical composition of the plaque.[8]

To assess left ventricular function a number of imaging modalities are available, being X-ray left ventriculography,[9] two (2D) and three-dimensional (3D) echocardiography,[10-11] blood pool imaging preferably by SPECT,[12] and MR imaging.[13,14]

The perfusion of the myocardial muscle can best be studied by thallium-201 and various technetium-99m preparations, again nowadays performed almost exclusively by SPECT imaging,[15] as well as by x-ray imaging techniques,[16,17] while the expectations are very high for contrast echocardiography and contrast MR imaging.[18,19]

It has been documented extensively that the purely visual interpretation of all of these images is subjective, and therefore subject to significant inter- and intra-observer variations, it is tedious and time-consuming. In particular, since most of the modern 3D approaches are associated with enormous amounts of digital data, it is clear that computer-supported approaches can help the cardiologists and radiologists in extracting objective and reproducible data from these imaging modalities. Although the practical realizations are still in their infancy for cardiologic applications, there is a definite need to combine the data from different imaging modalities, e.g. biplane x-ray and 3D IVUS; this field is called image fusion.

The goal of this chapter is to provide an overview of current approaches of quantitative image analysis using automated edge detection techniques and developed in our departments, for a few of these applications mentioned above, and to try to envision where these will go to in the near future. As the rate of development and the availability of new imaging technologies is extremely rapid, it is very difficult to make realistic long-term predictions.

Coronary anatomy

Quantitative coronary arteriography

Quantitative coronary arteriography (QCA) was developed in the seventies to quantify vessel vasomotion and the effects of drugs on the regression and progression of coronary artery disease.[20,21] Initially, vessel contours were traced manually on optically magnified cineframes, later supported by semi-automated edge detection approaches.[22,23] Two major clinical developments from the early 1980's which have grown exponentially since then have stimulated the use and interest in QCA: 1) the innovation and application in coronary recanalization techniques (PTCA, atherectomy, thrombolysis, stenting, laser, etc.), and 2) the increasing interest to study the effects of new drugs directed at the regression or no-growth of existing coronary artery disease, or the delay in the formation of new lesions.[24] Until recently these analytical approaches were used predominantly in clinical research trials with 35 mm cinefilm as the exclusive storage and exchange medium. In the mid-1980's, digital systems were introduced into the catheterization laboratory to support the angiographer with the interventional procedures. Initially, only single digital frames could be displayed for road map purposes, later followed by cine loops, and facilities for on-line QCA.[25] As a result of the continuous evolution of digital angiographic technology, it has largely become common practice that interventional procedures should only be carried out in a laboratory with digital facilities. On-line QCA has been used predominantly for the selection of the optimal sizes of the interventional devices, and for the assessment of the efficacy of the procedure. This application is likely to expand as health insurance companies and governments will follow with increasing interest the cost-benefit aspects of these expensive interventional procedures.

The general principles and characteristics of QCA analytical software packages can be illustrated using the CMS (Cardiovascular Measurement System, MEDIS, Nuenen, the Netherlands) algorithms developed in our laboratory.[22,23] Since these have been described extensively elsewhere, only a brief summary follows. For cinefilm applications, a region of interest (ROI) in a selected frame is magnified optically on the cine-projector, converted into video format and digitized (analog to digital conversion) by a frame grabber and stored in memory of the QCA-workstation. For a digital application, the ROI's are extracted from the digital matrix data and digitally zoomed to the correct matrix size using an interpolation approach.

To select the coronary segment to be analyzed, the user only needs to define with the computer mouse the start and end point of that segment. In the next step, an arterial pathline through the segment of interest is computed automatically.[22] The contour detection technique is based on the so-called Minimum Cost Analysis (MCA), which uses the weighted sum of the first and second derivative values applied to the brightness levels measured along scanlines perpendicular to the pathline. To correct for the limited resolution of the entire x-ray system, the MCA algorithm is carried out in two iterations based on an analysis of the point spread function of the imaging chain, which is of particular importance for the accurate measurement of small diameters as in coronary obstructions.

Calibration of the image data is performed on a non-tapering part of the contrast catheter following a similar MCA edge detection procedure as for the arterial segment. However, additional information is used in the edge detection process, knowing that this part of the catheter is characterized by parallel boundaries. From the left- and right-hand contours of the arterial segment, a diameter function is determined. From this calculated diameter function, many parameters are derived automatically, i.e. the site of maximal percent stenosis, the obstruction diameter, the corresponding automatically determined reference diameter, and the extent of the obstruction. Additionally derived parameters include obstruction symmetry, inflow and outflow angles, the area of the atherosclerotic plaque, and functional information. The results of the contour detection and the most important data are presented on the first result page (Figure 1A), while a complete overview of all the derived data is presented on the second result page (Figure 1B).

Complex vessel morphology

As explained above, the conventional or second generation contour detection technique is based on the MCA approach, which is very fast and robust for images which can vary significantly in image quality. This approach has demonstrated to operate very well in QCA as long as the contours are relatively smooth in shape. However, complex vessel morphology may occur post-coronary intervention, for example, when a dissection occurs. Also before intervention, obstructions with very sharp corners may be found. The MCA technique in its design is hampered in tracing very irregular and complex boundaries. To be able to adequately analyze such very irregular stenoses, we have developed a novel algorithm, the Gradient Field Transform (GFT®), which does not have the limitations of the MCA algorithm[26] (Figure 2).

The GFT has been validated extensively on phantom images and on digital coronary arteriograms.[26] Our experiences with the GFT indicate that this approach is advocated for the analysis of ostial lesions and of radiopaque stents. With the appropriate optical zooming (in an off-line configuration), the GFT is able to follow the outer boundaries of the stent struts and the contrast lumen in between the stent struts.

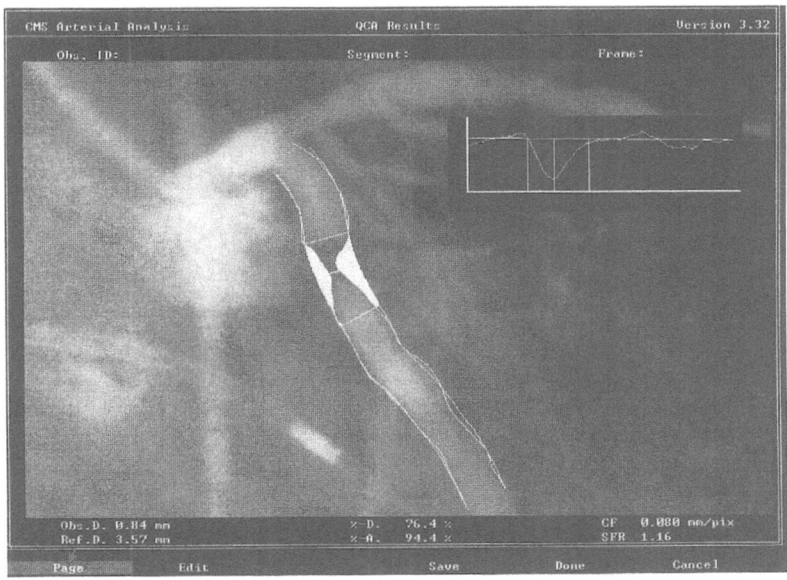

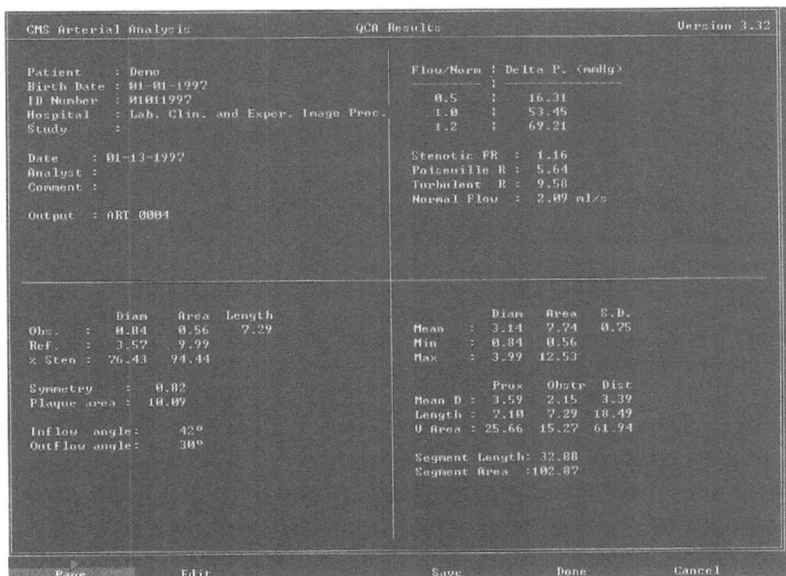

Figure 1. *Example of the first result page on the QCA-CMS, including the luminal contours, the reconstructed original vessel contours, plaque area (shaded) and the diameter function (Figure 1A). Figure 1B shows the second result page with all the derived absolute and relative QCA-parameters. The left upper quadrant contains the demographic data, the left lower quadrant the obstruction related data, the right upper quadrant the hemodynamic data, and the right lower quadrant data about the proximal, lesional and distal portions of the vessel segment.*

108

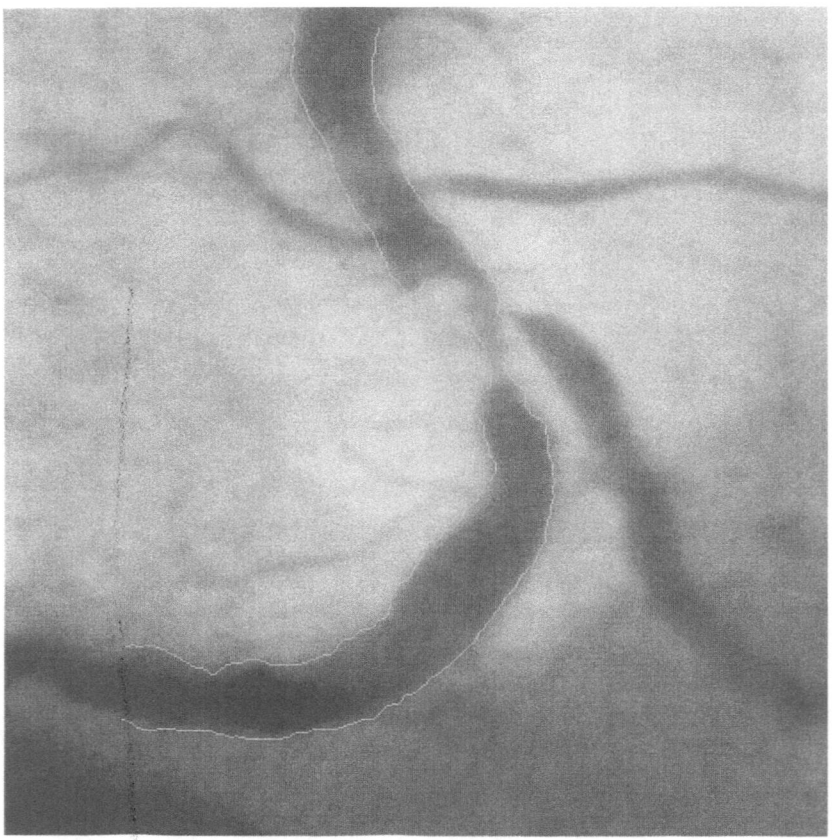

Figure 2. *Example of the outcome of the Gradient Field Transform analysis on a vessel segment with a complex stenosis. The shape changes in the proximal portion of the obstruction are very abrupt. Conventional approaches with the MCA algorithm would significantly underestimate the severity of the disease.*

Digital QCA

To the user the analysis of digital images on the QCA-CMS is basically not different from the analysis of cinefilm frames described above. One obvious difference with cinefilm is that digital zooming is used in the QCA analysis of the CD-R's, while optical zooming (approximately 2.3 fold) is used on cinefilm.

However, there are still a number of issues associated with digital QCA in general that need to be studied in great detail in the very near future. Questions have been raised whether the commonly used matrix size of 512 x 512 pixels and 8 bits of density resolution (256 gray levels) is really sufficient to appreciate the same fine details as visible on cinefilm. Should one use a matrix size of 1024 x 1024 by 12 bits in stead? Are there any differences in QCA results between these different media (cinefilm and digital) and matrix sizes? Although various QCA studies carried out in the past have confirmed that there were only minor, nonsignificant differences between digital and cinefilm, these were based on phantom and clinical studies of relatively smooth vessels. We have also shown that QCA from cinefilm is associated with a smaller random error (by 10 - 15 %) than from digital.[27] With modern interventional cardiology, however, the requirements for proper viewing of these small devices and the subsequent quantitative analysis have increased, and with these goals in mind these resolution issues need to be revisited.

Other major issues of difference between the conventional cinefilm and the modern digital approach are edge enhancement and image compression. Edge enhancement is one of the major reasons why digital images look so much appealing to the user: the images have been sharpened and the degree of enhancement is even user-customizable! However, it has been demonstrated quite clearly that edge enhancement has a definite affect on the results of QCA.[28] It was concluded from that study that the raw digital data, as produced by the x-ray equipment, *must be used* for QCA and archival purposes! This is in accordance with the DICOM-3 exchange standard.

In an attempt to limit the enormous amount of digital data associated with a catheterization procedure, the use of image compression techniques has been considered. Lossless techniques allow only a compression factor of two. To increase efficiency higher compression ratios are desired, which by definition become lossy, i.e. the original information cannot fully be recovered anymore. For these purposes the widely available Joint Photographic Experts Group (JPEG) techniques have been applied, although other modern compression schemes (e.g. Wavelets) may provide better results in the future. The highest acceptable lossy compression factor will be determined by the fact whether effects on the diagnostic interpretation of these images, and on the QCA results will still just not be noticeable. In a small pilot study on clinical images we have found that already at a JPEG compression factor of five, significantly increased random differences in QCA results were apparent although at unchanged systematic differences.[29] To come up with a widely acceptable standard, the Working Group 1 of the DICOM Standards Committee in which the ACC, ACR, NEMA and the ESC participate has set up a Compression Viability Study which will answer these remaining questions in the forthcoming years.

110

Digital review stations
We all have been so familiar with the 35 mm cinefilm (worldwide standard), that viewing of such a patient record all over the world does not represent any problem. With the introduction of the digital CD-R's, high quality digital viewers (also called 'digital Tagarno's') must become available. It is obvious that such new digital viewers should at least satisfy the same requirements as the conventional cinefilm projectors, and preferably even more. This sounds like a natural requirement nowadays, but the enormous amounts of digital data that need to be read from the CD-R's and displayed onto the computer screen at high frame speeds, requires top quality hardware and software and lots of computer memory. A number of such requirements are: 1) review of image runs in real time, i.e. at least at the acquisition speed (12.5-30 frames/s) and preferably even faster up to 100 frames/s as on a cinefilm projector and 2) display of a still image at the original resolution in a lossless format, while a small degree of lossy image compression may be allowed during the dynamic display of a run. Because these images are available in a digital format facilitates a number of features that are not available on the cineprojectors. Examples of these are 1) adjustment of contrast and brightness, 2) zooming in on a region-of-interest, 3) providing an overview of all the runs on a particular disk using the socalled thumbnails, 4) allowing two or more runs to be displayed at the same time in separate windows, e.g. two views of the same artery or left ventricle, or a baseline and follow-up run of some artery, and 5) of course, the availability of analytical software for QCA and quantitative left ventriculography.
The role of DICOM in the digital catheterization laboratory and an overview of digital review stations as of February 1996 was presented in reference 30. Although the development of digital review stations has continued actively thereafter, there certainly are major differences in the qualities, usefulness, price, etc. of all the workstations that are and will be made available commercially. We do expect to present an updated overview of the different digital workstation approaches later this year. To educate the cardiological community about DICOM, the Working Group 1 of the DICOM Standards Committee has published the so-called Primer.[31]

Future QCA directions
It must be clear that the DICOM-3 standard has been developed to exchange image data between machines from different vendors. It has never been meant to be an archive standard. The simplest archive of a digital laboratory is of course the same old shelf, now with the CD-R's on it in stead of the cinefilm boxes in the past. This may work for a small laboratory (e.g. less than 1000 cases/yr), but that is not exactly what we expect from a digital laboratory. For the medium- and large-volume laboratories automated

archives are preferred with different levels of access, for example an "on-line" short-term storage, a "near-line" long-term storage and an "off-line" storage. For an excellent overview, the reader is referred to reference 32. Furthermore, we do expect extensive networking of digital review stations with and without QCA packages in the catheterization laboratory. Of course, this network will be connected to the imaging network of the catheterization laboratories, thereby allowing images to be transferred to the cardiologist's office and also to referring hospitals. The selected images and the corresponding results can be saved on a central file server for later review and possibly reanalysis.

In terms of extension of analytical software packages, we anticipate further developments in the automated segmentation of parts of or the entire coronary tree from two preferably orthogonal views.[33,34] This will allow the selection of optimal views for selected coronary segments, and the assessment of the area at risk of the myocardial muscle.[35] For the near future, the integration with IVUS can be expected. This will be discussed under the section Image Fusion.

With so many different approaches and devices for coronary recanalization now available (balloons: compliant and noncompliant; long, medium and short; perfusion balloon; hybrid balloon; ultralow profile balloon; local drug delivery balloon; stents: slotted tube, coiled, self-expanding with or without biocompatible coatings, etc.), it is likely that on-line QCA and/or IVUS will be used increasingly to help guide the logical choice of technology, based on lesion morphology and location in the coronary tree.

Quantitative intravascular ultrasound

Intravascular ultrasound (IVUS) is able to provide real-time high resolution images of sections of the arterial wall, in contrast to x-ray arteriography that provides a shadow image (luminogram) of the entire lumen. IVUS has potentially a great strength in diagnostic and interventional procedures.[36] In the first application, IVUS is able to demonstrate the presence or absence of compensatory coronary artery enlargement, to assess the severity of intermediate lesions, to reveal occult left main disease, and angiographically 'silent' atherosclerosis. In interventional cardiology, IVUS may support the selection of the devices, i.e. rotablators in calcified lesions, and atherectomy devices in large plaque burden. The results of such procedures can be studied on-line, under the restrictions described later. In interventional cardiology, the lumen and the wall of a particular coronary segment are inspected visually by moving the intracoronary ultrasound catheter through the vessel. The global positioning of the catheter is guided by x-ray angiography. In this way the section with the narrowest lumen can be selected and analyzed quantitatively by using a manual caliper in its simplest approach, or by outlining the lumen and vessel wall contours in a more accurate approach. This will lead to the calculation of the percent cross-sectional area narrowing at that particular cross section, and minimal·and maximal diameters. However, the associated inter- and intra-observer variabilities have been mentioned as a definite limitation in the Section Introduction. Knowing how irregular in shape the cross sections in coronary arteries can be, it will be clear that simple contour detection approaches that are looking for more or less convex cross sections, will not work; a technique with characteristics as the earlier mentioned Gradient Field Transform is needed. Another approach of automated contour detection is the use of active shape models (snakes) for luminal boundary detection, which has been developed by Maurincomme et al.[37]

Since IVUS is in principle a tomographic technique, the catheter can be pulled back, while at the same time the images are being digitized and stored in computer memory. To assure that the pullback speed is constant, motorized pullback techniques have been developed. Because of the cardiac motion, the image acquisition for a pullback should be ECG-triggered. The individual cross-sections can be stacked in the computer memory and visualized. For visualization, at least two approaches have been developed, one being the display of the longitudinal cross-sections of the vessel segment in combination with the corresponding cross-sections, and the other one the 'clam-shell' view which requires image segmentation. Since the catheter does not provide information about its 3D trajectory of its pullback path, the vessel can only be reconstructed and displayed as a straight tube. Of course, in the far majority of the cases this will not be correct, thereby leading to highly incorrect luminal and plaque volumes. With pullback techniques, the catheter movement is sensed at its proximal site, but it is the distal tip that produces the images. In short, the following error sources can be identified in three-dimensional IVUS (Table 1). An excellent overview of the advantages and limitations of 3D IVUS imaging can be found in reference 38.

3D quantitative analysis
Since the image quality of the individual cross sections is limited due to the relatively low image resolution and image contrast, it is very difficult to develop a technique that is automated and robust in the individual cross sections. Therefore, one should try to make use of the continuity of the morphology in the individual cross sections. Li et al. have developed a very elegant and practical approach in this direction.[39] Their semi-automatic

Table 1. Limitations in 3D intravascular ultrasound

- translation and rotation of the catheter during pullback
  - . longitudinal movement due to cardiac motion
  - . angulation of the catheter due to curvature
  - . torsion of the catheter due to curvature
- acquisition planes are not parallel
- slice orientation may change during pullback
- acquisition and analysis time consuming and tedious
- automated quantitation still in its infancy

approach consists of three steps. First, two perpendicular cut planes which are parallel to the longitudinal axis are selected interactively. The second step is an interactive tracing procedure which defines the contours of the lumen and plaque in the longitudinal images. For each longitudinal image, two lumen and two media contours are traced. The third step is the contour detection in each cross-sectional image thereby using the information from the longitudinal contours. By transforming the contours from the two longitudinal planes to the transverse plane, four pre-defined points per contour become available for each cross-section. These points indicate the locations through which the contours should go in that particular cross section. The automated contour detection in the cross section again is based on the minimum cost (MCA) contour detection technique. Once the contours are available, the clinically relevant data such as the volumes of the lumen and the plaque can easily be calculated. Figure 3 shows the first results of our automatically determined luminal and vessel contours and derived quantitative data.

The approach that we have taken is somewhat similar. Our IVUS-CMS system is running under the Windows-NT operating system on a Pentium-Pro 200 processor computer. For the image processing, we have developed the MPIRE software package, that allows easy manipulation of images and integration with other software developed in our laboratory. A part of the contour detection approach is similar to that by Li et al.[39]; the IVUS-CMS system allows the user to select any longitudinal cross-section (more than two are allowed and they do not need to be perpendicular). The contour detection in the longitudinal images is based on the MCA approach. Recently, our MCA has been redesigned using C + + in an object-oriented approach. The advantage of the redesign is that it has become very flexible and therefore can be adapted very quickly to new applications. This redesigned MCA allows the incorporation of models and other knowledge, which makes the contour detection more robust. The approach by Li et al.[39]

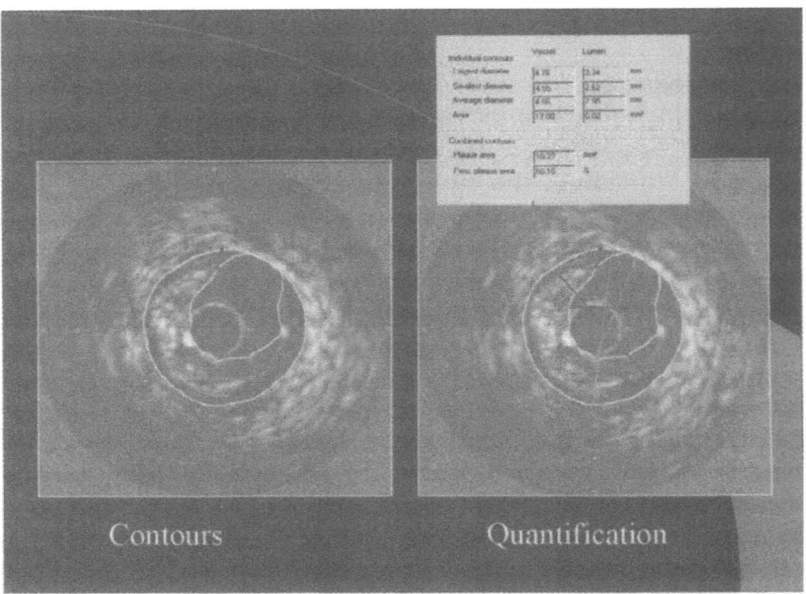

Figure 3. *First results of our automated contour detection approaches for the luminal and vessel boundaries in IVUS images.* (For colour plate of figure 3 see page 219)

is based on a matching technique, whereby the information of the contours drawn in a first frame, will be matched as best as possible to the subsequent frames. We intend to base the results from our contour detection on the local images properties and additional information from models and knowledge about IVUS images. The information from neighboring frames is only used to guide the positions and directions of the scanlines for the resampling of the images. In addition, a Gradient Field Transform-like approach will be developed and implemented allowing to detect irregularly shaped cross sections, especially for the lumen contour. In the 3D reconstruction, corrections need to be carried out for possible rotation of the catheter during pull-back, catheter movement as well as other error sources.

Future IVUS directions
It will be clear that IVUS is complementary rather than in competition with angiography. Angiography provides an overall, critically important roadmap, while IVUS goes to the appropriate address and tells the investigator what is happening in the vessel wall at that particular place. The stand-alone 3D IVUS reconstructions do not provide a reliable picture of the coronary vessel, since a simple straight tube model is assumed. Advanced registration of

biplane coronary angiography will be required to provide a 3D reconstruction of the vessel's pathline and the individual IVUS cross sections will be stacked and displayed relative to this pathline.[40] QCA and IVUS pre-intervention can help to decide which interventional device to use and its size. It can also teach all sorts of things about the local environment inside the artery, that will help make the case go better and quicker. Preliminary results indicate that IVUS may allow the automated assessment of plaque composition in terms of soft and hard/shadowed plaques based on texture descriptors and automated classification techniques.[41] It is also clear that not in all cases the combination of QCA and IVUS will be necessary. In some vessels it will suffice to use only QCA, in other only IVUS and in the remaining cases the combination. Clinical trials need to be designed to sort out these choices, taking into account that IVUS adds to the cost and the length of a procedure. Anyway, the angiogram will always be needed to guide the 3D reconstruction procedure. Large prospective trials are underway to address the effects of IVUS on device selection or the predictibility of long-term results; these will provide answers to the cost-benefit ratio of peri-interventional IVVS.[36]

Left ventricular function

In this section the analytical approaches for three imaging modalities, being x-ray angiography, echocardiography and MR imaging will be described, in the assessment of left ventricular function.

Quantitative x-ray left ventriculography

Over the past 20 to 25 years many different techniques have been developed for the quantitative analysis of left ventricular (LV) x-ray angiograms using automated contour detection algorithms.[42] None of these approaches has demonstrated to be ideal: each technique requires a certain amount of user-interaction in the definition of the structure to be detected, and corrections to the detected contours in a significant percentage of the cases.

We have continued to be intrigued by the idea to be able to analyze routinely generated x-ray ventriculograms without any or with a minimal amount of user-interaction. Our current philosophy is directed at a three-stage approach:

1. fully automated assessment of a model of the LV plus aorta from the LV angiogram by itself;

2. detection of the LV contours by resampling the image perpendicular to the model and by applying the MCA algorithm;

3. selection of the aortic valve positions and thereby cutting off the aorta. The first stage has been realized by the combination of two methods: a neural network approach and a pyramidal segmentation procedure. The neural network was trained on a total of approximately 250 LV investigations. For each image to be analyzed, a number of blurred images at various resolution levels (128x128, 64x64, 32x32 and 16x16 pixels) is generated; from these multi-resolution images, the original image is segmented into a number of regions. These regions are then labeled as the left ventricle or the background by using the model obtained by the neural network. This combination of both approaches thus results in a model of the LV plus the aorta.[43] Once an acceptable model has been generated, the execution of phase 2 is relatively trivial. Sofar the automated assessment of the two valve positions and the apex has been the most problematic; an initial experiment with a second neural network only for the recognition of these three points did not result in a sufficiently high success score. For that reason we have developed an intermediary practical approach, resulting in two packages, denoted Automated Left Ventricular (ALV) and Automated Multi-frame Ventricular (AMV).

For the assessment of LV ejection fraction based on the end-diastolic (ED) and end-systolic (ES) frames, the user indicates the two aortic valve points and the apex, followed by the automated detection of the LV contours using the neural network and pyramidal segmentation approaches (ALV approach). Also, the contour detection algorithm has the constraint that the LV contours must go through these valve and apex points. Once the contours are known, the standard wall motion models and ejection fraction measurements can be applied. For the frame-to-frame analysis (AMV), the user indicates the aortic valve points and the apex again in the first ED, the ES and the following ED frames. For the intermediate frames, these individual points are defined by interpolation by a nonlinear function. Next, the same contour detection algorithm as for the ALV approach can be applied to the individual frames with the additional constraint of continuity from frame to frame. From these data instantaneous and regional LV wall motion can be assessed.[42] Also, this provides the potential to correlate the instantaneous LV volumes with the corresponding pressure data, and thus the generation of pressure-volume (PV) loops. Current experiences have been very promising, also for routine clinical applications, with an analysis time for the entire process of approximately 10 seconds per frame.

Future expectations LV by x-ray
From our experiences it has become clear that additional information about

the shape and appearance of the left ventricle must be provided to approach a fully automated assessment of the LV contours. To achieve this, we have decided to develop a framework for automatic image interpretation based on a blackboard system. In this framework, segmentation is approached by representing image processing strategies as knowledge sources, and storing the results of these operations in a central data container, also referred to as a blackboard.

Examples of currently implemented knowledge sources are, among others, the earlier mentioned neural network and pyramidal segmentation approaches, but now with a 3D analyzing capability. By a 3D approach, all images over one cardiac cycle will be involved simultaneously in the pyramidal segmentation procedure. In addition, unsupervised segmentation approaches such as the fuzzy clustering technique, which labels the regions generated by the pyramidal segmentation method, will also be integrated in the blackboard system as a knowledge source. The course of activation of these knowledge sources is not defined a-priori, but evolves dynamically as each knowledge source can call on other knowledge sources and use processing results already present on the blackboard. In this way a number of possible segmentations are generated concurrently. An optimal segmentation can be obtained by comparing the different segmentation results to a model of a "normal" ventricle, which is also represented as a knowledge source. This segmentation then serves as a basis for more accurate boundary finding algorithms, like the previously mentioned MCA.

Quantitative echocardiography

Left ventricular echocardiography allows the real-time assessment of the wall motion of the heart.[10] The technique is harmless to the patient, relatively cheap, simple to use and widely spread. Most echocardiographic investigations are used for qualitative diagnostic purposes. In routine practice quantitative analysis of these images is hardly used because of the required manual contour tracing. Several approaches for automated analysis of the echocardiographic images have been described, varying from computer-assisted manual techniques, interactive methods and (semi-)automated methods.[44] Given the large quantities of images to be processed, preferably on a frame-by-frame basis, the (semi-)automated methods are naturally of greater interest. However, their practical utility has remained limited sofar, also due to the fact that the image quality is very variable in routine practice. Echocardiographic exercise protocols have been used for the assessment of ischemia-induced changes in wall motion under pharmacologic (e.g. dobutamine) or physical stress conditions.[45] To detect wall motion abnormalities, regional endocardial wall motion (contrary to the total lumen area) must be followed over one or more cardiac cycles.

Stimulated by these potential clinical applications, we have developed and validated the Echocardiographic Workstation (ECHO-CMS).[46,47] In the following paragraphs the basic principles of ECHO-CMS and the results from an intermediate evaluation study will be presented, as well as our future developments.

Basic principles

ECHO-CMS consists of a standard powerful workstation (Pentium, 200 MHz) with a frame grabber for the digitization of the video sequences, a single high resolution color monitor and a computer mouse for user-interaction. Echocardiographic images can be provided in digital format (e.g. from a magneto-optical disk unit or network), or digitized from an analog video source (e.g. a video cassette recorder (VCR) or the video output of an echoscanner). The ECHO-CMS analytical software has been implemented as a MS-Windows application, so that a known, standardized and versatile user-interface could be created, allowing the user to control the analytical process in a user-friendly, intuitive manner. Furthermore, this provides the possibility for direct interchange of data with standard applications as Excel, Word, and PowerPoint for further statistical processing, reporting and presentation.

ECHO-CMS supports both automated contour detection and manual tracing in the echocardiographic images.[48] In addition, manual correction of otherwise automatically detected contours is always possible, as well as the application of such single corrections over multiple images. The automated contour detection process for a sequence of frames can be initialized in a number of ways: 1) by manually defining the centerpoint of a fixed model, such as a circle in short-axis views, 2) by manually defining two valve points and the apex in any long-axis cross-section followed by the generation of an elliptical model through these points, 3) by manually drawing one or two contours, etc. The actual contour detection process is based upon the MCA algorithm. In short, the contour detection procedure works as follows. From the user input (points or contours) and the phase information, contour models are generated for each image. Models incorporate expected spatial position of the contour, gray value profiles and shape constraints. From any manually defined or corrected contours, contour shape and gray value pattern information is integrated into the models. Perpendicular to the local directions of the models, a large number of scanlines of limited length is defined. For each point of each scanline, a cost value is defined based on a weighted sum of matched gray values, edge strength (first derivative values of the brightness profile along and perpendicular to the scanline) and model information, such as distance from the model, etc. Finally, an optimal contour is searched for through all the points belonging to the cost matrix using dynamic programming techniques. Different smoothness constraints can be applied here. For detection in sequences spanning multiple heart beats, the contours detected in key frames like ES and ED can be used as a model for the detection in the intermediate frames. Figure 4 is an example of the display of the ECHO-CMS with automatically derived contours.

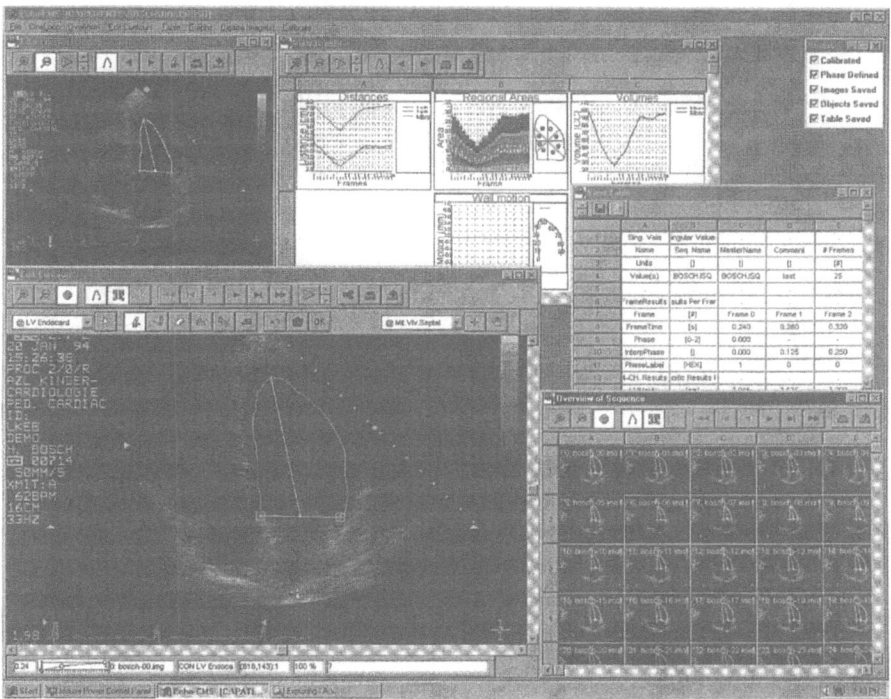

Figure 4. Example of the computer display of the ECHO-CMS with multiple windows open showing automatically detected contours on a frame-by-frame basis, the working window with one of the frames, plots with derived volumetric, distance and wall motion data, and part of the automatically filled data spread sheet.

Validation study on short-axis images

An initial evaluation study on an early version of the ECHO-CMS was carried out in 20° patient studies (10 transthoracic, 10 transesophageal echocardiography) with short-axis cross-sections taken at the papillary level. VHS video tapes were selected from routinely obtained patient materials from different hospitals in the Netherlands, so that a wide range of echocardiographic equipment, image quality, pathologies and operator settings were represented.

From each patient study, 16 consecutive images covering the first part of one cardiac cycle were digitized by ECHO-CMS at a matrix size of 256x256 pixels and stored for later manual and automated analysis of the endocardial contours. After a period of 6 weeks the manual and automated analyses were repeated by the first observer on two patient studies (1 TEE, 1 TTE) and by a second observer. From all these data the inter- and intra-observer variabilities could be derived. The systematic errors in the areas calculated within the contours were defined by the average value of the signed differences between corresponding measurements. The random errors were defined by the standard deviations of these differences.

In summary, the following results were obtained: in 82% of the 320 contours no direct manual corrections were required.[46] The average analysis time per patient study for the MANUAL procedures was 25 minutes, of which 18½ minutes were required for manual tracing and carrying out necessary corrections. The average AUTO analysis time was 5½ minutes, of which 1½ minutes were used for corrections. Regression analysis gave the following result: AUTO = 1.01 * MAN + 5.58%, r = 0.989, SEE (standard error of the estimate) = 0.08 for N = 320 contours. The following inter- and intra-observer variabilities were found:

	Intra-observer		Inter-observer	
	AUTO	MAN	AUTO	MAN
Systematic errors	1.74%	2.91%	1.97%	8.44%
Random errors	4.18%	8.54%	4.95%	5.45%

On the basis of these results it could be concluded that 1) ECHO-CMS provides automatically detected contours which are very similar to manually traced outlines, which served as the gold standard, 2) ECHO-CMS is five to ten times faster than the manual tracing procedure, and 3) ECHO-CMS is characterized by reduced inter- and intra-observer variabilities as compared to manual tracings. This makes ECHO-CMS a useful tool for clinical echocardiographic research studies.

Evaluations on 4-chamber and 2-chamber images

In a study carried out at the Cardiology Department of the University Hospital of Maastricht with a newer version of ECHO-CMS with improved contour detection, 2-chamber and 4-chamber views were acquired of a total of 22 patients. Automated scoring of wall motion abnormalities based on ECHO-CMS analyses was compared to eyeball scoring (13-segment model, 5-grade scale). It was concluded that the infarct location (either anterior or inferior) was correct in 82% of the cases, while the difference in wall motion scoring was less than two grades in 84% of the segments.

In a recent study carried out at the cardiology department of the Free University Hospital with the latest version of the ECHO-CMS, 2-chamber and 4-chamber views were acquired of 135 infarct patients; per patient either 4 or 6 heart beats were analyzed. The acquisitions were done at 3 days and 3 months after the infarct. For each beat, 2 contours were drawn manually (ED and ES); all other contours were detected automatically. Where necessary, manual corrections to the otherwise automatically detected contours and subsequent redetections were applied until the luminal deliniation was considered accurate. Analysis of the first set of 53 patient studies of this population, revealed that of a total of 7024 contours, only 12.3% were drawn or had to be corrected (88% generated automatically).[47]

Future ECHO-CMS directions

In the near future we will extend the ECHO-CMS with the appropriate acquisition and analysis modules to facilitate the analysis of stress echo images. This is an area where the automated contour detection could provide more objective and reproducible results than possible by visual interpretation, if and only if the contour detection is sufficiently robust. It is our belief that the current version of the MCA plus the use of matching techniques will allow such analyses. To be able to analyze images of lesser quality as well, we are in the phase of developing a knowledge-guided image processing infrastructure based again on a black board architecture. By this approach, all kinds of different knowledge sources, e.g. geometric models, fuzzy clustering, texture measures, etc., will be able to contribute to the final result. In the near future, contrast echo and 3D echocardiographic analyses will be supported. Needless to say that from a technical point of view, the support of digital imaging, DICOM exchange and network communication will play a dominant role in the developments to come.

Quantitative magnetic resonance imaging

Nearly all aspects of cardiovascular function and flow can be quantified nowadays with fast MR imaging techniques. Conventional and breath-hold cine MR imaging allows the precise and highly reproducible assessment of global and regional left ventricular function. Since MR imaging provides a three-dimensional data set for quantification of ventricular volumes and mass, it can be expected to have improved accuracy and inter-study reproducibility as compared to the results currently obtained from echocardiography.[49,50] Recently, segmented, fast cine MR imaging has been introduced to improve the time efficiency of functional evaluation of ventricular dimensions and function.[51,52] With this technological improvement, it has become possible to acquire multiple images at one particular anatomical level during a breath-hold period of about 16 seconds. It takes approximately 5 to 8 minutes to obtain a series of such images at the multiple levels encompassing the complete left ventricle, resulting in a complete 3D data set.

More dedicated exams such as myocardial perfusion analysis using intravascular contrast agents,[53] or analysis of truly 3D myocardial motion using MR tagging techniques[54,55] may be used additionally to provide more detailed analysis of the ventricular performance.

Until today, MR imaging for cardiac evaluation has not found widespread application in the clinical environment. Quantitative image analysis by simple manual tracing of contours is a very time-consuming and tedious procedure and may be seen as an important obstacle for the application of MR in routine clinical practice. Reliable automated or semi-automated image analysis approaches are required to overcome these limitations.

In the following paragraphs a short description is given of the underlying methods and validation results of the methods developed at our laboratory, which have been integrated in a software package, MASS®, implemented on a SUN workstation[56,57] and to be ported to the Windows-NT environment. Our approach to the automated detection of endocardial and epicardial contours follows a model-based technique and is directed to the definition of the endocardial and epicardial contours in all the phases and slices of an imaging study. The amount of user-interaction required to obtain reliable contours has been limited, and is minimal in case the images are of sufficient quality. Using this algorithm, automated analysis of an imaging study can be completed in less than 20 minutes, while completely manual tracing of the endocardial and epicardial outlines in each of the images, would take 3-4 hours depending on the number of images and the image quality.

The contour detection of a series of short-axis cross sections starts by searching for circular objects in the imaging slices to find the approximate center of the left ventricle. Using the detected centerpoint, epicardial contours are found in the first phase and subsequently in the remaining phases using a frame-to-frame contour detection procedure. This frame-to-frame epicardial contour detection procedure is based on matching of line profiles which are positioned perpendicularly to the model contour (derived from the first phase) and then automatically positioned at the corresponding tissue transitions in other phases within the same slice level.

After the epicardial contours have been found the detection of endocardial contours is initiated. During this detection the search region is limited to the area inside the available epicardial contours. A first estimate of the endocardial contour is found using an optimal thresholding technique. The final endocardial contour is found using the strengths of the gray value changes in a small neighborhood of the initial estimate using an MCA approach.

From the contours describing the endocardial and epicardial border of the myocardium, ventricular volume and global and regional function parameters can be derived, including ED and ES volumes, ejection fraction (EF), stroke volume (SV) and LV mass. Since multiple phases are acquired within the cardiac cycle, also the dynamic changes in left ventricular volume may be studied. These dynamic processes can be described by the peak ejection rate (PER) and peak filling rate (PFR), as well as by their time offsets (TPER and TPFR, respectively). The MASS analytical package was evaluated on MR imaging studies from 10 infarct patients and 10 healthy volunteers.[57]

As MR imaging provides excellent depiction of the epicardial borders of the myocardium, not only wall motion, but also regional and instantaneous wall thickening and thinning, can be derived. It has been shown that wall thickening analysis is more sensitive to the detection of dysfunctional myocardium than wall motion analysis.[58] However, since 2D methods are confined to measurements within individual 2D images, the implicit assumption is made that the myocardial wall itself is always perpendicular to the acquisition plane. Because of the ellipsoidal cardiac geometry this assumption is rarely true, even when true short-axis images are obtained, particularly near the apex. Planar, 2D wall thickness methods will therefore inevitably overestimate true wall thickness in a systematic manner. However, the myocardial boundaries of a multi-slice, multi-phase MR image acquisition contain 3D shape information which may be used to prevent these systematic and random overestimations.

A relatively uncomplicated algorithm, which is a straightforward extension to the 2D centerline method, was developed at our institution.[59] This new 3D wall thickness calculation method allows the measurement of wall thickness perpendicular to the myocardial wall by correcting the overestimation present in the 2D centerline method for each individual centerline chord based on the angle between the local normal vector to the myocardial wall and the horizontal slice. The improved accuracy and precision of this 3D approach was demonstrated very clearly in a phantom and a clinical study.[59]

Three-dimensional displays are used to offer a good 3D perception of the shape of the ventricle as seen from different viewing angles. Cine loops displaying the 3D-images of the ventricle in different phases within the cardiac cycle provide insight in patterns of myocardial contraction and relaxation. In addition, functional data such as wall thickness or wall motion can be projected onto the 3D-displays using color-coding of the ventricular surface. By using standardized color coding schemes based on normal ranges computed from a large population of healthy volunteers, the location, size and severity of myocardial abnormalities can easily be derived from such a display. Computation of a single display takes less than one second on a standard SUN Sparc 20 workstation. Pre-computed displays for a complete cardiac cycle can be displayed in real-time. Figure 5 is an example of such a functional 3D display and the user-interface of the MASS package.

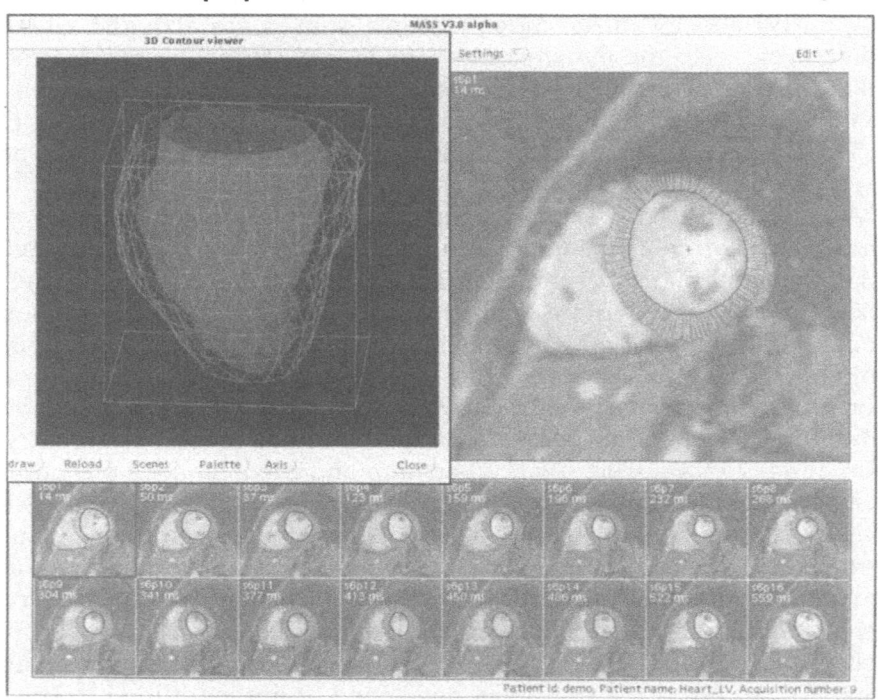

Figure 5. Computer display of the MASS analytical software package. The small images along the bottom represent the individual frames over a cardiac cycle at a certain anatomic level. The endo- and epicardial contours were detected automatically. From the contours in all the frames and slices, a 3D model can be reconstructed that can also be used as a functional display representing e.g. regional wall thickening/thinning. (For colour plate of figure 5 see page 219)

Velocity mapping

Velocity encoded cine MR imaging (VEC-MRI), also called MR flow velocity mapping, is another MR imaging technique which plays an important role in the evaluation of ventricular performance.[60] VEC-MRI is a non-invasive method that provides accurate two-dimensional velocity maps anywhere in the cardiovascular system at high temporal resolution. VEC-MRI can be applied during the same MR examination in conjunction with other MR acquisitions, to provide measurements of stroke volume of both ventricles, quantification of valvular regurgitation, assessment of flow through the atrio-ventricular valves and coronary artery flow reserve.

Application of VEC-MRI to the proximal portion of the ascending aorta allows the assessment of left ventricular systolic function by evaluating the flow over a complete cardiac cycle. Such a study requires a VEC-MRI acquisition in the transversal plane crossing the ascending aorta. The left ventricular stroke volume can be measured by integrating the flow over a complete cardiac cycle.

For an accurate assessment of volume flow, contours describing the lumen of the vessels have to be obtained in the images. Manual contour tracing is still the most commonly used analysis method. The in-plane motion of the greater vessels and changes in shape of the vessel cross section over the cardiac cycle require the user to trace the luminal border of the vessel in each individual phase of the MR examination. To overcome these practical limitations, an automated analysis method FLOW® was developed in our department to automatically detect the required contours in each of the cardiac phases.[61] This algorithm operates on the standard cine MR images which are obtained during a VEC-MRI acquisition. It takes care of the small changes in spatial position from frame to frame, as well as of the deformations in the vessel's cross sections. For further details, please, refer to.[61]

The automated analytical package FLOW® was validated on flow velocity maps from a study population of 12 healthy volunteers (three men) with normal ECG and no history of cardiac malfunction. The FLOW® quantification package ran on a commercially available SUN Sparc 20 workstation (Sun Microsystems, Mountain View, CA). The time required for manual analysis was 5-10 minutes, and for automated analysis less than 10 seconds. No statistically significant differences were found between the results of manual and automated analyses. The mean difference between automated and manually assessed SV was 0.78 ml (SD 1.99 ml). The intra-observer variability was 0.65 ml for manual analysis and 0.58 ml for automated analysis; the intra-observer variability was 0.99 ml for manual analysis and 0.90 ml for automated analysis.

Future LV MR imaging directions
Recent progress in MR imaging of the coronary arteries and myocardial perfusion imaging with contrast media, along with the further development of fast imaging sequences, suggest that MR imaging could evolve into a single technique ("one stop shop") for the evaluation of many aspects of heart disease. The reduction in MR acquisition times indicates that it may

become feasible to carry out a comprehensive MR examination within an acceptable time period. As a result, even more images will be obtained during an MR examination and the need for automated or semi-automated image analysis software will only further increase. The noninvasive visualization of the coronary arteries would be a major step forward for two reasons: 1) for the noninvasive diagnosis of coronary artery disease either for screening or in patients at high risk; and 2) for repeated examinations after coronary interventions, e.g. PTCA or bypass surgery. At the current state of the technique, only the proximal one- to two-thirds of the coronary arteries can be visualized reliably, and due to its anterior location close to the surface coil, the right coronary artery is best suited for imaging.[62] However, the spatial resolution is currently still insufficient to assess the degree of coronary atherosclerosis present with sufficient accuracy. Further developments in both hardware and acquisition techniques are necessary to approximately double the spatial resolution. Optimized ('phased array' or 'synergy') heart coils, as well as a near to complete elimination of breathing motion artifacts are needed to achieve this goal. In the mean time, significant progress is expected on automated segmentation by incorporating an anatomical model of the thoracic content based on hyperquadric shape descriptors into the segmentation process.[63] Furthermore, we will see significant developments in the field of 3D visualization, including endoscopic-like presentations, of MR angiographic applications in the larger, peripheral vessels.[64]

Image fusion

Sofar we have addressed the current and future approaches for the different image modalities. With all the data available in digital format, it will be clear, that attempts will be made towards image fusion. One of the most apparent applications, is the image fusion of coronary arteriography and QCA, and intracoronary ultrasound and quantitative coronary ultrasound. As was described earlier, at present 3D reconstructions of coronary vessels are generated from IVUS by stacking up ECG-gated and segmented IVUS frames of a pullback sequence. This simplified approach always results in straight vessel reconstructions, and therefore, provides an incorrect representation of bended and tortuous coronary arteries. From two biplane x-ray views, the pathlines of the relevant coronary segment, can be traced by well-known pathline tracer techniques. Subsequently, the 3D course of the vessel can be reconstructed three-dimensionally assuming that the correct geometric data of the x-ray gantries are available. The IVUS cross-sectional images can then be displayed around this 3D pathline, thereby providing a realistic view of the reconstructed coronary segment and allowing more accurate calculations of luminal and plaque volumes. Figure 6 illustrates the basic concepts of this data fusion approach (with permission from reference 65). It should be recognized that the catheter, in general, will twist during the pullback procedure. Prause and Sonka et al. have elegantly demonstrated that robust algorithms for the definition of the pullback path and the estimation of the IVUS catheter twist during pullback can be developed.[65]

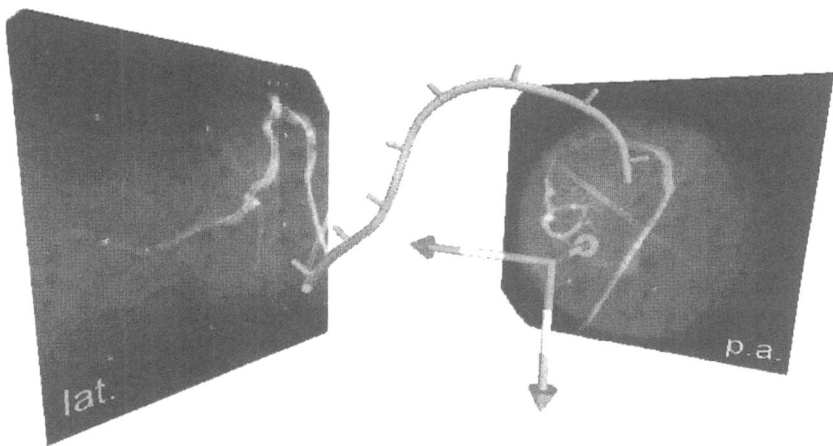

Figure 6. Biplane contrast angiogram of right coronary artery in a cadaveric pig heart with 3-D reconstructed catheter centerline. Short vectors indicate the orientation of IVUS images along the pullback as derived by sequential triangulation; note the clockwise twist from front to back. One unit of the axes equals 10 mm in the real world (with permission from reference 65).

Acknowledgement

The authors wish to acknowledge the financial support by MEDIS Medical Imaging Systems, Nuenen and the Technology Foundation, Utrecht (project no's LGN92.1706, LGN22.2781, LGN44.3419) both in the Netherlands in the research and development of the different quantitative image analysis approaches.

References

1. Johnson MR. Principles and practice of coronary angiography. In: Marcus Cardiac Imaging. DJ Skorton, HR Schelbert, GL Wolf, BH Brundage (Eds.). W.B. Saunders Company, Philadelphia, 1996:220-51.
2. Plokker HWTh. Coronary arteriography. Limitations and unresolved issues. Int J

Cardiac Imaging 1995;11(Suppl.1):49-51.

3. Brundage BH. What is the current role of ultrafast CT in coronary imaging? In: Cardiovascular Imaging. JHC Reiber, EE van der Wall, Eds., Kluwer Academic Publishers, Dordrecht, 1996:531-44.

4. van Rossum AC, Post JC. To which extent can the coronary artery tree be imaged and quantified with the current MR technology? In: Cardiovascular Imaging. JHC Reiber, EE van der Wall (Eds.). Kluwer Academic Publishers, Dordrecht, 1996:301-14.

5. Duerinckx AJ. Advantages and limitations of coronary MR angiography. In: Cardiovascular Imaging. JHC Reiber, EE van der Wall (Eds.). Kluwer Academic Publishers, Dordrecht, 1996:357-65.

6. Manning WJ. Current and future applications of magnetic resonance coronary angiography. In: Cardiovascular Imaging. JHC Reiber, EE van der Wall (Eds.). Kluwer Academic Publishers, Dordrecht, 1996:329-55.

7. Di Mario C, Fitzgerald PJ, Colombo A. New developments in intracoronary ultrasound. In: Cardiovascular Imaging. JHC Reiber, EE van der Wall (Eds.). Kluwer Academic Publishers, Dordrecht, 1996:257-75.

8. Römer TjJ. Raman spectroscopy during catheterization: the chemical composition of the plaque. This book, Chapter 11.

9. Sheehan FH. Principles and practice of contrast ventriculography. In: Marcus Cardiac Imaging. DJ Skorton, HR Schelbert, GL Wolf, BH Brundage (Eds.). W.B. Saunders Company, Philadelphia, 1996:164-87.

10. Weyman AE. Principles and practice of Echocardiography. Lea & Febiger, Philadelphia, 2nd edition, 1994.

11. Marwick ThH. Current status of stress echocardiography for the diagnosis of myocardial ischemia and viability. In: Advances in Imaging Techniques in Ischemic Heart Disease. EE van der Wall, ThH Marwick, JHC Reiber (Eds.). Kluwer Academic Publishers, Dordrecht, 1995:83-99.

12. Gibbons RJ, Miller TD. Equilibrium radionuclide angiography. In: Marcus Cardiac Imaging. DJ Skorton, HR Schelbert, GL Wolf, BH Brundage (Eds.). W.B. Saunders Company, Philadelphia, 1996:941-62.

13. van der Wall EE, Vliegen HW, de Roos A, Bruschke AVG. Magnetic resonance imaging in coronary artery disease. Circulation 1995;92:2723-39.

14. Holman ER, Buller VGM, de Roos A et al. Detection and quantification of dysfunctional myocardium by magnetic resonance imaging. A new three-dimensional method for quantitative wall-thickening analysis. Circulation 1997;52:924-31.

15. van der Wall EE. Current status of myocardial perfusion scintigraphy. In: Advances in Imaging Techniques in ischemic heart disease. EE van der Wall, ThH Thomas, JHC Reiber (Eds.). Kluwer Academic Publishers, Dordrecht, 1995:1-16.

16. Reiber JHC, Koning G, van der Zwet PMJ et al. Assessment of myocardial flow reserve with the DCI. Medica Mundi 1993;38:81-8.

17. Wolters MJA. Densitometric assessment of regional myocardial perfusion. Doctoral thesis. Leiden University, 1997.

18. Thomas JD. Contrast ultrasound for assessment of myocardial perfusion: promise and pitfalls. In: Advances in imaging techniques in ischemic heart disease. EE van der Wall, ThH Thomas, JHC Reiber (Eds.). Kluwer Academic Publishers, Dordrecht, 1995:101-11.

19. Jerosch-Herold M, Wilke N. MR first pass imaging: quantitative assessment of transmural perfusion and collateral flow. Int J Cardiac Imaging 1997:14:205-18.

20. Gensini GG, Kelly AE, Da Costa BCB, Huntington PP. Quantitative angiography: the measurement of coronary vaso-motility in the intact animal and man. Chest 1971;60:522-30.
21. Brown BG, Bolson E, Frimer M, Dodge HT. Quantitative coronary arteriography. Estimation of dimensions, hemodynamic resistance, and atheroma mass of coronary artery lesions using the arteriograms and digital computation. Circulation 1977;55:329-37.
22. Reiber JHC, Serruys PW, Kooijman CJ et al. Assessment of short-, medium-, and long-term variations in arterial dimensions from computer-assisted quantitation of coronary cineangiograms. Circulation 1985;71:280-8.
23. Reiber JHC. An overview of coronary quantitation techniques as of 1989. In: Quantitative Coronary Arteriography. JHC Reiber, PW Serruys (Eds.). Kluwer Academic Publishers, Dordrecht, 1991:55-132
24. Bruschke AVG, Reiber JHC, Lie KI, Wellens HJJ (Eds.). Lipid-lowering therapy and progression of coronary atherosclerosis. Kluwer Academic Publishers, Dordrecht, 1996.
25. Reiber JHC, van der Zwet PMJ, Koning G et al. Accuracy and precision of quantitative digital coronary arteriography: observer-, short-, and medium-term variabilities. Cath Cardiovasc Diagn 1993;28:187-98.
26. van der Zwet PMJ, Reiber JHC. A new approach for the quantification of complex lesion morphology: The Gradient Field Transform: Basic principles and validation results. JACC 1994;24:216-24.
27. Reiber JHC, von Land CD, Koning G et al. Comparison of accuracy and precision of quantitative coronary arterial analysis between cinefilm and digital systems. In: Progress in quantitative coronary arteriography. JHC Reiber, PW Serruys (Eds.). Kluwer Academic Publishers, Dordrecht, 1994:67-85.
28. van der Zwet PMJ, Reiber JHC. The influence of image enhancement and reconstruction on quantitative coronary arteriography. Int J Cardiac Imaging 1995;11:211-21.
29. Koning G, Baretta P, Zwart P, Reiber JHC. Effect of lossy image compression on QCA results. Circulation 1995;82(Suppl.I):I-22 (Abstract).
30. Goedhart B, Reiber JHC. The role of DICOM in the digital catheterization laboratory. In: Cardiovascular Imaging. JHC Reiber, EE van der Wall (Eds.). Kluwer Academic Publishers, Dordrecht, 1996:171-84.
31. Digital Cardiac Imaging in the 21st century: A Primer. ThE Kennedy, SE Nissen, R Simon, JD Thomas, PL Tilkemeier (Eds.). The Cardiac and Vascular Information Working Group, American College of Cardiology, Bethesda, Maryland, USA, 1997.
32. Cusma JT, Bashore TM. The digital catheterization laboratory - is it practical today? In: Cardiovascular Imaging. JHC Reiber, EE van der Wall (Eds.). Kluwer Academic Publishers, Dordrecht, 1996:157-70.
33. Dumay ACM. Image reconstruction from biplane angiographic projections. Doctoral thesis, Delft University of Technology, 1992.
34. Wahle A, Wellnhofer E, Mugaragu I, Sauer HU, Oswald H, Fleck E. Assessment of diffuse coronary artery disease by quantitative analysis of coronary morphology based upon 3-D reconstruction from biplane angiograms. Trans Med Imaging 1995;14:230-41.
35. Seiler C, Kirkeeide RL, Gould KL. Basic structure-function relations of the epicardial coronary vascular tree; basis of quantitative coronary arteriography for diffuse coronary artery disease. Circulation 1992;85:1987-2003.

36. Görge G, Ge J, Haude M et al. Intravascular ultrasound for evaluation of coronary arteries. Herz 1996;21:78-89.

37. Maurincomme E, Finet G, Reiber JHC, Savalle L, Magnin I. Quantitative intravascular ultrasound imaging: evaluation of an automated approach. J Am Coll Cardiol 1995;25:354A (Abstract).

38. Maurincomme E, Finet G. What are the advantages and limitations of three-dimensional intracoronary ultrasound imaging? In: Cardiovascular Imaging. JHC Reiber, EE van der Wall (Eds.). Kluwer Academic Publishers, Dordrecht,1996:243-255.

39. Li W, Bom N, von Birgelen C, van der Steen TFW, de Korte CL, Gussenhoven EJ, Lancée CL. State of the art in ICUS quantitation. In: Cardiovascular Imaging. JHC Reiber, EE van der Wall (Eds.). Kluwer Academic Publishers, Dordrecht, 1996:79-92.

40. Evans JL, Ng K-H, Wiet SG et al. Accurate three-dimensional reconstruction of intravascular data - spatially correct three-dimensional reconstructions. Circulation 1996;93:567-76.

41. Zhang X, Sonka M (Personal communication).

42. Reiber JHC, Serruys PW, Slager CJ. In: Quantitative coronary and left ventricular cineangiography: methodology and clinical applications. Martinus Nijhoff Publishers, Dordrecht, 1986.

43. van der Zwet PMJ, Koning G, Reiber JHC. Left ventricular contour detection. A fully automated approach. Comput Cardiol 1992:359-62.

44. Sher DB, Revankar S, Rosenthal S. Computer methods in quantitation of cardiac wall parameters from two-dimensional echocardiograms: a survey. Int J Cardiac Imaging 1992;8:11-26.

45. Marwick ThH. Current status of stress echocardiography for the diagnosis of myocardial ischemia and viability. In: Advances in imaging techniques in ischemic heart disease. EE van der Wall, ThH Marwick, JHC Reiber (Eds.). Kluwer Academic Publishers, Dordrecht, 1995:83-99.

46. Bosch JG, Savalle LH, van Burken G, Reiber JHC. Evaluation of a semiautomatic contour detection approach in sequences of short-axis two-dimensional echocardiographic images. J Am Soc Echocardiogr 1995;8:810-21.

47. Nijland F, Kamp O, Verhorst PMJ, de Voogt WG, Visser CA. Impact of myocardial viability on left ventricular size and function following acute myocardial infarction. Abstract submitted to AHA, 1997.

48. Bosch JG, Reiber JHC, van Burken G, Savalle L, Maurincomme E, Helbing WA. Automated contour detection and acoustic quantification. Eur Heart J 1995;16(Suppl.J):35-41.

49. Sakuma H, Fujia N, Foo TKF et al. Evaluation of left ventricular volume and mass with breath-hold cine MR imaging. Radiology 1993;188:377-80.

50. Young AA, Kramer CM, Ferrari VA, Axel L, Reichek N. Three dimensional left ventricular deformation in hypertrophic cardiomyopathy. Circulation 1994;90:854-67.

51. Kramer CR, Lima JAC, Reichek N et al. Regional differences in function within noninfarcted myocardium during left ventricular remodelling. Circulation 1993;88:1279-88.

52. Lamb HJ, Doornbos J, van der Velde EA, Kruit MC, Reiber JHC, de Roos A. Echo-panar MRI of the heart on a standard sytem: validation of measurement of left ventricular function and mass. JCAT 1996;20:942-9.

53. Wilke N, Simm C, Zhang J et al. Contrast-enhanced first pass myocardial perfusion imaging: correlation between myocardial blood flow in dogs at rest and during hyperhemia. Magn Res Med 1993;29:485-97.

54. Maier SE, Fischer SE, McKinnon GC, Hess OM, Krayenbuehl HP, Boesigner P. Evaluation of left ventricular segmental wall motion in hypertrophic cardiomyopathy with myocardial tagging. Circulation 1992;86:1919-28.

55. Bayar R, Shapiro EO, Graves WL et al. Quantification and validation of left ventricular wall thickening by a three-dimensional volume element magnetic resonance imaging approach. Circulation 1990;81:297-307.

56. van der Geest RJ, Jansen E, Buller VGM, Reiber JHC. Automated detection of left ventricular epi- and endocardial contours in short-axis MR images. Comput Cardiol 1994:33-6.

57. van der Geest RJ, Buller VGM, Jansen E et al. Comparison between manual and automated analysis of left ventricular volume parameters from short axis MR images. J Comput Assist Tomogr (in press).

58. Azhari H, Sidemen S, Weiss JL et al. Three-dimensional mapping of acute ischemic regions using MRI: wall thickening versus motion analysis. Am J Physiol 1990;259 (Heart Circ Physiol 28):H1492-H503.

59. Buller VGM, van der Geest RJ, Kool MD, Reiber JHC. Accurate three-dimensional wall thickness measurement from multi-slice short-axis MR imaging. Comput Cardiol 1995:245-8.

60. Szolar DH, Sakuma H, Higgins CB. Cardiovascular application of magnetic resonance flow and velocity measurements. J Magn Res Imag 1996;6:78-89.

61. van der Geest RJ, Buller VGM, Reiber JHC. Automated quantification of flow velocity and volume in the ascending and descending aorta using MR flow velocity mapping. Comput Cardiol 1995:29-32.

62. Scheidegger MB, Stuber M, Boesiger P, Hess OM. Coronary artery imaging by magnetic resonance. Herz 1996;21:90-6.

63. Lelieveldt BPF, van der Zwet PMJ, van der Geest RJ, Reiber JHC. Anatomical modelling with CSG-trees consisting of hyperquadric shape primitives. Comp Aided Geometric Design (submitted).

64. Davis CP, Ladd MEB, Romanowski BJ, Wildermuth S, Knoplioch JF, Debatin JF. Human aorta: preliminary results with virtual endoscopy based on three-dimensional MR imaging data sets. Radiology 1996;199:37-40.

65. Prause GPM, DeJong SC, McKay CR, Sonka M. Towards a geometrically correct 3-D reconstruction of turtuous coronary arteries based on biplane angiography and intravascular ultrasound. Int J Cardiac Imag 1997 (in press).

Is Hypertriglyceridemia Always a Risk Factor?

Frits H.A.F. de Man, Mariëtte J.V. Hoffer, Augustinus H.M. Smelt, Jan A. Gevers Leuven, Arnoud van der Laarse

Summary

The concept that hypertriglyceridemia is a risk factor for CHD has been disputed by epidemiological data that showed that an elevated plasma triglyceride concentration is not an independent risk factor of CHD. However, more insight in the heterogeneity of triglyceride-rich lipoproteins and the increased knowledge of lipoprotein metabolism have contributed to the growing notion that accumulation of cholesterol-rich VLDL and chylomicron remnants constitutes an atherogenic risk. An elevated plasma triglyceride concentration associated with obesity, low HDL-cholesterol concentration, dense small LDL particles, insulin resistance and prolonged postprandial lipemia bears a high risk of CHD. In the present chapter, we review the metabolic derangements of triglyceride-rich lipoproteins in hypertriglyceridemia. Endogenous hypertriglyceridemia is a multifactorial disease. Genetic as well as exogenous factors predispose subjects to the development of the characteristic lipoprotein abnormalities. Mutations in the LPL- and apoC-III gene are important genetic factors, whereas increased amounts of visceral fat and insulin resistance are principal exogenous factors that contribute to the expression of hypertriglyceridemia. Several studies have demonstrated that overproduction of triglycerides and an impaired catabolism contribute to the hypertriglyceridemia. An increased supply of glucose and free fatty acids contributes to overproduction of very low density lipoproteins, thereby increasing the burden of triglyceride-rich lipoproteins on the common lipolytic pathway at the level of lipoprotein

133

E.E. van der Wall et al. (eds.), Vascular Medicine, 133-160.
© 1997 *Kluwer Academic Publishers.*

lipase. Low lipoprotein lipase activity and increased amounts of lipolysis-inhibiting free fatty acids further impair lipolysis. When dietary measures and hypoglycemic agents have failed to achieve acceptable lipid levels, lipid-lowering drugs should be advised. Fibric acids are the drugs of choice because of their significant improvement of lipid, lipoprotein and fibrinogen levels.

Normal metabolism of triglycerides

Transport of triglycerides (TG) is carried out by chylomicrons from the intestine (exogenous route) and very low density lipoproteins (VLDL) from the liver (endogenous route), designated triglyceride-rich lipoproteins or TRL. TRL are large particles which consist of a lipid core of predominantly TG and a small amount of cholesteryl esters (CE) with an outer layer of phospholipids, free cholesterol and apolipoproteins.

Exogenous route
Chylomicrons are synthesized in intestinal cells. After a meal, the ingested fat is mostly absorbed as monoglycerides. These monoglycerides are esterified to triglycerides inside the intestinal cell. Assembly of TG with apoB-48, A-I, A-II and A-IV results in chylomicron formation. The intestinal apoB isoform, apoB48, is the structural protein of chylomicrons. A newly discovered protein, microsomal triglyceride transfer protein (MTP) functions as the obligatory protein in the co-translational transfer of lipids into nascent chylomicrons in intestinal cells, or VLDL in hepatocytes.[1] The chylomicrons are secreted into the lymph and enter the systemic circulation via the thoracic duct. They receive C and E apolipoproteins from HDL in exchange for apoA-I. The enzyme lipoprotein lipase (LPL) plays a key role in the catabolism of TRL. LPL is produced by various parenchymal tissues and binds to heparan sulphate chains on the luminal surface of capillary endothelium. Apolipoproteins have active roles in the lipolytic process. ApoC-II interacts directly with LPL and activates the enzyme. ApoB and apoE have heparan-binding sites and are thought to interact with the heparan sulphate chains.[2] The heparan sulphate-bound LPL extends into the bloodstream to bind TRL. To allow interaction in vivo of TRL with endothelium-bound LPL and subsequent lipolysis, the particle has to reside transiently at the proteoglycan-LPL complex as is shown in Figure 1. Apolipoproteins are considered to play a role in this process. ApoE has been found to bind to proteoglycans.[3,4] Recently, we addressed this issue by studying the binding and lipolysis of VLDL samples with different apoE-mutations by proteoglycan-bound LPL in vitro.[5] We demonstrated that VLDL,

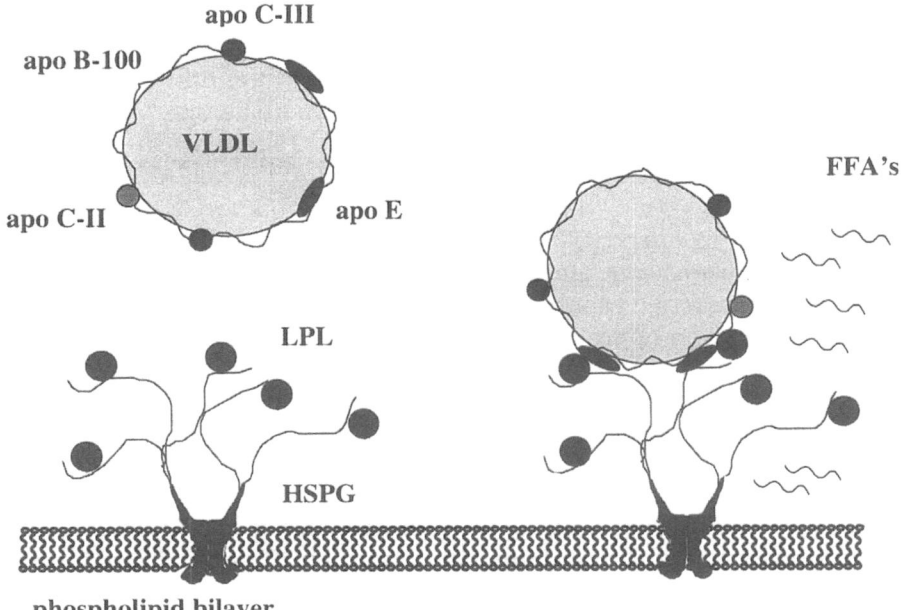

Figure 1. Schematic presentation of lipolysis of TRL: LPL binds to heparan sulphate chains on the luminal surface of capillary endothelium. The heparan sulphate-bound LPL extends into the bloodstream to bind TRL. Apolipoproteins mediate the interaction between the TRL and proteoglycan-LPL complex. ApoC-II, apoE and apoB have been shown to contain LPL-binding or heparin-binding sites and are thought to stimulate the interaction, whereas apoC-III has been shown to be an important inhibitor of this binding process. After LPL has bound to apoC-II, attached to the surface of the particle, hydrolysis of triglycerides occurs and fatty acids are liberated in the circulation. The reduction in size of the TRL and the accumulation of lipolysis products (particularly fatty acids) reduce its affinity to the proteoglycan-LPL complex and the particle dissociates from the endothelium.

carrying mutant apoE, displayed a decreased lipolysis by HSPG-bound LPL due to a defective binding of these lipoproteins to the HSPG-LPLcomplex. However, Rensen et al.[6] elegantly showed that apoE-enrichment of artificial chylomicrons inhibited *in vivo* and *in vitro* lipolysis in a dose-dependent way. We speculate that apoE variants display decreased lipolysis rates due to 1) increased amounts of LPL-inhibiting apoE, and 2) defective binding capacity of lipoproteins to the HSPG-LPL complex. With regard to the function of apoE, it is suggested that enrichment of TRL with apoE during lipolysis results in dissociation of the TRL from HSPG-bound LPL, subsequently leading to avid uptake of the TRL remnants by apoE-specific lipoprotein receptors.[6] Also apoC-II and apoB have been shown to contain LPL-binding sites and may be involved in this interaction. After LPL has bound to apoC-II, attached to the surface of the particle, hydrolysis of triglycerides occurs and fatty acids are liberated in the circulation. Many LPL molecules are thought to act simultaneously on the chylomicron, holding the particle firmly at the endothelial binding sites. It is not clear how the particle dissociates from the endothelium, but it is thought that both the reduction in size and the accumulation of lipolysis products, particularly fatty acids, reduce its affinity to the surface.[7,8] After "digestion" of the chylomicron by LPL, a smaller cholesterol-rich remnant remains which will subsequently be eliminated by specific mechanisms that are reviewed below. In addition, there is evidence that in normolipidemic man, direct removal of large chylomicron remnants from the plasma compartment occurs.[9,10] Conversion to small remnants is therefore not a prerequisite for elimination from the circulation.

The uptake mechanism of chylomicron remnants (CR) has received a lot of attention recently. The low density lipoprotein (LDL) receptor participates in the clearance of CR.[11] However, in vitro and in vivo studies do not provide evidence for an exclusive role of the LDL receptor (LDL-R) in this process.[12,13] This is illustrated by the fact that animals and humans who are homozygous for LDL-R mutations show normal CR catabolism.[14-16] Several in vitro and in vivo studies have provided evidence that the LRP is involved in the remnant removal.[17] An intriguing finding was the fact that chylomicrons are taken up by the liver only after lipolysis by LPL.[18] This binding-enhancing effect was not dependent on lipolysis, but was due to the structural properties of LPL itself. Endothelium-bound proteoglycans play an important role in this process. It is thought that proteoglycans serve to concentrate LPL-lipoprotein complexes on the cell surface, thereby enhancing their interaction with the LRP.[19]

Endogenous route

The endogenous triglyceride transport is mediated by TRL from the liver. These hepatic TRL, known as VLDL, contain apoB-100 as structural protein, while chylomicrons contain the structural protein apoB-48. The flow of fatty acids, liberated by LPL and derived from peripheral adipose tissue, is partly assimilated by extra-hepatic tissues. However, a substantial amount of fatty acids, either bound to albumin or still present in the remnant particles, is taken up by the liver and reesterified to VLDL triglycerides in the hepatocyte. Upon secretion, nascent VLDL contain apoB-100 as well as apoE and apoC as structural proteins. More apoE and apoC become associated to VLDL immediately after secretion. The initial phase of VLDL metabolism resembles that of chylomicrons: hydrolysis of carried triglycerides by LPL. After hydrolysis, cholesterol- and apoE-enriched remnants remain (IDL, intermediate density lipoproteins). The hepatic clearance of IDL particles is mediated by the LDL-R.[20] The IDL particles interact with the LDL-R via apoE and/or apoB. A high concentration of apoE on the surface of the remnant particle results in high affinity binding and rapid removal by the LDL-R. In man, the LRP may be involved in IDL clearance as well.[16] Part of the IDL particles is processed to LDL particles by LPL and perhaps HL.[21]

Interrelations between triglyceride-rich lipoproteins and other lipoproteins
High density lipoproteins play an important role in the metabolism of TRL. They serve as a storage pool of apolipoproteins including apoE and apoC. When TRL enter the circulation, they receive apoC-II and apoE from HDL, facilitating lipolysis and remnant removal. During lipolysis of TRL, surface fragments are delivered to HDL, adding a substantial contribution to the HDL pool.[22,23] Accordingly, the effectiveness of TRL catabolism has been shown to correlate positively with HDL-C concentrations.[24,25] Small, protein-rich HDL particles (HDL-3) initiate reverse cholesterol transport, accepting free cholesterol from peripheral cells.[26,27] Subsequently, the cholesterol is esterified by lecithin:cholesterol acyltransferase (LCAT). In plasma, cholesterylester transfer protein (CETP) mediates the transfer of triglycerides and surface fragments from lipoproteins to HDL-3 in exchange for CE, creating a lipid-enriched intermediate HDL particle.[26] Subsequent esterification by lecithin:cholesterol acyltransferase (LCAT) completes conversion of HDL-3 to HDL-2. This exchange of lipids is most pronounced in the postprandial phase. HDL-2 is reconverted into HDL-3 by the action of hepatic lipase on the hepatic membranes. In this process, HDL cholesterol is adsorbed by the hepatocyte membrane, completing one route of reverse cholesterol transport. The second route, represented by the transferred CE inside apoB-containing lipoproteins, is completed when the remnant particles are degraded by the liver.
LDL particles are produced as end products of VLDL metabolism. Because LDL particles are deprived of the majority of apoE, associated to the precursor IDL particles, its affinity to the LDL-R is relatively lower than that of other apoB-containing lipoproteins, resulting in a long residence time of approximately 3 days. Eventually, the LDL particle binds to the LDL-R in the liver and extra-hepatic tissues and is degraded. There is evidence for lipid transfer between TRL and LDL particles.[23] Schaefer et al. demonstrated that during in vitro lipolysis of chylomicrons, particle constituents were transferred to LDL density.[23] In man, TG enrichment of LDL depends on interactions with determinants of the removal pathways of TRL.[28,29] LDL particle size is determined in part by genetic factors including CETP, the apoAI-CIII-AIV gene cluster, and the LDL-R locus.[30]

Epidemiological and clinical evidence for an association between plasma triglyceride concentration and coronary heart disease (CHD)

Although plasma triglyceride concentration has not attracted the epidemiological attention as a risk factor for CHD to the same extent as plasma cholesterol, LDL-cholesterol and HDL-cholesterol concentrations, several groups have emphasized the epidemiological evidence of an association between plasma triglyceride concentration and CHD.[31-34] The controversial issue of this association is caused by the fact that an increased plasma triglyceride concentration is often seen in combination with a decreased HDL-cholesterol concentration and an increased concentration of small dense LDL particles. In multivariate statistical models the association between plasma triglyceride concentration and CHD becomes insignificant after adjustment for covariates, which has led to the conclusion that an elevated plasma triglyceride levels is not an independent risk factor for CHD. In a report from the Framingham Heart Study, Abbott et al.[35] pointed out that, when 2 items are associated both statistically and metabolically, the current mathematical models will grossly underestimate the contribution to risk of one of the items, thus representing a misapplication of the statistical models. By scoring the incidence of coronary artery disease during 14 years of the Framingham Study, Castelli[33] demonstrated that in the lowest HDL-cholesterol tertile (men: < 1.03 mmol/l; women < 1.29 mmol/l) the group of subjects in the highest triglyceride tertile (men > 1.57 mmol/l; women > 1.34 mmol/l) had a 4 times higher incidence of CHD for men and a 10 times higher incidence for women than those in the lowest triglyceride tertile (men > 1.02 mmol/l; women > 0.90 mmol/l).

In the Helsinki Heart Study and the PROCAM study it was demonstrated that the combination of high triglyceride and low HDL-cholesterol represents the most unfavorable lipoprotein pattern with respect to risk of future CHD.[36,37] In a recently published meta-analysis of 17 population-based prospective studies, Hokanson and Austin[34] calculated relative risks (RR) and 95% confidence intervals (CI) and standardized these figures with respect to a 1 mmol/l increase in triglyceride (Figure 2). For men and women the univariate RRs for fasting plasma triglyceride levels were 1.32 (95% CI 1.26-1.39) and 1.76 (95% CI 1.50-2.07), respectively. Adjustment of HDL-cholesterol and other risk factors (if provided in the published reports, these other risk factors include age, total cholesterol, LDL-cholesterol, smoking, body mass index, and blood pressure) attenuated these RRs to 1.14 (95% CI 1.05-1.28) and 1.37 (95% CI 1.13-1.66), respectively. These authors conclude from this meta-analysis that fasting triglyceride level in plasma is a risk factor for CHD for men and women in the general population, independent of HDL-cholesterol.

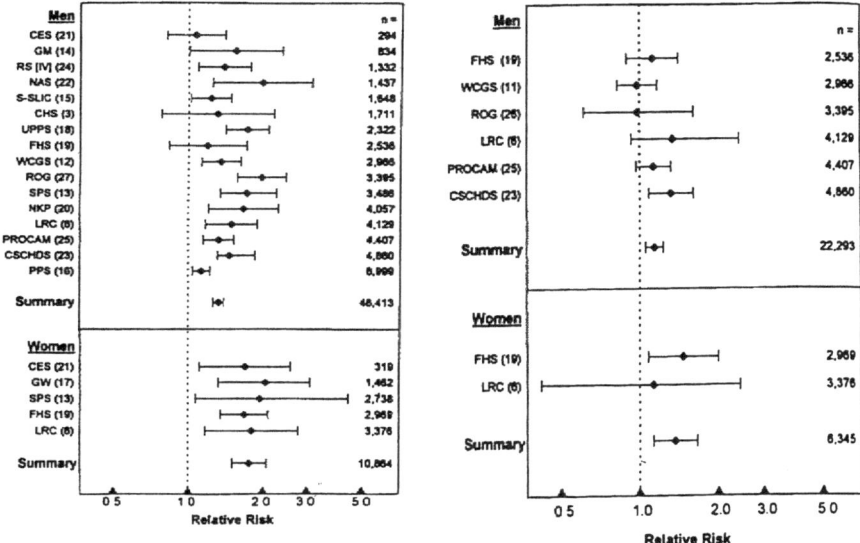

Figure 2. Left: Univariate relative risk estimates and 95% confidence intervals for the association between incident cardiovascular disease and a 1 mmol/l increase in triglyceride level, by gender. Relative risk values are presented on the x-axis on a logarithmic scale. The y-axis lists 21 studies included in the meta-analysis, and the summary relative risk. Right: Multivariate-adjusted relative risk estimates and 95% confidence intervals for the association between incident cardiovascular disease and a 1 mmol/l increase in triglyceride level, by gender, for the studies that adjusted for HDL-cholesterol level. Relative risk values are presented on the x-axis on a logarithmic scale. The y-axis lists 8 studies included in the meta-analysis, and the summary relative risk (reprinted with permission by Rapid Science Publishers Ltd, from[34]).

Also in case-control studies it was shown that an elevated concentration of total triglycerides or VLDL-triglycerides in plasma is the best discriminant between subjects with and without CHD.[38,39] In a cross-sectional angiographic study, plasma triglyceride (in addition to LDL), HDL-2 and HDL-3 cholesterol proved independently predictive of the extent of coronary atherosclerosis.[40] Others presented evidence that small VLDL remnants were associated with the presence or severity of CHD.[41-43] VLDL remnants were found to predict progression of coronary atherosclerosis, as well as clinical events occurring up to 7 years later in a prospective study using quantitative coronary angiography at 2-year intervals.[44] Accordingly, in the MARS study triglyceride-rich lipoproteins, particularly small VLDL, have been identified as being the most important lipoprotein to predict progression of coronary atherosclerosis in patients with mild-to-moderate coronary lesions.[45] Although there is debate about the atherogenic potential of chylomicrons and normal buoyant VLDL particles, it is generally accepted that VLDL remnants and chylomicron remnants are atherogenic. Several groups have presented evidence that postprandial lipoproteins, and particularly chylomicron remnants, contribute to the risk of CHD[46-50] or to the risk of carotid atherosclerosis.[51]

Causes of endogenous hypertriglyceridemia

The oldest case-report of hypertriglyceridemia entitled "pure milk on the blood" dates from 1641, when it was originally described by the Dutch physician Nicolaes Tulp (1593-1674), who was famous as the demonstrator in Rembrandt's painting "The anatomical lesson of Dr Nicolaes Tulp".[52] In accordance with the current perspective that hypertriglyceridemia is a risk factor for cardiovascular disease, Tulp makes the connection between the milky serum of this obese patient and premature atherosclerosis. The typical patient with hypertriglyceridemia is moderately obese and insulin-resistant. The frequency of hypertension and gout is several fold higher than in a normal population. These features are frequently found in hypertriglyceridemic individuals but can also be encountered in the general population. A more specific and visible clinical feature are the eruptive xanthomas. Although typical xanthomas are found only in the minority of HTG patients, these lesions are pathognomonic for a severe hypertriglyceridemia (type V hyperlipoproteinemia (HLP)). The most dangerous complication of HTG is acute pancreatitis.

Hypertriglyceridemia is a complex multifactorial disease. Genetic factors as well as exogenous factors are believed to contribute to the expression of hypertriglyceridemia. Although several genetic factors for HTG have been identified, frequently no cause is found.

Genetic factors

With regard to the genetic predisposition, the lipoprotein lipase (LPL) gene has received a lot of attention as it is considered to be the key enzyme in triglyceride catabolism. The human LPL gene is located on chromosome 8 and consists of 10 exons. The mature LPL protein consists of 448 amino acids. Several functional domains have been identified, including a catalytic domain and binding sites for heparan sulphate proteoglycans and apoC-II. Amino acid substitutions have been found in most of the exons in the LPL gene. Homozygosity for a functional LPL mutation is rare and is associated with LPL deficiency and gross hypertriglyceridemia with fasting chylomicronemia.[53] Few data are available on the prevalence of heterozygous LPL mutations. Mailly et al.[54] studied the prevalence of the LPL (Asp9-Asn) mutation in a randomly selected English-Scottish population of subjects without CAD. In this large population, 25 heterozygotes and 2 homozygotes were found yielding an average frequency of 3.5%. In the carrier group plasma triglyceride levels were increased by 24% as compared to the noncarriers, while plasma cholesterol levels were not different. In patients with HTG and combined HLP, the prevalence of the LPL (Asp9-Asn) mutation was increased about 2-fold. In addition, Minnich et al.[55] performed a study to assess the prevalence of four common LPL point mutations in exon 5 in a French-Canadian population of patients with endogenous HTG (type IV and V HLP). Interestingly, 15-20% of the patients proved to be carrier of one of these four LPL mutations while in the normolipidemic control group no carriers could be identified. Syvänne et al.[56] recently published an elegant study describing two Finnish families with the LPL (Asn291-Ser) mutation. The carriers showed higher triglycerides (+ 154%) and lower post-heparin LPL activities (-23%) than noncarrying family members. More than half of the carriers (9/16) were hypertriglyceridemic. This study makes two important points: First, not all carriers express lipid disturbances. And second, LPL activities are only mildly decreased in the heterozygous state. Therefore it appears that LPL mutations predispose subjects to the development of HTG but other genetic and/or environmental factors are required for the expression of HTG.

ApoC-III is an important inhibitor of LPL. In transgenic mice, overexpression of apoC-III causes hypertriglyceridemia whereas the induction of apoC-III deficiency by means of knock-out mice is associated with reduced triglyceride-levels and resistance to diet-induced hyperlipidemia.[57,58] The apoC-III gene has therefore been regarded as an important candidate gene in hyperlipoproteinemias. The apoC-III encoding gene is located in the APOAI-CIII-AIV gene cluster on chromosome 11. Numerous studies have demonstrated a strong relationship between the Sst1 restriction length polymorphism (RFLP) and the occurrence of hypertriglyceridemia.[59-63] A recent study by Surguchow et al.[64] performed in a sample of the ARIC population demonstrated a frequency of the S2 allele of 14.2% in those with high TG levels and 5.2% in those with normal TG levels. These results are in accordance with our data. In a well-defined population of patients with endogenous hypertriglyceridemia from the outpatient lipid clinic of the Leiden University Hospital, the Sst1 RFLP was 3-fold more common than in a normolipidemic control population.[63] Although the Sst1 RFLP of all candidate genes has shown the best correlation with hypertriglyceridemia so far, its significance remains a matter of dispute. Since the Sst1 polymorphic site is located in the 3' untranslated region of the APOC-III gene, it is considered not to influence transcription or function of apoC-III, but merely indicative of a second, as yet unknown, mutation related to hypertriglyceridemia.

The promoter region of the apoC-III is an important regulatory element of apoC-III transcription. Dammerman et al.[61] demonstrated that a combination of five polymorphic sites in the apoC-III promoter associates with an increased risk of hypertriglyceridemia. Hoffer et al.[63] studied the -455 and -482 RFLP in a group of patients with HTG from the outpatient lipid clinics in Leiden. Interestingly, an increased frequency was observed in the HTG group as compared to a normolipidemic control group. This result indicates that the promoter region of the apoC-III gene may be involved in the expression of HTG. How variations in the promoter region of apoC-III can be linked to HTG was reported by Li et al.[65] They performed a study to determine if the variant promoter DNA sequence would cause a change in transcriptional activity of the apoC-III gene. Interestingly, they demonstrated loss of the, normally suppressive, activity of insulin on apoC-III transcription. It was hypothesized that the regulatory dysfunction of insulin on the variant apoC-III promoter region may lead to an increased apoC-III production and subsequently hypertriglyceridemia. Whether this *in vitro* observation bears clinical significance remains to be determined by future research.

An other gene that may be involved in the pathogenesis of HTG is the APOE gene. Although the effect of apoE on lipolysis remains a matter of dispute, its central role in receptor-mediated lipoprotein removal is generally accepted. Mutations in (or in the vicinity of) the receptor-binding domain (aa 130 - aa 150) result in dominantly heritable forms of familial dyslipidemia or type III HLP, which is characterized by the accumulation of remnant lipoproteins[66,67] (for review, see[68]). Theoretically, mutations in the C-terminal region of the APOE gene, which contains the heparin binding (aa 214 - aa 236) and lipid-binding region (aa 246 - aa 266) may result in a defective lipolysis and subsequent HTG. Several studies have demonstrated an association between C-terminal mutations and HTG.[68,69] Recently, we studied the occurrence of apoE mutations in a population of HTG patients from the lipid clinics at the Leiden University Hospital.[70] Interestingly, in 2 out of 62 HTG patients a rare apoE mutation could be demonstrated: the apoE5(Pro^{84}-Arg;Cys^{112}-Arg) and the apoE3(Cys^{112}-Arg; Arg^{251}-Gly) mutation. These mutations were not encountered in a large control population (n = 2014) of 35-yr. old males from three different parts of the Netherlands. Additional analysis of first-degree relatives suggested an association between these apoE mutations and HTG. In addition, the apoE allele frequency distribution in the HTG group was markedly different from the control group. These data suggest that mutations in the APOE gene, as well as the apoE genotype, contribute to the expression of HTG.

Exogenous factors
Patients with endogenous hypertriglyceridemia generally present insulin resistance, characterized by high fasting insulin and normal or mildly

elevated glucose concentrations. In addition to the elevated cardiovascular risk of dyslipidemia, high fasting insulin concentrations appear to be an independent predictor of ischemic heart disease in men.[71] Although the debate continues as to which comes first: dyslipidemia or insulin resistance, there is growing evidence that hyperinsulinemia precedes the lipid abnormalities. Mykkänen et al.[72] reported in a prospective study that hyperinsulinemia preceded dyslipidemia in an eldery population during a 3.5 year follow-up. Several factors are involved in the development of insulin resistance. First, the mass of abdominal visceral adipose tissue plays a key role in insulin resistance.[73] Adipose tissue lipase, also designated as hormone sensitive lipase, are thought to mobilize FFA which are used in preference to glucose. So, glucose levels rise together with insulin levels resulting in the biochemical features of insulin resistance. Second, diets rich in saturated fat can induce insulin resistance. A recent study by Hunnicutt et al.[74] showed that chronic exposure of isolated adipocytes to saturated fatty acids in vitro induced insulin resistance. And third, smoking has been demonstrated to induce hyperinsulinemia although the underlying mechanism is not understood.[75] The characteristic lipid abnormalities in insulin resistance include increased plasma triglyceride levels, decreased HDL cholesterol and presence of small dense LDL. Both overproduction and decreased clearance of VLDL are responsible for the lipid derangements. The high levels of insulin and glucose stimulate hepatic VLDL production, designated as the substrate driven VLDL overproduction (Figure 3).[76,77] In addition, the elevated FFA levels inhibit VLDL lipolysis by a negative feedback mechanism.[8] Post-heparin LPL-activity is decreased in patients with insulin resistance, as was recently shown by Knudsen et al.[78] in first-degree relatives of NIDDM patients. Probably, there is a direct effect of insulin resistance on the expression of LPL. In conclusion, hyperinsulinemia is an important factor involved in the development of hypertriglyceridemia.

Secondary causes of hypertriglyceridemia

A wide variety of secondary causes of hyperlipoproteinemia have been identified.[79] It is crucial in the clinical evaluation of the hyperlipidemic patient to exclude the most important causes of hyperlipoproteinemia since it has a major effect on the type of treatment. For example, hyperlipoproteinemia associated with hypothyroidism is very resistant to lipid-lowering drugs. The only effective therapy is adequate treatment of the underlying disease. The most important causes of secondary hypertriglyceridemia are summarized in the following paragraph.

144

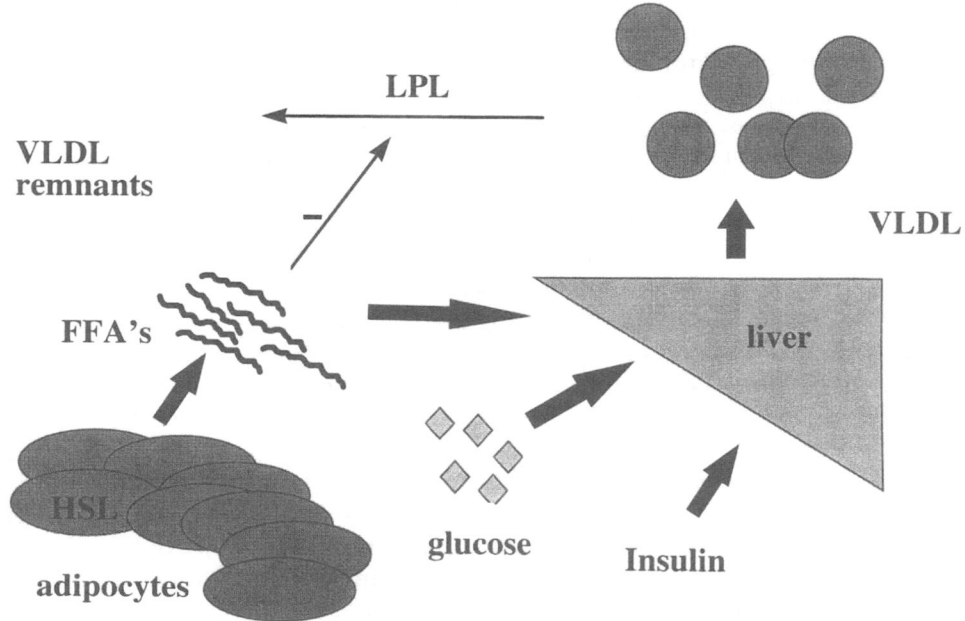

Figure 3. *Schematic presentation of the VLDL metabolism in insulin resistance: An increased amount of visceral fat plays a central role in the development of dyslipidemia in insulin resistant states. Adipose tissue lipase mobilizes increased amounts of FFA which are metabolized in preference to glucose. Therefore, the glucose and insulin levels rise, which stimulate the VLDL production by the liver. The elevated FFA levels also contribute to the VLDL overproduction. In addition, FFAs inhibit lipolysis by a negative feedback mechanism. The catabolism of TRL is further impeded by a low LPL activity and glycative modification of apolipoproteins. Thus, both VLDL overproduction and an impaired catabolism contribute to the dyslipidemia, associated with insulin resistance.*

Alcohol

Immoderate alcohol consumption is associated with hypertriglyceridemia. Several mechanisms have been identified. First, alcohol consumption is known to stimulate the synthesis of endogenous lipoproteins. This is probably due to the fact that ethanol is metabolized in preference to fatty acids as source of energy. The accumulating fatty acids may be used for the production of triglycerides and incorporated in VLDL particles. Second, ethanol consumption may be associated with reduced lipolysis of TRL by LPL.[80] Pownall et al.[81] demonstrated that addition of alcohol to a fat load significantly increased the postprandial lipemia. It is obvious that HTG patients who drink high amounts of alcohol should stop drinking as the alcohol is the primary cause of their lipid derangements. What to advise for the patient with endogenous HTG who drinks less than 4 units a day which is considered to be "normal"? We addressed this issue recently by studying the effect of dietary counseling in patients with endogenous HTG.[82] The only changes in dietary intake that correlated with improvement of TG levels were weight reduction and limitation of alcohol intake. So, limitation of alcohol intake seems obligatory in every patient with HTG, even if drinking habits are normal.

Diabetes mellitus

Poorly controlled diabetes mellitus (type I and type II) is associated with a high incidence of hyperlipidemia and premature atherosclerosis. If type I diabetes (insulin-dependent diabetes mellitus, or IDDM) is accurately treated, lipid and lipoprotein levels generally are within the normal range. The same applies to the insulin-resistant type, designated as type II or non-insulin dependent diabetes mellitus (NIDDM).[83] One of the most common lipid abnormalities in NIDDM is hypertriglyceridemia and low HDL cholesterol. The LDL cholesterol levels are normal or mildly elevated. The HTG is due to both overproduction of TRL and decreased catabolism. With regard to the overproduction, an increased supply of glucose and free fatty acids contributes to overproduction of very low density lipoproteins, increasing the burden of triglyceride-rich lipoproteins on the common lipolytic pathway at the level of lipoprotein lipase. Low lipoprotein lipase activity and increased amounts of lipolysis-inhibiting free fatty acids further impair lipolysis of postprandial lipoproteins. In addition, glycation of apolipoproteins (apoC-II, apoB and apoE) are considered to impair lipolysis and receptor-mediated lipoprotein catabolism.[84] Correction of the lipid abnormalities in NIDDM is advisable since it may contribute to attenuation of the risk on premature atherosclerosis. When dietary measures and hypoglycemic agents have failed to achieve acceptable lipid levels, lipid-lowering drugs should be advised. Fibric acids and HMG-CoA reductase inhibitors are the drugs of choice. The clinical efficacy of statin therapy was recently confirmed in a subgroup analysis of diabetic subjects from the 4S-study.[85] Secondary prevention of CAD with simvastatin treatment resulted in a 60% reduction of coronary events in this high-risk group. Whether an aggressive lipid-lowering treatment is indicated in the primary prevention of CAD in diabetics remains to be established.

Hypothyroidism

Hypothyroidism is a frequent cause of hyperlipidemia. Previous studies have shown that 5 - 10% of all hyperlipidemic subjects demonstrate apparent or subclinical hypothyroidism.[86-88] Therefore, it is recommendable to screen all patients with hyperlipidemia for hypothyroidism (thyroid stimulating hormone and thyroxin). Hypothyroidism is not associated with a specific hyperlipidemia but can express different phenotypes. Although hypothyroidism has been associated with a decreased LPL activity and decreased LDL catabolism, the exact pathophysiological mechanism is not fully understood. Adequate treatment of the thyroid disease rapidly improves the lipid derangements.

Liver/renal disease

Liver disease may lead to lipid derangements in several ways. Cholestasis leads to hyperlipidemia when biliary lipids leak into the plasma. This may result in severe hypercholesterolemia and even the presence of cutaneous xanthomas. Interestingly, a rare lipoprotein can be identified in these subjects: lipoprotein X or Lp-X. This LDL-like particle does not contain apoB and contains high amounts of unesterified cholesterol. Inflammation of liver tissue can also lead to hyperlipidemia. However, in case of advanced hepatic disease, lipid levels tend to fall due to a reduced lipoprotein synthesis. Treatment of liver disease related hyperlipidemia is difficult since most drugs are metabolized by the liver and bear a potential risk for the remaining liver function. In addition, fibric acids should not be given in case of cholelithiasis. Renal failure is associated with hyperlipidemia and premature atherosclerosis. A decreased LPL activity is thought to be the basic pathophysiological defect in patients with chronic renal failure. This typically results in hypertriglyceridemia, low HDL cholesterol levels and small dense LDL. A renal transplantation is advisable, however, the extensive use of steroids and other drugs often sustains a mild hyperlipidemia. The nephrotic syndrome, characterized by albuminuria > 3 g/day, is also associated with hyperlipidemia. It is thought that the hypoalbuminemia leads to increased hepatic production of albumin that is accompanied passively by an increased lipoprotein synthesis. Improvement of the proteinuria by adequate therapy is associated with normalization of the hyperlipidemia.

Medication

Many drugs are known to affect plasma lipid levels. One of the most important drugs that interfere with the lipoprotein metabolism are the steroids. Corticosteroid usage causes slight increase in serum lipid levels in normal individuals. However, in subjects prone to the development of hyperlipidemia, e.g. E2 homozygotes, corticosteroid therapy may result in a marked hyperlipidemia. Induction of insulin resistance is thought to be the underlying mechanism. Also hormone preparations such as oral contraceptives may cause HTG.[89] On the other hand, postmenopausal hormone replacement has been reported to improve plasma lipid levels. Many effects have been reported on different hormones in different age groups. Some of these effects are positive, some are negative, but the message is that hormones can effect lipid levels and it would be recommendable to discontinue hormone therapy in a hyperlipidemic patient to evaluate the drug effect. Beta blocking agents are known to elevate triglyceride levels and decrease HDL cholesterol levels mildly. There is no difference between the older aselective and newer class of selective beta blockers. With regard to hypertension treatment in primary prevention of CAD, beta blocking agents should be replaced by alpha blockers, ACE inhibitors or calcium channel blockers if hyperlipidemia is present. In case of secondary prevention of CAD, prescription of beta blockers in combination with platelet inhibitors and lipid-lowering drugs seems advisable. Other drugs that affect lipid levels include retinoic acid, cyclosporin, and amiodarone.

Mechanisms of atherogenicity of triglycerides

There is ongoing debate about the atherogenic potential of VLDL. Skeptics believed that VLDL particles were too large to penetrate the arterial wall. These rumours were silenced when Rapp et al.[90] demonstrated the presence of VLDL and VLDL remnants in atherosclerotic plaques. Over one third of the total cholesterol content of plaques were found to be derived from VLDL and VLDL remnants. In addition, macrophages are known to bind and internalize TRL-triglycerides. In this process, the macrophages can transform into "foam cells", a feature that is considered to play a central role in atherogenesis. Interestingly, VLDL from HTG patients proved to induce a several fold higher accumulation of lipids in macrophages as compared to VLDL isolated from normolipidemic individuals.[91] In conclusion, high concentrations of TRL may initiate and potentiate atherogenesis 1) by penetration of the endothelium into the plaque and 2) by foam cell formation.
Hypertriglyceridemia is not only a derangement of the larger triglyceride-rich lipoproteins. It affects the entire lipoprotein metabolism and beyond. All classes of lipoproteins show abnormal size, lipid contents and apolipoprotein distribution. The primary affected class, namely the VLDL are relatively large, triglyceride-enriched and cholesterol-depleted. The apolipoprotein distribution shifts towards high apoC-III amounts, a condition which is associated with delayed lipolysis and decreased receptor-mediated lipoprotein catabolism. The LDL particles in hypertriglyceridemia are typically small, dense and persistent. This atherogenic LDL pattern is a consequence of the overwhelming presence of TRL. Triglycerides are transported by CETP from the TRL to the other lipoproteins, e.g. LDL and HDL. These acceptor lipoproteins become enriched in triglycerides and relatively depleted of cholesteryl esters (CE). The CE are shuttled back to the TRL. As the LDL particles circulate for several days, they become progressively lipolysed

which results in small LDL particles. These small dense LDL are prone to oxidative modification. There is overwhelming evidence that this LDL type is potentially atherogenic. Austin et al.[92] demonstrated that small dense LDL particles were associated with a 3-fold increased risk of CHD.

The same mechanism is seen in the HDL fraction. In HTG states, triglycerides are transported to HDL in exchange for CE. This results in large, buoyant HDL-2 which simply have no more space to accept free cholesterol from peripheral tissues. The HDL cholesterol concentration decreases, which is known to be associated with an increased risk for CHD. Thus, the reverse cholesterol transport becomes saturated. The CE which originally were derived from peripheral tissues and were meant to be removed by the liver, end up in the potentially atherogenic, apoB-containing lipoproteins. In conclusion, the abundance of triglycerides saturates the normal lipoprotein removal pathways and the reverse cholesterol transport becomes impaired. These mechanisms may contribute to the accelerated atherosclerosis in hypertriglyceridemic patients.

Lipid values are determined in fasting subjects only. However, the general patient who consumes three meals a day spends most of the day and night in a postprandial phase. The postprandial lipid metabolism is receiving a lot of attention recently. The postprandial TG rise has been found to be highly dependent on the fasting TG levels. The higher the fasting TG concentration, the longer and higher is the postprandial TG concentration. Therefore, all HTG states are associated with a disturbed postprandial TG metabolism. Although most people think that only chylomicrons are found in the first hours after a meal, Cohn et al.[93] demonstrated that both intestinally and hepatically derived TRL contribute to the triglyceride rise after ingestion of a meal. An exaggerated postprandial lipidemia in HTG patients may contribute to the increased risk of CHD, since there is evidence that a disturbed postprandial TRL metabolism has atherogenic potential, as Zilversmit already postulated in 1979.[94] This has been overlooked for a long time, since most epidemiological studies of CHD examined fasting subjects only. Several studies support the concept that an exaggerated alimentary lipidemia predisposes to coronary artery disease (CAD). Karpe et al.[25] compared the postprandial lipoprotein metabolism between healthy subjects and patients with CAD, and demonstrated an impaired postprandial lipoprotein metabolism in the patient group. Moreover, experimental and clinical studies have demonstrated that TRL remnants are atherogenic.[47,95,96] Illustrative is the remnant removal disease, also called familial dysbetalipoproteinemia, which is due to insufficient ligand activity of apoE-2 to apoE-dependent lipoprotein receptors. This genetic lipid disorder, characterized by massive accumulation of remnant particles, leads to premature atherosclerotic disease. Remnants have been shown to exert their atherogenic effect in two ways. First, accumulation of remnants at the vascular endothelium leads to cholesterol deposition in the vessel wall and transforms macrophages into foam cells. Secondly, remnants have a direct cytotoxic effect on vessel wall cells, which in accordance with the response-to-injury-hypothesis, promotes atherogenesis. HDL protects against this cytotoxic effect. However, in the HTG patient, an abnormal HDL-subclass distribution and low HDL cholesterol levels are generally encountered. We infer from these observations that a prolonged postprandial exposure of the vessel wall to remnant particles, in combination with low plasma levels of HDL-C, may lead to accelerated atherogenesis.

Most hypertriglyceridemic patients demonstrate insulin resistance, a phenomenon that appears to precede the dyslipidemia. Although insulin resistance is associated with a wide variety of biochemical alterations, high fasting insulin concentrations appear to be an independent predictor of ischemic heart disease in men.[71] The biochemical variations indicate a clustering of cardiovascular risk factors. Characteristic features are: low HDL cholesterol, high TG, small dense LDL, obesity, insulin resistance and hypertension. High triglyceride levels are frequently accompanied by insulin resistance,[97] which Reaven[98] designated as "syndrome X", characterized by high triglyceride and low HDL-cholesterol levels, increased insulin resistance, and hypertension. The combination of these metabolic alterations has been given the name "insulin resistance syndrome" emphasizing the role of insulin resistance as the underlying mechanism.[99] Some years earlier, Kaplan[100] suggested that this syndrome begins with central obesity, followed by dyslipidemia, insulin resistance, and hypertension, all combining to form the "deadly quartet". Austin et al.[92] have shown that patients with nonfatal myocardial infarction had LDL-cholesterol levels similar to those of control subjects, but were three times as likely to have a larger number of small, dense LDL particles, the so-called pattern B. Subjects with pattern B were also more obese and had higher triglyceride levels and lower HDL-cholesterol levels.

It is generally accepted that the hemostatic and fibrinolytic system play an important role in the occurrence of atherosclerosis and acute cardiovascular syndromes.[101] It is also known that dyslipidemias can affect both counterbalancing systems. The most prominent changes in hypertriglyceridemia are increased factor VIIc and PAI-1 activity.[102,103] Both have shown a positive correlation with plasma triglyceride levels. Silveira et al.[104] demonstrated activation of factor VII after a fat-rich meal, emphasizing the relation between factor VII activation and TRL. PAI-1 is an important inhibitor of the fibrinolytic degradation of thrombus by t-PA. The finding that PAI-1 is increased in HTG indicates that the fibrinolytic capacity is decreased. Also other derangements of the hemostatic system have been reported in HTG patients. Plasma fibrinogen levels, known to be an important predictor of CAD, are increased.[105] Tissue factor pathway inhibitor (TFPI) levels, an important inhibitor of the clotting system, are decreased in HTG.[103] These changes in the hemostatic system indicate a pro-thrombotic state in hypertriglyceridemic patients. Future research is needed to identify the metabolic links between hemostasis and lipoprotein metabolism.

Treatment

Life style changes

Environmental factors are considered to play an important role in the expression of hypertriglyceridemia. Therefore, dietary and life-style measures are first-line strategy in these patients. In the Netherlands, the following dietary guidelines are applied: 1) Total fat < 30 % of energy intake, 2) Saturated fat < 10% of energy intake, 3) Dietary cholesterol < 300 mg/d, and 4) Calorie reduction if body mass index > 25 kg/m^2. Recently, we studied the short-term effects of dietary counseling in 43 patients with endogenous HTG.[82] Both at intake and 12 weeks after dietary counseling, blood samples were taken and dietary intake was assessed by a trained dietician. By means of a dietary history method and a computerized food table, the nutrient content of the diet was calculated. Total energy, total fat and saturated fat intake decreased whereas the intake of polyunsaturated fat increased in response to dietary counseling. In accordance with the reported improvement of dietary habits, an average weight reduction of 2 kg was observed after 12 weeks of diet. Corresponding changes in plasma lipids and lipoproteins are shown in the following Table:

(mmol/l)	Chol	TG	VLDL-Chol	VLDL-TG	LDL-Chol	HDL-Chol
Before diet	9.3	16.8	6.2	16.5	2.69	0.62
During diet	7.9	11.3	4.0	9.4	3.03	0.68
Change (%)	- 14 %	- 32 %	- 35 %	- 43 %	+ 13 %	+ 10 %

Regression analysis was performed to determine which dietary changes correlate with TG reduction. Only weight reduction (r = 0.36, p < 0.05) and limitation of alcohol intake (r = 0.56, p < 0.001) showed a correlation with TG reduction. This study demonstrates that short-term dietary counseling is effective in reducing VLDL concentrations in endogenous HTG subjects. Unlike shifts in dietary compounds towards a more "healthy", balanced diet, weight loss and reduction of alcohol intake appear to be most effective in improving lipid and lipoprotein levels in endogenous hypertriglyceridemia.

Fish oil

Diets enriched in polyunsaturated fatty acids and poor in saturated fatty acids reduce both triglyceride and total cholesterol levels. In the Zutphen Study, Kromhout et al.[106] demonstrated that habitual fish consumers (who eat, on average, 33 g of fish per day) had lower triglyceride levels (by 26%) and a lower IDL-triglyceride level (by 38%) than controls (who eat, on average, 2 g of fish per day). The content of the n-3 polyunsaturated fatty acids (PUFAs), eicosapentaenoic acid and docosahexaenoic acid, of the phospholipids of circulating lipoproteins was significantly higher among the habitual fish consumers than in controls. Patients with hypertriglyceridemia who receive large doses of n-3 PUFAs from fish oil have substantially reduced plasma triglyceride levels because of decreased triglyceride synthesis in the liver.[107] When patients with hypertriglyceridemia were given fish oil (5 g per day) for 6 weeks, total triglyceride, VLDL-triglyceride, VLDL-cholesterol and total cholesterol concentrations in serum decreased by 54%, 56%, 40% and 15%, respectively. Serum LDL-cholesterol and HDL-cholesterol concentrations increased by 23% ($p < 0.05$) and by 14% (n.s.), respectively, and the LDL-cholesterol/HDL-cholesterol ratio did not change.[108] An adverse effect of fish oil was the increased susceptibility to oxidation of LDL and VLDL, which was correlated with the increased number of double bonds in PUFAs of LDL and VLDL. Therefore, fish oil should not be used in patients with HTG until its effectiveness has been established in clinical trials.

Nicotinic acid

Nicotinic acid treatment reduces plasma triglyceride and total cholesterol levels by decreasing the hepatic synthesis of VLDL-triglycerides. This effect of the drug on the liver is considered to be due to a reduced flow of circulating FFAs to the liver for triglyceride synthesis, which is caused by an inhibited mobilization of adipose tissue triglycerides. The nicotinic acid induced decrease in plasma triglyceride levels is associated with an increase in HDL-cholesterol levels. A 6-week treatment with nicotinic acid (4 g daily) produced lowering of total triglyceride (by 49%), VLDL-triglycerides (by 54%), and LDL-cholesterol (by 20%) and increase of HDL-cholesterol (by 45%). This therapy caused only minor changes in fatty acid composition of circulating lipoproteins.[109] A derivative of nicotinic acid, acipimox, is better tolerated than plain nicotinic acid. In 31 non-diabetic patients with hypertriglyceridemia acipimox (250 mg, 3 times daily) was as potent as nicotinic acid (3 g per day) in reducing VLDL-triglycerides and increasing HDL-cholesterol. The glucose area under the curve after a glucose load (75 g p.o.) was not significantly affected by acipimox, whereas nicotinic acid increased this area significantly, especially the late glucose response.[110] An interesting finding by Noma et al.[111] is a lowering of serum Lp(a) concentration by α-tocopheryl nicotinate (200 mg, 3 times daily), particularly in those with elevated Lp(a) levels before treatment. Although this group of drugs is effective in improving lipid levels in patients with HTG, a substantial number of subjects discontinue medication because of side-effects. Since there are other effective triglyceride-lowering drugs available, nicotinic acid therapy should be restricted to patients with severe hypoalphalipoproteinemia (improvement of HDL-cholesterol).

HMG-CoA reductase inhibitors

HMG-CoA reductase inhibitors have been proposed as the therapy of choice for patients with a combined hyperlipidemia.[112] However, in patients with endogenous hypertriglyceridemia, statin therapy is not advised since LDL-cholesterol levels are normal or subnormal. A new and potent statin, atorvastatin, has been reported to suppress VLDL levels and may therefore be effective in patients with endogenous HTG. Bakker Arkema et al.[113] reported a study with atorvastatin in patients with endogenous HTG. Atorvastatin was well tolerated and improved the lipid and lipoprotein levels in these patients significantly. At highest dosage (1 dd 80 mg), the following changes were observed: total triglycerides -46%, LDL-cholesterol -41%, VLDL-cholesterol -58% and HDL-cholesterol +12%. In contrast to some other triglyceride-lowering drugs, fibrinogen and PAI-1 levels were not affected. Thus, atorvastatin seems a good candidate drug for the treatment of HTG.

Fibrates

Fibric acid derivates, or fibrates, are considered to be the drugs of choice in the treatment of endogenous hypertriglyceridemia. Although there are only a limited number of intervention trials available, fibrates have been reported to be effective in the prevention of CAD in high risk patients.[114,115] In the Stockholm ischemic Heart Disease Secondary Prevention Study, the group treated with clofibrate and niacin had a sharp and significant reduction in the rate of mortality from CHD, which was strongly and significantly correlated with the reduction in triglyceride levels but not with the reduction in cholesterol levels.[116] In the Helsinki Heart Study, the reduction in CHD resulting from gemfibrozil therapy was largely localized to the subgroup of patients with high TG (≥ 2.3 mmol/l) and a ratio of LDL-cholesterol to HDL-cholesterol of ≥ 5.0.[117] Their effects are mediated by activation of nuclear receptors (PPAR's) that influence the transcription of several target genes involved in lipoprotein metabolism.[118] Fibrates increase the transcription of LPL and decrease the transcription of apoC-III resulting in an increased triglyceride catabolism. A wide variety of fibrates is available, however, the most popular ones (with regard to safety, efficacy and tolerability) are bezafibrate (bezalip retard®, 1 dd 400 mg), ciprofibrate (modalim®, 1 dd 100 mg) and gemfibrozil (lopid®, 2 dd 600 mg). Impressive improvements in serum lipid and lipoprotein levels have been reported in response to fibrate treatment: TG reductions of 40-70%, elevation of HDL-C of 5-20%, improvement of the LDL-subclass distribution and lowering of the serum cholesterol/HDL-C ratio by 25 %.[119-121] In addition, beneficial changes have also been reported on insulin resistance, fibrinogen and other components of the hemostatic system.[122,123] The differences between the fibrates are small.[124]

References

1. Wetterau JR, Aggerbeck LP, Bouma ME et al. Absence of microsomal triglyceride transfer protein in individuals with abetalipoproteinemia. Science 1992;258:999-1001.
2. Mahley RW, Hussain MM. Chylomicron and chylomicron remnant metabolism. Curr Opin Lipidol 1991;2:170-6.
3. Olivecrona G, Olivecrona T. Triglyceride lipases and atherosclerosis. Curr Opin Lipidol 1995;6:291-305.
4. Goldberg IJ. Lipoprotein lipase and lipolysis: central roles in lipoprotein metabolism and atherogenesis [Review]. J Lipid Res 1996;37:693-707.
5. de Man FH, de Beer F, van der Laarse A, Smelt AHM, Gevers Leuven JA, Havekes LM. Impaired lipolysis of very low density lipoproteins in type III hyperlipoproteinemia. J Am Coll Cardiol 1997:160A.
6. Rensen PCN, van Berkel TJ. Apolipoprotein E effectively inhibits lipoprotein lipase-mediated lipolysis of chylomicron-like triglyceride-rich lipid emulsions *in vitro* and *in vivo*. J Biol Chem 1996;271:14791-9.
7. Saxena U, Witte LD, Goldberg IJ. Release of endothelial cell lipoprotein lipase by plasma lipoproteins and free fatty acids. J Biol Chem 1989;264:4349-55.
8. Peterson J, Bihain BE, Bengtsson Olivecrona G, Deckelbaum RJ, Carpentier YA, Olivecrona T. Fatty acid control of lipoprotein lipase: a link between energy metabolism and lipid transport. Proc Natl Acad Sci USA 1990;87:909-13.
9. Redgrave TG. Carlson LA. Changes in plasma very low density and low density lipoprotein content, composition, and size after a fatty meal in normo- and hypertriglyceridemic man. J Lipid Res 1979;20:217-29.
10. Berr F. Characterization of chylomicron remnant clearance by retinyl palmitate label in normal humans. J Lipid Res 1992;33:915-30.
11. Cabezas MC, de Bruin TW, Kock LA et al. Simvastatin improves chylomicron remnant removal in familial combined hyperlipidemia without changing chylomicron conversion. Metabolism 1993;42:497-503.
12. Choi SY, Fong LG, Kirven MJ, Cooper AD. Use of an anti-low density lipoprotein receptor antibody to quantify the role of the LDL receptor in the removal of chylomicron remnants in the mouse in vivo. J Clin Invest 1991;88:1173-81.
13. Szanto A, Balasubramaniam S, Roach PD, Nestel PJ. Modulation of the low-density-lipoprotein-receptor-related protein and its relevance to chylomicron-

remnant metabolism. Biochem J 1992;288:791-4.

14. Kita T, Goldstein JL, Brown MS, Watanabe Y, Hornick CA, Havel RJ. Hepatic uptake of chylomicron remnants in WHHL rabbits: a mechanism genetically distinct from the low density lipoprotein receptor. Proc Natl Acad Sci USA 1982;79:3623-7.

15. Hoeg JM, Demosky SJJ, Gregg RE, Schaefer EJ, Brewer HBJ. Distinct hepatic receptors for low density lipoprotein and apolipoprotein E in humans. Science 1985;227:759-61.

16. Rubinsztein DC, Cohen JC, Berger GM, Van der Westhuyzen DR, Coetzee GA, Gevers W. Chylomicron remnant clearance from the plasma is normal in familial hypercholesterolemic homozygotes with defined receptor defects. J Clin Invest 1990;86:1306-12.

17. Willnow TE, Sheng Z, Ishibashi S, Herz J. Inhibition of hepatic chylomicron remnant uptake by gene transfer of a receptor antagonist. Science 1994;264:1471-4.

18. Willnow TE, Armstrong SA, Hammer RE, Herz J. Functional expression of low density lipoprotein receptor-related protein is controlled by receptor-associated protein in vivo. Proc Natl Acad Sci U S A 1995;92:4537-41.

19. Mulder M, Lombardi P, Jansen H, van Berkel TJ, Frants RR, Havekes LM. Low density lipoprotein receptor internalizes low density and very low density lipoproteins that are bound to heparan sulfate proteoglycans via lipoprotein lipase. J Biol Chem 1993;268:9369-75.

20. Windler EE, Kovanen PT, Chao YS, Brown MS, Havel RJ, Goldstein JL. The estradiol-stimulated lipoprotein receptor of rat liver. A binding site that mediates the uptake of rat lipoproteins containing apoproteins B and E. J Biol Chem 1980;255:10464-71.

21. Zambon A, Torres A, Bijvoet S et al. Prevention of raised low-density lipoprotein cholesterol in a patient with familial hypercholesterolaemia and lipoprotein lipase deficiency. Lancet 1993;341:1119-21.

22. Redgrave TG, Small DM. Quantitation of the transfer of surface phospholipid of chylomicrons to the high density lipoprotein fraction during the catabolism of chylomicrons in the rat. J Clin Invest 1979;64:162-71.

23. Schaefer EJ, Wetzel MG, Bengtsson G, Scow RO, Brewer HB Jr., Olivecrona T. Transfer of human lymph chylomicron constituents to other lipoprotein density fractions during in vitro lipolysis. J Lipid Res 1982;23:1259-73.

24. Patsch JR, Prasad S, Gotto AM Jr., Patsch W. High density lipoprotein2. Relationship of the plasma levels of this lipoprotein species to its composition, to the magnitude of postprandial lipemia, and to the activities of lipoprotein lipase and hepatic lipase. J Clin Invest 1987;80:341-7.

25. Karpe F, Bard JM, Steiner G, Carlson LA, Fruchart JC, Hamsten A. HDLs and alimentary lipemia. Studies in men with previous myocardial infarction at a young age. Arterioscler Thromb 1993;13:11-22.

26. Eisenberg S. High density lipoprotein metabolism. J Lipid Res 1984;25:1017-58.

27. Castro Cabezas M, Van Heusden GP et al. Reverse cholesterol transport: relationship between free cholesterol uptake and HDL3 in normolipidaemic and hyperlipidaemic subjects. Eur J Clin Invest 1993;23:122-9.

28. Austin MA, King MC, Vranizan KM, Krauss RM. Atherogenic lipoprotein phenotype. A proposed genetic marker for coronary heart disease risk. Circulation 1990;82:495-506.

29. DeFronzo RA, Ferrannini E. Insulin resistance. A multifaceted syndrome responsible for NIDDM, obesity, hypertension, dyslipidemia, and atherosclerotic cardiovascular disease. Diabetes Care 1991;14:173-94.

30. Rotter JI, Bu X, Cantor RM et al. Multilocus genetic determinants of LDL particle size in coronary artery disease families. Am J Hum Genet 1996;58:585-94.

31. Austin MA. Plasma triglyceride as a risk factor for coronary heart disease. The epidemiologic evidence and beyond [see comments]. Am J Epidemiol 1989;129:249-59.

32. Austin MA. Plasma triglyceride and coronary heart disease. Arterioscler Thromb 1991;11:2-14.

33. Castelli WP. Epidemiology of triglycerides: a view from Framingham. Am J Cardiol 1992;70:3H-9H.

34. Hokanson JE, Austin MA. Plasma triglyceride level is a risk factor for cardiovascular disease independent of high-density lipoprotein cholesterol level: a meta-analysis of population-based prospective studies. J Cardiovasc Risk 1996;3:213-9.

35. Abbott RD, Garrison RJ, Wilson PW, Castelli WP. Coronary heart disease risk: the importance of joint relationships among cholesterol levels in individual lipoprotein classes. Prev Med 1982;11;131-41No.

36. Tenkanen L, Pietila K, Manninen V, Manttari M. The triglyceride issue revisited. Findings from the Helsinki Heart Study. Arch Intern Med 1994;154:2714-20.

37. Heinrich J, Balleisen L, Schulte H, Assmann G, van de Loo J. Fibrinogen and factor VII in the prediction of coronary risk. Results from the PROCAM study in healthy men. Arterioscler Thromb 1994;14:54-9.

38. Hamsten A, Walldius G, Dahlen G, Johansson B, de Faire U. Serum lipoproteins and apolipoproteins in young male survivors of myocardial infarction. Atherosclerosis 1986;59:223-35.

39. Barbir M, Wile D, Trayner I, Aber VR, Thompson GR. High prevalence of hypertriglyceridaemia and apolipoprotein abnormalities in coronary artery disease. Br Heart J 1988;60:397-403.

40. Drexel H, Amann FW, Beran J et al. Plasma triglycerides and three lipoprotein cholesterol fractions are independent predictors of the extent of coronary atherosclerosis. Circulation 1994;90:2230-5.

41. Tatami R, Mabuchi H, Ueda K et al. Intermediate-density lipoprotein and cholesterol-rich very low density lipoprotein in angiographically determined coronary artery disease. Circulation 1981;64:1174-84.

42. Steiner G, Schwartz L, Shumak S, Poapst M. The association of increased levels of intermediate-density lipoproteins with smoking and with coronary artery disease. Circulation 1987;75:124-30.

43. Krauss RM, Lindgren FT, Williams PT et al. Intermediate-density lipoproteins and progression of coronary artery disease in hypercholesterolaemic men. Lancet 1987;2:62-6.

44. Phillips NR, Waters D, Havel RJ. Plasma lipoproteins and progression of coronary artery disease evaluated by angiography and clinical events. Circulation 1993;88:2762-70.

45. Hodis HN, Mack WJ, Azen SP et al. Triglyceride- and cholesterol-rich lipoproteins have a differential effect on mild/moderate and severe lesion progression as assessed by quantitative coronary angiography in a controlled trial of lovastatin. Circulation 1994;90:42-9.

46. Simpson HS, Williamson CM, Olivecrona T et al. Postprandial lipemia, fenofibrate

and coronary artery disease. Atherosclerosis 1990;85:193-202.

47.   Groot PH, van Stiphout WA, Krauss XH et al. Postprandial lipoprotein metabolism in normolipidemic men with and without coronary artery disease. Arterioscler Thromb 1991;11:653-62.

48.   Karpe F, Steiner G, Uffelman K, Olivecrona T, Hamsten A. Postprandial lipoproteins and progression of coronary atherosclerosis. Atherosclerosis 1994;106:83-97.

49.   Karpe F, Tornvall P, Olivecrona T, Steiner G, Carlson LA, Hamsten A. Composition of human low density lipoprotein: effects of postprandial triglyceride-rich lipoproteins, lipoprotein lipase, hepatic lipase and cholesteryl ester transfer protein. Atherosclerosis 1993;98:33-49.

50.   Patsch JR, Miesenbock G, Hopferwieser T et al. Relation of triglyceride metabolism and coronary artery disease. Studies in the postprandial state. Arterioscler Thromb 1992;12:1336-45.

51.   Ryu JE, Howard G, Craven TE, Bond MG, Hagaman AP, Crouse JR. Postprandial triglyceridemia and carotid atherosclerosis in middle-aged subjects. Stroke 1992;23:823-8.

52.   Erkelens DW, de Bruin TW, Castro Cabezas M. Tulp syndrome. Lancet 1993;342:1536-7.

53.   Brunzell JD. Familial lipoprotein lipase deficiency and other causes of the chylomicronemia syndromes. In: Scriver RS, Beaudet AL, Sly WS, Valle D, eds. The Metabolic Basis of Inherited Diseases. New York: McGraw-Hill Book Co, 1995:1913-2.

54.   Mailly F, Tugrul Y, Reymer PW et al. A common variant in the gene for lipoprotein lipase (Asp9-->Asn). Functional implications and prevalence in normal and hyperlipidemic subjects. Arterioscler Thromb Vasc Biol 1995;15:468-78.

55.   Minnich A, Kessling A, Roy M et al. Prevalence of alleles encoding defective lipoprotein lipase in hypertriglyceridemic patients of French Canadian descent. J Lipid Res 1995;36:117-24.

56.   Syvanne M, Antikainen M, Ehnholm S et al. Heterozygosity for ASN(291)SER mutation in the lipoprotein lipase gene in two Finnish pedigrees: Effect of hyperinsulinemia on the expression of hypertriglyceridemia. J Lipid Res 1996;37:727-38.

57.   Ito Y, Azrolan N, O'Connell A, Walsh A, Breslow JL. Hypertriglyceridemia as a result of human apo CIII gene expression in transgenic mice. Science 1990;249:790-3.

58.   Maeda N, Li H, Lee D, Oliver P, Quarfordt SH, Osada J. Targeted disruption of the apolipoprotein C-III gene in mice results in hypotriglyceridemia and protection from postprandial hypertriglyceridemia. J Biol Chem 1994;269:23610-6.

59.   Henderson HE, Landon SV, Michie J, Berger GM. Association of a DNA polymorphism in the apolipoprotein C-III gene with diverse hyperlipidaemic phenotypes. Hum Genet 1987;75:62-5.

60.   Aalto Setala K, Kontula K, Sane T, Nieminen M, Nikkila E. DNA polymorphisms of apolipoprotein A-I/C-III and insulin genes in familial hypertriglyceridemia and coronary heart disease. Atherosclerosis 1987;66:145-52.

61.   Dammerman M, Sandkuijl LA, Halaas JL, Chung W, Breslow JL. An apolipoprotein CIII haplotype protective against hypertriglyceridemia is specified by promoter and 3' untranslated region polymorphisms. Proc Natl Acad Sci USA 1993;90:4562-6.

62.   Zeng Q, Dammerman M, Takada Y, Matsunaga A, Breslow JL, Sasaki J. An apolipoprotein CIII marker associated with hypertriglyceridemia in Caucasians also

confers increased risk in a west Japanese population. Hum Genet 1995;95:371-5.

63. Hoffer MJ, Sijbrands EJ, De Man FH, Smelt AHM, Frants RR. Different associations between polymorphisms in the APOC3 gene and distinct types of hypertriglyceridemia. (Submitted).

64. Surguchov AP, Page GP, Smith L, Patsch W, Boerwinkle E. Polymorphic markers in apolipoprotein C-III gene flanking regions and hypertriglyceridemia. Arterioscler Thromb Vasc Biol 1996;16:941-7.

65. Li W, Dammerman M, Smith JD, Metzger S, Breslow JL, Leff T. Common genetic variation in the promoter of the human apo CIII gene abolishes regulation by insulin and may contribute to hypertriglyceridemia. J Clin Invest 1995;96:2601-5.

66. de Knijff P, van den Maagdenberg AM, Stalenhoef AF et al. Familial dysbetalipoproteinemia associated with apolipoprotein E3-Leiden in an extended multigeneration pedigree. J Clin Invest 1991;88:643-55.

67. Smit M, de Knijff P, van der Kooij Meijs E et al. Genetic heterogeneity in familial dysbetalipoproteinemia. The E2(lys146----gln) variant results in a dominant mode of inheritance. J Lipid Res 1990;31:45-53.

68. de Knijff P, van den Maagdenberg AM, Frants RR, Havekes LM. Genetic heterogeneity of apolipoprotein E and its influence on plasma lipid and lipoprotein levels. [Review]. Hum Mutat 1994;4:178-94.

69. Zhao SP, van den Maagdenberg AM, Vroom TF et al. Lipoprotein profiles in a family with two mutants of apolipoprotein E: possible association with hypertriglyceridaemia but not with dysbetalipoproteinaemia. Clin Sci 1994;86:323-9.

70. De Man FH, de Knijff P, de Beer F et al. ApoE allele frequencies and apoE mutations in endogenous hypertriglyceridemia. Atherosclerosis 1997:S34.

71. Despres JP, Lamarche B, Mauriege P et al. Hyperinsulinemia as an independent risk factor for ischemic heart disease. N Engl J Med 1996;334:952-7.

72. Mykkanen L, Kuusisto J, Haffner SM, Pyorala K, Laakso M. Hyperinsulinemia predicts multiple atherogenic changes in lipoproteins in elderly subjects. Arterioscler Thromb 1994;14:518-26.

73. Despres JP. Dyslipidaemia and obesity. Baillieres Clin Endocrinol Metab 1994;8:629-60.

74. Hunnicutt JW, Hardy RW, Williford J, McDonald JM. Saturated fatty acid-induced insulin resistance in rat adipocytes. Diabetes 1994;43:540-5.

75. Eliasson B, Attvall S, Taskinen MR, Smith U. The insulin resistance syndrome in smokers is related to smoking habits. Arterioscler Thromb 1994;14:1946-50.

76. Taskinen MR. Insulin resistance and lipoprotein metabolism. Curr Opin Lipidol 1995;6:153-60.

77. Coppack SW, Evans RD, Fisher RM et al. Adipose tissue metabolism in obesity: lipase action in vivo before and after a mixed meal. Metabolism 1992;41:264-72.

78. Knudsen P, Eriksson J, Lahdenpera S, Kahri J, Groop L, Taskinen MR. Changes of lipolytic enzymes cluster with insulin resistance syndrome. Botnia Study Group. Diabetologia 1995;38:344-50.

79. Stone NJ. Secondary causes of hyperlipidemia. Med Clin North Am 1994;78:117-41.

80. Knudsen P, Murtomaki S, Antikainen M, Ehnholm S, Taskinen MR, Ehnholm C. Lipoprotein lipase gene mutations in Finish hypertriglyceridemic patients. In: 1996:

81. Pownall HJ. Dietary ethanol is associated with reduced lipolysis of intestinally derived lipoproteins. J Lipid Res 1994;35:2105-13.

82. De Man FH, de Beer F, Smelt AHM et al. Short-term effects of dietary counselling in patients with endogenous hypertriglyceridemia. Atherosclerosis 1997:S26.

83. De Man FH, Cabezas MC, Van Barlingen HH, Erkelens DW, de Bruin TW. Triglyceride-rich lipoproteins in non-insulin-dependent diabetes mellitus: postprandial metabolism and relation to premature atherosclerosis. Eur J Clin Invest 1996;26:89-108.

84. Kortlandt W, Erkelens DW. Glycation and lipoproteins. Diab Nutr Metab 1993;6:231-9.

85. Haffner SM. The Scandinavian Simvastatin Survival Study (4S) subgroup analysis of diabetic subjects: implications for prevention of coronary heart disease. Diabetes Care 1997;20:469-71.

86. Series JJ, Biggart EM, O'Reilly DS, Packard CJ, Shepherd J. Thyroid dysfunction and hypercholesterolaemia in the general population of Glasgow, Scotland. Clin Chim Acta 1988;172:217-21.

87. Ball MJ, Griffiths D, Thorogood M. Asymptomatic hypothyroidism and hypercholesterolaemia. J R Soc Med 1991;84:527-9.

88. Glueck CJ, Lang J, Tracy T, Speirs J. The common finding of covert hypothyroidism at initial clinical evaluation for hyperlipoproteinemia. Clin Chim Acta 1991;201:113-22No.

89. Gevers Leuven JA. Sex steroids and lipoprotein metabolism. Pharmacol Ther 1994;64:99-126.

90. Rapp JH, Lespine A, Hamilton RL et al. Triglyceride-rich lipoproteins isolated by selected-affinity anti-apolipoprotein B immunosorption from human atherosclerotic plaque. Arterioscler Thromb 1994;14:1767-74.

91. Gianturco SH, Bradley WA, Gotto AM Jr. Morrisett JD, Peavy DL. Hypertriglyceridemic very low density lipoproteins induce triglyceride synthesis and accumulation in mouse peritoneal macrophages. J Clin Invest 1982;70:168-78.

92. Austin MA, Breslow JL, Hennekens CH, Buring JE, Willett WC, Krauss RM. Low-density lipoprotein subclass patterns and risk of myocardial infarction. JAMA 1988;260:1917-21.

93. Bagdade JD, Lane JT, Subbaiah PV, Otto ME, Ritter MC. Accelerated cholesteryl ester transfer in noninsulin-dependent diabetes mellitus. Atherosclerosis 1993;104:69-77.

94. Zilversmit DB. Atherogenesis: a postprandial phenomenon. Circulation 1979;60:473-85.

95. Simons LA, Dwyer T, Simons J et al. Chylomicrons and chylomicron remnants in coronary artery disease: a case-control study. Atherosclerosis 1987;65:181-9.

96. Floren CH, Albers JJ, Bierman EL. Uptake of chylomicron remnants causes cholesterol accumulation in cultured human arterial smooth muscle cells. Biochim Biophys Acta 1981;663:336-49.

97. Steiner G. Hypertriglyceridemia and carbohydrate intolerance: interrelations and therapeutic implications. Am J Cardiol 1986;57:27G-30G.

98. Reaven GM. Banting lecture 1988. Role of insulin resistance in human disease. Diabetes 1988;37:1595-607.

99. Haffner SM, Valdez RA, Hazuda HP, Mitchell BD, Morales PA, Stern MP. Prospective analysis of the insulin-resistance syndrome (syndrome X). Diabetes 1992;41:715-22.

100. Kaplan NM. The deadly quartet. Upper-body obesity, glucose intolerance, hypertriglyceridemia, and hypertension. Arch Intern Med 1989;149:1514-20.

101. Meade TW, Mellows S, Brozovic M et al. Haemostatic function and ischaemic heart disease: principal results of the Northwick Park Heart Study. Lancet 1986;2:533-7.
102. Assmann G, Schulte H. The importance of triglycerides: results from the Prospective Cardiovascular Munster (PROCAM) Study. Eur J Epidemiol 1992;8 Suppl.1:99-103.
103. Zitoun D, Bara L, Basdevant A, Samama MM. Levels of factor VIIc associated with decreased tissue factor pathway inhibitor and increased plasminogen activator inhibitor-1 in dyslipidemias. Arterioscler Thromb Vasc Biol 1996;16:77-81.
104. Silveira A, Karpe F, Blomback M, Steiner G, Walldius G, Hamsten A. Activation of coagulation factor VII during alimentary lipemia. Arterioscler Thromb 1994;14:60-9.
105. Benderly M, Graff E, Reicher Reiss H, Behar S, Brunner D, Goldbourt U. Fibrinogen is a predictor of mortality in coronary heart disease patients. The Bezafibrate Infarction Prevention (BIP) Study Group. Arterioscler Thromb Vasc Biol 1996;16:351-6.
106. Kromhout D, Katan MB, Havekes LM, Groener A, Hornstra G, de Lezenne Coulander C. The effects of 26 years of habitual fish consumption on serum lipid and lipoprotein levels (The Zutphen study). Nutr Metab Cardiovasc Dis 1996;6:65-71.
107. Harris WS. Fish oils and plasma lipid and lipoprotein metabolism in humans: a critical review. J Lipid Res 1989;30:785-807.
108. Hau MF, Smelt AH, Bindels AJ et al. Effects of fish oil on oxidation of very low density lipoprotein in hypertriglyceridemic patients. Arterioscler Thromb Vasc Biol 1996;16:1197-202.
109. Wahlberg G, Walldius G, Efendic S. Effects of nicotinic acid on glucose tolerance and glucose incorporation into adipose tissue in hypertriglyceridaemia. Scand J Clin Lab Invest 1992;52:537-45.
110. Tornvall P, Walldius G. A comparison between nicotinic acid and acipimox in hypertriglyceridaemia--effects on serum lipids, lipoproteins, glucose tolerance and tolerability. J Intern Med 1991;230:415-21.
111. Noma A, Maeda S, Okuno M, Abe A, Muto Y. Reduction of serum lipoprotein(a) levels in hyperlipidaemic patients with alpha-tocopheryl nicotinate. Atherosclerosis 1990;84:213-7.
112. Grundy SM, Vega GL. Two different views of the relationship of hypertriglyceridemia to coronary heart disease. Implications for treatment. Arch Intern Med 1992;152:28-34.
113. Bakker Arkema RG, Davidson MH, Goldstein RJ et al. Efficacy and safety of a new HMG-CoA reductase inhibitor, atorvastatin, in patients with hypertriglyceridemia. JAMA 1996;275:128-33.
114. Frick MH, Elo O, Haapa K et al. Helsinki Heart Study: primary-prevention trial with gemfibrozil in middle-aged men with dyslipidemia. Safety of treatment, changes in risk factors, and incidence of coronary heart disease. N Engl J Med 1987;317:1237-45.
115. Ericsson CG, Hamsten A, Nilsson J, Grip L, Svane B, de Faire U. Angiographic assessment of effects of bezafibrate on progression of coronary artery disease in young male postinfarction patients. Lancet 1996;347:849-53.
116. Carlson LA, Rosenhamer G. Reduction of mortality in the Stockholm Ischaemic Heart Disease Secondary Prevention Study by combined treatment with clofibrate and nicotinic acid. Acta Med Scand 1988;223:405-18.

117. Manninen V, Tenkanen L, Koskinen P et al. Joint effects of serum triglyceride and LDL cholesterol and HDL cholesterol concentrations on coronary heart disease risk in the Helsinki Heart Study. Implications for treatment [see comments]. Circulation 1992;85:37-45.
118. Auwerx J, Schoonjans K, Fruchart JC, Staels B. Transcriptional control of triglyceride metabolism: fibrates and fatty acids change the expression of the LPL and apo C-III genes by activating the nuclear receptor PPAR. Atherosclerosis 1996;124 Suppl:S29-37.
119. Bastow MD, Durrington PN, Ishola M. Hypertriglyceridemia and hyperuricemia: effects of two fibric acid derivatives (bezafibrate and fenofibrate) in a double-blind, placebo-controlled trial. Metabolism 1988;37:217-20.
120. Vessby B, Lithell H. Interruption of long-term lipid-lowering treatment with bezafibrate in hypertriglyceridaemic patients. Effects on lipoprotein composition, lipase activities and the plasma lipid fatty acid spectrum. Atherosclerosis 1990;82:137-43.
121. Yang CY, Gu YH, Xie YH al. Effect of gemfibrozil on very low density lipoprotein composition and low density lipoprotein size in patients with hypertriglyceridemia or combined hyperlipidemia. Atherosclerosis 1996;126:105-16.
122. Almer LO, Kjellstrom T. The fibrinolytic system and coagulation during bezafibrate treatment of hypertriglyceridemia. Atherosclerosis 1986;61:81-5.
123. Petrogiannopoulos C, Zaharof A, Labropoulos L, Tzoumani A, papageorgiou N, Poulikakos J. The influence of gemfibrozil on plasma fibrinogen levels in patients with primary hypertriglyceridemia. In: 1996:
124. Tikkanen MJ. Fibric acid derivates. Curr Opin Lipidol 1992;3:29-33.

HYPERLIPIDEMIA AND ATHEROSCLEROSIS IN APOE TRANSGENIC MICE

Louis M. Havekes, Bart J.M. van Vlijmen, Miek C. Jong, Pieter H.E. Groot, Ko Willems van Dijk and Marten H. Hofker

Summary

Patients with Familial Dysbetalipoproteinemia (FD) are characterized by elevated plasma levels of VLDL- and chylomicron-remnant lipoproteins concomitant with a strongly increased risk for atherosclerosis. Even in healthy people of industrialized societies the plasma levels of remnant lipoproteins is rather high, since people live under non-fasting conditions during most of their life-span. It is commonly assumed therefore that in the Western societies increased levels of remnant lipoproteins is a main contributor to the high risk of atherosclerosis.
The aim of our research is to investigate the environmental and genetic factors that influence the remnant lipoprotein metabolism. A better insight in the mechanism of remnant lipoprotein metabolism will eventually lead to new strategies in lowering the prevalence of heart and vessel diseases, the main cause of death in Western societies.

Plasma lipid levels in APOE*3-Leiden transgenic mice

Since humans are heterogeneous in both genetic and environmental background (nutrition), we decided to perform our studies with the use of transgenic mice. However, since mice display very low plasma lipid levels and the metabolism of remnant lipoproteins is very rapid, we decided first to generate transgenic mice carrying the gene for human APOE*3-Leiden.

E.E. van der Wall et al. (eds.), Vascular Medicine, 161-173.
© 1997 *Kluwer Academic Publishers.*

APOE*3-Leiden is known to inhibit remnant clearance, which is a prerequisite for studying remnant metabolism in mice. Three different APOE*3-Leiden transgenic lines were generated with different levels of expression of the transgene. The high expressing line (#2) shows hyperlipidemia, whereas a low expressor (#195) did not show a clear phenotype (Table 1). After feeding high cholesterol and fat containing diets the high expressor line #2 displayed a severe hypercholesterolemia (confined to the VLDL/LDL-sized fraction), whereas the low expressor #195 only showed a very weak hypercholesterolemia, indicating that the response to dietary treatment is related to the level of transgene expression.

By crossbreeding these APOE*3-Leiden transgenic mice (#2, #195 and control) with homozygous apoE-deficient mice, we obtained APOE*3-Leiden transgenic mice with a reduced level of endogenous apoE.[1] It appeared that a reduction of endogenous (wild type) apoE in APOE*3-Leiden transgenic mice leads to a more severe phenotype, not after feeding chow diet, but upon feeding cholesterol (Table 1). Analysis of the lipoprotein profiles of these mice showed that the increased plasma cholesterol levels is confined to the VLDL/LDL-sized lipoprotein fraction.

Atherosclerosis in APOE*3-Leiden transgenic mice

Upon feeding cholesterol containing diets the VLDL lipoprotein fraction accumulating in the plasma was highly enriched in cholesterol as compared to VLDL from chow fed animals. Increased cholesterol to triglyceride ratios in the VLDL fraction is commonly assumed to be atherogenic and also occurs in patients with familial dysbetalipoproteinemia. We wondered, therefore, whether cholesterol feeding leads to atheroscleroses in the mice of line #2. Feeding cholesterol to mice of line #2 indeed resulted in the development of atherosclerotic lesions near the aortic arch as shown after staining with oil red O (Figure 1). Microscopic analysis of cross sections of the aortic root near the valves clearly showed atherosclerotic plaques developed after 6 months of cholesterol feeding (Figure 2). Quantifications of these atherosclerotic lesion areas in cross sections of the aortic arch showed that in the APOE*3-Leiden mice the lesion area is 5 to 10 times greater than in control mice and increasing with increasing cholesterol exposure, which is a multiplication of plasma cholesterol level and duration of the cholesterol level (Figure 3). We calculated a strong correlationship between plasma cholesterol exposure and lesion size ($r = 0.85$).[2]

Table 1. The effect of dietary treatment on plasma lipid levels in APOE*3Leiden mice

Mouse line	SRM-A		HFC Diet	
	Cholesterol	Triglycerides	Cholesterol	Triglycerides
	mmol/l		mmol/l	
control	1.8 ± 0.2	0.4 ± 0.1	2.8 ± 0.2	0.1 ± 0.1
#195	2.3 ± 0.2[a]	0.7 ± 0.2[a]	3.9 ± 0.2[a]	0.2 ± 0.1[a]
#2	2.7 ± 0.5[a]	1.7 ± 0.5[a]	9.9 ± 1.4[a]	2.7 ± 0.6[a]
control,apoE(+/-)	1.8 ± 0.2	0.2 ± 0.1[a]	3.0 ± 0.6	0.1 ± 0.1
#195,apoE(+/-)	2.4 ± 0.3[a]	0.7 ± 0.2[a]	4.9 ± 0.6[ab]	0.4 ± 0.2[ab]
#2,apoE(+/-)	2.6 ± 0.5[a]	1.5 ± 0.6[a]	15.8 ± 4.8[ab]	5.7 ± 2.5[ab]

SRM-A, standard rat/mouse A diet; HFC, mild high fat/cholesterol, containing 15 %,cocoa butter and 0.25% cholesterol. Values are the mean serum levels ± S.D. of at least 12 mice. Mice were fed the HFC diet for 8 weeks. [a]Significant difference (P<0.05) as compared with control mice on the same diet, using non-parametric Mann-Witney test. [b]Significant difference (P<0.05) as compared with same transgenic line with two Apoe genes on the same diet, using nonparametric Mann-Whitney test

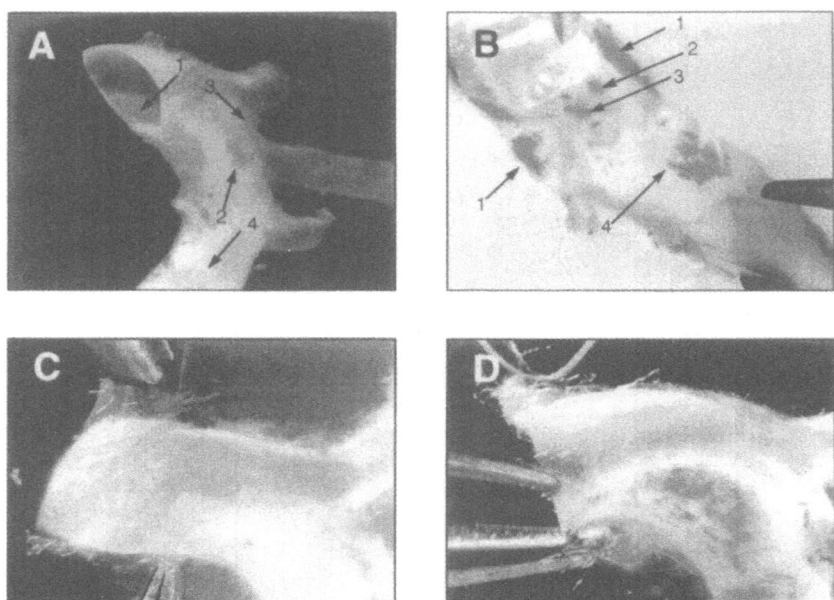

Figure 1. Atherosclerosis in the aortic arch of APOE*3Leiden mice, after feeding HFC diet for 3 months. A, Photomicrograph of the oil red O-stained aortic arch. B, Photomicrograph of the same aortic arch as shown in A, after opening longitudinally along the inner curvature. C and D, En face view of the aortic arch of a control mouse and an APOE*3Leiden mouse, respectively, after 3 months of feeding HFC diet. (For colour plate of figure 1 see page 220)

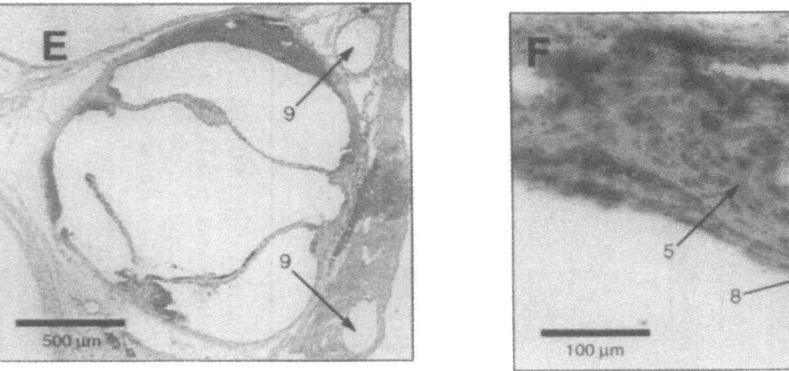

Figure 2. Photomicrographs of a cross section of the aortic root of APOE*3Leiden mice, after feeding HFC diet for 3 months. Slide was stained with oil red O and hematoxylin. F, higher magnification of the lesion shown in E. Note the presence of many lipid foam cells (arrow 5), as well as large amounts of extracellular lipid in the core of the lesion (arrow 6). Also note the dark blue deposits (arrow 7), indicative of calcification and oil red O-positive spindle shaped cells (arrow 8). Note also that the proximal coronary arteries do not show any sign of lesion development (arrows 9). (For colour plate of figure 2 see page 220)

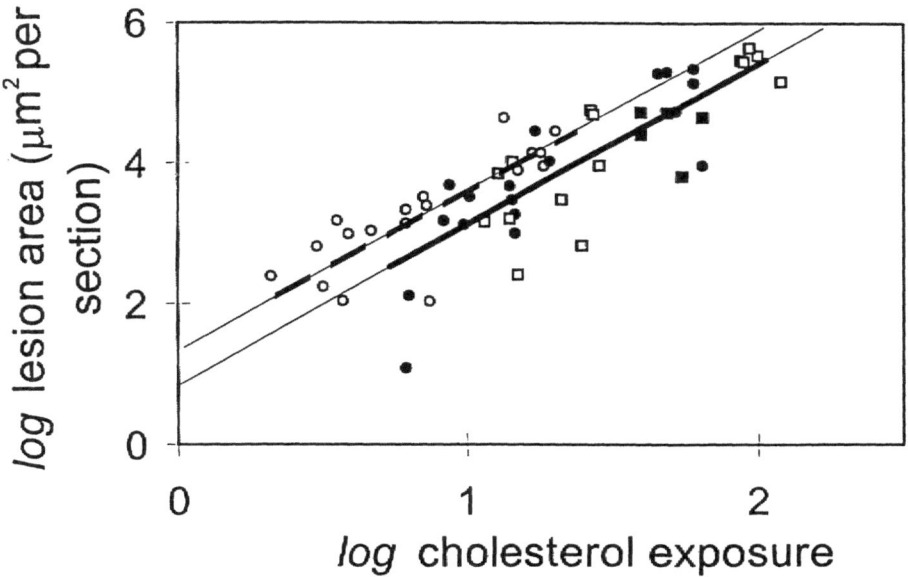

Figure 3. *Log transformed data of cholesterol exposure and lesion area of APOE*3Leiden transgenic mice fed with different diets for different periods of time.*

Effect of age and gender on plasma lipid levels in APOE*3-Leiden transgenic mice

As presented in Table 2, at young age transgenic mice showed higher plasma cholesterol and triglyceride levels (with an optimum at 45 days of age) than at older age (>100 days). This phenomenon was more pronounced in males than in females. We hypothesized that the transient hyperlipidemia in young animals is due to a relatively greater flux of nutrients which is needed during rapid growth. Since these transgenic mice have a reduced rate of clearance of remnant lipoproteins (due to the introduction of the binding defective apoE3-Leiden protein), an increased production of either hepatic VLDL or intestinal chylomicrons will lead to an extra response in plasma lipid levels.

This hypothesis is sustained by VLDL turnover experiments.[3] In young transgenic mice the fractional catabolic rate was reduced as compared to non-transgenic young mice (1.45 ± 0.34 vs 3.94 ± 1.22 pools/hour), whereas the VLDL synthetic rate was similar for both animals. This implies that the APOE*3-Leiden transgene indeed inhibits the clearance of VLDL remnant liporoteins, as expected. We also found that young transgenic mice indeed have a significantly higher VLDL production rate than older mice

Table 2. The effect of age and gender on plasma lipid levels in APOE*3Leiden mice

Mouse	Age (days)	SRM-A		HFC Diet	
		Cholesterol	Triglycerides	Cholesterol	Triglycerides
		mmol/l		*mmol/l*	
control ♂	45	2.5 ± 0.5	1.5 ± 1.0	3.8 ± 0.4	0.9 ± 0.2
control ♀	45	1.8 ± 0.2[a]	0.8 ± 0.2[a]	3.2 ± 0.1	0.7 ± 0.1
#2 ♂	45	4.5 ± 1.3[b]	4.0 ± 1.0[b]	10.8 ± 2.6[b]	4.9 ± 1.5[b]
#2 ♀	45	2.8 ± 0.3[ab]	2.8 ± 0.6[ab]	9.1 ± 1.7[ab]	4.5 ± 1.0[b]
control ♂	>100	1.9 ± 0.2	0.4 ± 0.1	3.2 ± 0.7	0.6 ± 0.2
control ♀	>100	1.8 ± 0.2	0.5 ± 0.2	2.5 ± 0.2[a]	0.3 ± 0.1[a]
#2 ♂	>100	2.1 ± 0.3[b]	1.4 ± 0.2[b]	7.3 ± 0.8[b]	1.3 ± 0.1[b]
#2 ♀	>100	2.5 ± 0.5[b]	2.0 ± 0.4[ab]	10.0 ± 1.5[ab]	1.6 ± 0.3[ab]

SRM-A, standard rat/mouse A diet; HFC, mild high fat/cholesterol, containing 15% cocoa butter and 0.25% cholesterol. Values are the mean serum levels ± S.D. of at least 12 mice. Mice wer fed the HFC diet for 8 weeks. [a]$P < 0.05$, indicating significant difference between male and female mice of the same genetic background on the same diet, using non-parametric Mann-Whitney test. [b]$P < 0.05$, indicating significant difference between APOE*3-Leiden and control mice of the same sex and on the same diet, using nonparametric Mann-Whitney test

$(4.24 \pm 0.95$ vs 2.45 ± 1.05 μg apoB/hour/gr body weight), as measured by VLDL-apoB turnover experiments. Similar results were found following a rise in plasma triglyceride levels after injection with Triton WR1339.

Female APOE*3-Leiden mice display significantly higher plasma cholesterol and triglyceride levels than males, when fed hyperlipidemic diets (Table 3). In line with this, injection of both male and female transgenic mice with estrogen leads to an enhanced plasma lipid level, whereas injection of APOE*3-Leiden mice with testosterone showed the opposite (Table 3). Lipoprotein profile analysis showed that this effect of sex steroid hormone on plasma lipid levels is confined to the VLDL/LDL sized lipoprotein fraction. By Triton WR 1339 injection experiments we were able to show that estrogens increase the hepatic production of VLDL, whereas testosterone administration had no effect on VLDL production. We also found by VLDL-apoB turnover studies that in female mice the VLDL rate of synthesis is increased as compared to male mice $(2.13 \pm 0.79$ vs 1.65 ± 0.34 μg apoB/hour/gr body weight), and that administration of estrogen to male mice also leads to an increased VLDL synthesis.

In male mice without hormone treatment the fractional catabolic rate is equal to that in female mice without treatment. After injecting male mice with testosterone, however, the fractional catabolic rate increased. We have experimental evidence that an increased VLDL clearance in male APOE*3-Leiden mice is the result of an inhibited expression of the APOE*3-Leiden transgene in these mice.

Thus, the increase in plasma lipid levels by estrogen is due to an increase in hepatic VLDL production followed by a lower fractional catabolic rate of VLDL, whereas the hypolipidemic effect of testosterone can be explained by an increased fractional catabolic rate.

Dominant and recessive forms of Familial Dysbetalipoproteinemia

As found with Familial Dysbetalipoproteinemia (FD) patients, mutant forms of apoE can lead to an impaired clearance of remnant lipoproteins from the circulation. FD, however, can be inherited either as a recessive or as a dominant trait. The recessive inheritance pattern occurs in FD patients carrying the APOE*2(Arg-158→Cys) mutation. Although about 1% of the population is homozygous for this defective APOE*2 allele, only a small percentage (4%) of these homozygous carriers develop hyperlipidemia, indicating that secondary metabolic or genetic factors are required for clinical expression of the disease. Several rare mutations show a dominant inheritance pattern, including the APOE*3-Leiden mutation. But, also in the case of the dominantly inherited forms of FD, additional environmental and

Table 3. The effect of hormone treatment on plasma lipid levels in APOE*3Leiden mice

Sex	Treatment	cholesterol			triglycerides		
			mmol/liter				
Males	Placebo	6.2	±	1.2	2.3	±	0.3
	Estradiol decanoate (100 μg/mouse)	6.7	±	0.3	4.5	±	0.6[a]
	Testosterone decanoate (1250 μg/mouse)	5.1	±	0.7	2.6	±	0.4
Females	Placebo	9.4	±	1.5	3.3	±	0.7
	Estradiol decanoate (100 μg/mouse)	10.6	±	1.5	5.1	±	0.7[a]
	Testosteron decanoate (1250 μg/mouse)	6.6	±	1.1[a]	2.3	±	0.3[a]

Mice were fed high cholesterol high fat diets (HFC). Total cholesterol and triglyceride values are the mean serum levels ± SD of five APOE*3-Leiden transgenic mice per group. [a]$P < 0.05$, indicating the difference between hormone and placebo treated groups of mice of the same sex, using nonparametric Mann-Whitney tests genetic factors do modulate the severity of the disease.

To characterize the biochemical mechanisms underlying the different modes of inheritance associated with the different apoE mutants, we compared APOE*3Leiden mice with mice carrying the APOE*2 allele.[4] As presented in Table 4, APOE*3-Leiden mice show significantly elevated levels of serum cholesterol levels as compared to non-transgenic mice (see also line #2 in Table 1). This increase in serum cholesterol was confined to the VLDL/LDL-sized lipoprotein fractions (not shown). On the regular chow diet (SRM-A), APOE*2 transgenic mice did not show elevated serum cholesterol levels as compared to non-transgenic mice.[5]

On a high/fat cholesterol diet, APOE*3-Leiden transgenic mice had a two-fold higher serum cholesterol level as compared to non-transgenic mice, which was mainly due to increased levels of VLDL/LDL-sized lipoproteins (not shown). In contrast, serum cholesterol levels in cholesterol fed APOE*2 transgenic were similar to non-transgenic mice. Hence, in the presence of the mouse *Apoe* gene, APOE*2 transgenic mice are normolipidemic, even under dietary stress, whereas APOE*3-Leiden transgenic mice develop (diet-induced) hypercholesterolemia. This implies that in mice the APOE*3-Leiden and APOE*2 mutation behave as a dominant and recessive mutation, respectively, as they do in humans.

These findings allowed us to investigate the mechanisms underlying the dominant and recessive forms of FD. For studying the *in vivo* functional properties of the mutant apoE forms in the absence of a functional mouse *Apoe* gene, APOE*2 and APOE*3-Leiden transgenic mice were cross-bred with *Apoe-/-* mice to deficiency in endogenous mouse apoE (designated as APOE*2·*Apoe-/-* and APOE*3-Leiden·*Apoe-/-* mice, respectively). On a regular SRM-A diet, the expression of the APOE*3-Leiden transgene resulted in an almost complete rescue of the extremely hypercholesterolemic phenotype usually found in *Apoe-/-* mice (Table 4). However, APOE*2·*Apoe-/-* mice were severely hypercholesterolemic and, in addition, showed a relatively mild hypertriglyceridemia.[6]

To study the underlying mechanism of the different hyperlipoproteinemias in the SRM-A fed female *Apoe-/-*, APOE*3-Leiden·*Apoe-/-* and APOE*2·*Apoe-/-* mice, *in vivo* VLDL-apoB kinetic studies were performed. Mice were injected with autologous ^{125}I-labeled VLDL, and the ^{125}I-apoB disappearance from the circulation was determined. VLDL-apoB clearance rate was clearly reduced in all apoE transgenic mice (Table 5) in the order: wild type >> APOE*3-Leiden·*Apoe-/-* and APOE*2·*Apoe-/-* > *Apoe-/-* mice. In vitro competition binding studies using VLDL samples from the respective mice showed that reduced VLDL-apoB clearance was completely parallel with a reduced binding of these lipoproteins to the LDL receptor.

To investigate whether an increase in VLDL production also contributes to

Table 4. The effect of the human APOE*3-Leiden and the APOE*2 transgene on serum lipid levels in APOE transgenic mice with or without the wild type mouse Apoe alleles

		endogenous Apoe genotype			
		Apoe+/+		Apoe-/-	
diet	APOE transgene	Cholesterol	Triglycerides	Cholesterol	Triglycerides
		mmol/l	mmol/l	mmol/l	mmol/l
SRM-A	-	2.1 ± 0.2	0.5 ± 0.2	23.6 ± 5.0	0.5 ± 0.3
SRM-A	APOE*3-Leiden	2.7 ± 0.5‡	0.8 ± 0.4	3.6 ± 1.5‡	0.3 ± 0.2
SRM-A	APOE*2	2.1 ± 0.2§	0.6 ± 0.2	16.5 ± 2.9‡§	2.4 ± 0.8‡§
HFC/0.5%	-	6.5 ± 1.1	0.1 ± 0.0	nd	nd
HFC/0.5%	APOE*3-Leiden	13.7 ± 2.5‡	0.2 ± 0.1‡	nd	nd
HFC/0.5%	APOE*2	6.8 ± 1.5§	0.1 ± 0.1‡	nd	nd

Female mice of 2-3 months of age were fed a SRM-A diet or a HFC diet for 4 weeks. Total serum cholesterol and triglycerides are the mean ± S.D. of 4-7 mice in case of mice with the Apoe+/+ background or 15-18 mice in case of the Apoe-/- background.
‡P<0.05, significantly different from non-transgenic mice fed the same diet, using nonparametric Mann-Whitney tests.
§P<0.05, indicating significant difference between APOE*3-Leiden and APOE*2 transgenic mice on the same diet and the same Apoe genotype, using nonparametric Mann-Whitney tests.

the observed accumulation of VLDL-sized lipoproteins, we determined hepatic VLDL-triglyceride production rate directly from serum triglyceride increase after injection of Triton WR 1339.[7] *Apoe-/-* and APOE*3-Leiden·*Apoe-/-* mice had a significant two-fold reduction in hepatic VLDL triglyceride production rate as compared to wild type mice, whereas APOE*2·*Apoe-/-* mice had a hepatic VLDL production rate comparable to wild type mice (Table 5).

The above described results thus indicate that the accumulation of VLDL-sized lipoproteins in APOE*2·*Apoe-/-* mice was due to a strong decreasing effect on VLDL clearance, as a consequence of a defect of apoE2 to bind to the LDL receptor. In contrast, the mild accumulation of VLDL-sized lipoproteins observed in APOE*3-Leiden·*Apoe-/-* mice seems to be due to a mildly reduced VLDL clearance that is partly compensated by a reduction in VLDL production rate.

Discussion

By introducing mutant human APOE genes, mice develop hyperlipidemia as compared to wild type mice. In these mice the elevated plasma cholesterol levels are confined to the VLDL/LDL lipoprotein fractions. Mutant apoE transgenic mice are sensitive to cholesterol feeding as far as their plasma cholesterol levels are concerned and are highly sensitive to atherosclerosis development. We have shown that in these mice the rate of atherosclerosis development is strongly correlated to plasma cholesterol levels. In addition, the plasma VLDL and LDL levels are strongly dependent on the rate of VLDL production. With our apoE transgenic mice we generated a suitable animal model system for studying the effect of diets and drugs on both hyperlipidemia and atherosclerosis development.[8-10]

Since APOE*3-Leiden and APOE*2 appeared to behave as a dominant and recessive mutation, respectively, in transgenic mice as well as they do in humans, we conclude that the differential expression of FD associated with these apoE mutants can also be studied in mice. It is striking that in mice the E2E2 genotype displays a complete penetrance of hyperlipoproteinemia, which is in strong contrast to humans, where E2E2 homozygosity exhibits a low penetrance for hyperlipidemia (4%). Further analyses of the differences between humans and mice in this respect might help in finding the factors involved in VLDL remnant clearance, a process which is commonly assumed to be of major importance in the western societies regarding the risk of development of early atherosclerosis. More specifically, these analyses might help to find major aggravating factors involved in the clinical expression of FD.

Table 5. VLDL-apoB fractional catabolic rates (FCR) and in vivo hepatic VLDL triglyceride production rate (PR) in APOE*3-Leiden and APOE*2 transgenic mice without endogenous mouse Apoe alleles

mouse	VLDL-apoB FCR	VLDL-triglyceride PR
	pool/hr	*mmol/hr/kg mouse*
wild type	22.1 ± 3.4[‡]	0.136 ± 0.044[‡]
Apoe-/-	3.2 ± 0.7[*]	0.076 ± 0.023[*]
APOE*3-Leiden·*Apoe-/-*	6.1 ± 1.9[*],[‡]	0.077 ± 0.017[*]
APOE*2·*Apoe-/-*	4.0 ± 0.5[*],[‡]	0.128 ± 0.027[‡]

After 5 hour fasting period SRM-A fed female mice were injected 10 µg of autologous labeled ^{125}I-labeled VLDL protein. ^{125}I-apoB(100+48) disappearance from circulation was determined and FCR was calculated. For determining hepatic VLDL production rate fasted SRM-A fed female mice were injected with Triton WR1339. Fasted serum triglycerides were determined just before injection (0 min) and at 30 and 60 min after Triton injection. Production of hepatic triglyceride production rate was calculated from the slope of the curve and is expressed as mmol/h/kg mouse. Values are the mean ± SD of 6-7 mice per group.
*$P < 0.05$, significantly different from mice with the wild type mouse *Apoe* allele, using nonparametric Mann-Whitney tests.
[‡]$P < 0.05$, significantly different from *Apoe-/-* mice, using nonparametric Mann-Whitney tests.

References

1. van den Maagdenberg AMJM, Hofker MH, Krimpenfort PJA et al. Transgenic mice carrying the apolipoprotein E3-Leiden gene exhibit hyperlipoproteinemia. J Biol Chem 1993;268:10540-5.
2. van Vlijmen B, van den Maagdenberg AMJM, Gijbels MJJ et al. Diet-induced hyperlipoproteinemia and atherosclerosis in apolipoprotein E3-Leiden transgenic mice. J Clin Invest 1994;93:1403-10.
3. Havekes LM, van Vlijmen B, Frants R, Hofker M. Rare mutations in the ApoE gene and their effect on chylomicron and VLDL remnant metabolism in familial dysbetalipoproteinemic patients and in transgenic mice. In: Multiple risk factors in Cardiovascular Disease, ed. by A. Yamamoto, Churchill Livingstone Japan, Tokyo, 1994 pp. 167-71.
4. Havekes LM, van Vlijmen BJM, van Ree JH, Frants RR, Hofker MH. Effect of expression of apoE mutants in transgenic mice. In: Atherosclerosis X. Eds. Woodford FP, Davignon J, and Sniderman A. 1995; pp. 656-61.
5. van Vlijmen BJM, van 't Hof HB, Mol MJTM et al. Modulation of very low density lipoprotein production and clearance contributes to age and gender dependent hyperlipoproteinemia in apolipoprotein E3-Leiden transgenic mice. J Clin Invest 1996;97:1184-92.
6. Groot PHE, van Vlijmen BJM, Benson GM et al. Quantitative assessment of aortic atherosclerosis in apoE3Leiden transgenic mice and its relationship to serum cholesterol exposure. Arterioscler Thromb Vasc Biol 1996;16:926-33.
7. Jong MC, Dahlmans VEH, van Gorp PJJ et al. Both lipolysis and hepatic uptake of very low density lipoproteins are impaired in transgenic mice co-expressing human apolipoprotein E*3Leiden and human apolipoprotein C1. Arterioscler Thromb Vasc Biol 1996;16:934-40.
8. Havekes LM, van Vlijmen BJM, Jong MC, Groot PHE, Frants RR, Hofker MH. The metabolism of VLDL remnants in APOE*3-Leiden transgenic mice. In: Drugs affecting lipid metabolism: Risk factors and future directions. Eds. Gotto AM, Paoletti R, Smith LC, Catapano AL, and Jackson AS. Medical Science Symposia Series 1996; 10: pp. 263-70.
9. van Vlijmen BLM, van Ree JH, Frants RR, Hofker MH, Havekes LM. Elevated levels of chylomicron- and VLDL remnants leads to atherosclerosis in apoE transgenic mice. Z Gastroenterology 1996;34:113-5.
10. van Vlijmen BJM, Willems van Dijk K, van 't Hof HB et al. In the absence of endogenous mouse apolipoprotein E, apolipoprotein E*2(Arg158→Cys) transgenic mice develop more severe hyperlipoproteinemiathan apolipoprotein E*3-Leiden transgenic mice. J Biol Chem 1996;271:30595-602.

RAMAN SPECTROSCOPY DURING CATHETERIZATION: A MEANS OF VIEWING PLAQUE COMPOSITION

Tjeerd J. Römer, James F. Brennan III

Summary

The progression and regression of atherosclerotic plaques appear to be related to the amount and type of lipids that accumulate in the intima of arteries.[1-3] Recent studies have shown that plaque composition, rather than size or volume, determines whether an arterial narrowing will rupture and cause an acceleration of clinical symptoms.[4,5] Clearly, an instrument is needed that can determine *in situ* the chemical composition of atherosclerotic lesions objectively and accurately. Raman spectroscopy is a powerful technique, capable of providing detailed, quantitative information about the chemical composition of arterial wall non-destructively. Such an instrument would be useful to clinicians and researchers in many applications, such as predicting plaque rupture and selecting proper therapeutic interventions. In this chapter, a review is given of the basic principles and potential applications of Raman spectroscopy.

Introduction

Raman spectroscopy is a promising technique that can be used to characterize the chemical composition of biological tissue.
A Raman spectrum of a given molecule is unique, which makes Raman spectroscopy ideal for detecting, identifying and diagnosing diseases that involve gross chemical changes in tissue, such as atherosclerosis.[6-9] Raman

175

E.E. van der Wall et al. (eds.), Vascular Medicine, 175-196.
© 1997 *Kluwer Academic Publishers.*

spectra of arterial tissue can be obtained by processing the collected light that is scattered from an artery as it is illuminated with a laser beam. With sensitive laboratory spectroscopic equipment, quality spectra can be collected in less than a second, and most spectral features are visible in spectra collected in only a few seconds via optical fiber catheters.[10,11] Since Raman spectroscopy is non-destructive, one can collect spectra of the tissue *in situ*, which can be processed to provide quantitative information about the chemical composition of an arterial wall.[12,13] This information has been used to identify histopathological and histomorphological features of the atherosclerotic process.[14] Certainly, Raman spectroscopy has the potential of providing diagnostic capabilities that are not available with current medical techniques.

A Raman spectrum contains a wealth of information about the scattering material so it is not surprising that thousands of uses have been found for this spectroscopic technique. For instance, Raman spectroscopy can provide information about the structure of specific molecules and has been used to study various molecular configurations.[15,16] Chemical processes can be remotely and actively monitored via optical fibers in hostile or inaccessible locations,[17,18] and trace elements can be detected for environmental, medical, or industrial purposes. Raman spectroscopy is also a powerful tool for determining the biological components and their chemical concentrations in human tissues.[9,12,13] Its ability to identify diseased tissue is under study by several research groups. Raman spectra have been obtained from eye lenses,[19,20] viruses,[21] teeth and bone,[22,23] single living cells,[24,25] living salmon sperm,[26] DNA,[21,24,27] etc. Numerous of studies have been published about chemical and biological processes analyzed with Raman spectroscopy.

Although the Raman effect was discovered in the 1920s, it was difficult to apply, because one needed strong light sources and sensitive light detection equipment. Little sustained interest was aroused by the promising practical aspects of the Raman effect until the advent of lasers. Biological and clinical applications of Raman techniques wanted additional technology innovations, since instruments were needed that were convenient to use and collected spectral information rapidly. In addition, Raman signal size was severely limited by the need to work at excitation intensities sufficiently low to avoid damage to biological samples. Early work employed near-infrared (NIR) Fourier Transform Raman systems or systems based on scanning photomultiplier tubes to collect spectra. However, at acceptable excitation powers the sensitivity of such systems is limited by detector dark current, and long data collection times, typically tens of minutes, are required to accumulate spectra with acceptable signal-to-noise ratios.

Silicon-based CCD detectors have dramatically improved the instrumentation used to measure Raman spectra. The high sensitivity and negligible dark noise of these detectors have permitted spectra to be measured orders of magnitude faster than with single-channel techniques. However, in materials such as biological tissue the Raman effect is often obscured by strong background fluorescence. In order to reduce this, recent investigators have used excitation wavelengths in the NIR range, 700 to 850 nm, where fluorescence is significantly reduced and silicon CCDs are still sensitive to the Raman scattered light (850 to 1000 nm). The remaining background fluorescence can then be removed with software to yield useful Raman spectra, which are limited by the shot-noise of the background.[10]

Raman spectroscopy is reproducible, objective and thus independent of intra- and inter-observer variability. Cardiovascular studies with Raman spectroscopy have been performed *in vitro* with arterial tissue, but successful *in vivo* measurements have been impeded by the high background noise generated by scattering within the optical fibers used to construct intravascular Raman probes. Methods of reducing this background signal are under investigation by several research groups.[28] Recent developments indicate that adequate reduction of background signal is feasible. Once these methods are perfect, it should be possible to collect Raman spectra *in vivo*. This review addresses some of our studies of arterial tissue with Raman spectroscopy. We will focus on our work with human coronary arteries. We provide a brief explanation of the Raman effect and direct the interested reader to the many texts written on the subject if more information is desired. A short biography of Prof C.V. Raman is also given. We collected thousands of spectra of arterial tissue in various stages of disease and noted that the spectral features of different chemical components comprising the artery were distinct and clearly visible in the spectra. We modeled the coronary artery spectra with spectra of these arterial compounds and used the results of the model to quantify the chemical composition of arterial wall. The relative weights of lipids and calcium salts were extracted, and their amounts were seen to vary with the type and extent of atherosclerotic disease in the arterial wall, illustrating that Raman spectroscopy can provide *in situ* histopathology. We also investigated how deep Raman spectroscopy can detect cholesterol deposits in arterial wall to define the capacity of Raman spectroscopy to detect subsurface lesions.

The applications in cardiology of Raman spectroscopy techniques will be probably widespread. We will present some exploratory studies that illustrate some possible uses of this new diagnostic technique. This technique combined with intravascular ultrasound may be used to map the chemical composition of an arterial wall. We also show how Raman spectroscopy can provide a detailed chemical map of atherosclerotic lesions developed in transgenic mice, which may be used to monitor and evaluate the effects of lipid lowering agents on plaque progression and regression.

The Raman effect

The vibrations and rotations between atoms within a molecule can occur only at discrete frequencies. This point may seem odd given typical daily observations, as if we are driving from Amsterdam to Leiden at only 10 km/hr, 20 km/hr, 30 km/hr, etc. and not at any speed between these decade intervals. But the motions of molecules do occur at only fixed intervals that are determined by factors such as the micro-environment of the molecule and the masses and attractive forces of the atoms. Quantum physics has explained satisfactorily this unexpected phenomenon, and interested readers are referred to the many books written about the topic.[29-31] These molecular motions store energy, like the flywheel on a gasoline engine stores energy. Since a molecule's internal motions are quantized, a molecule can absorb or emit energy in only discrete units as it changes from one vibrational state to another.

Light also consists of discrete packets of energy called photons. The energy of a photon is inversely proportional to the wavelength of the light; an ultraviolet photon at a wavelength of 244 nm has more energy than an infrared photon at a wavelength of 900 nm. When a molecule radiatively changes state, the wavelength of the light that is emitted or absorbed during the transition changes by a discrete amount corresponding to the change in stored energy of the molecule. Since different molecules have distinct internal configurations, they have unique frequencies of internal motion and thus can be identified by their spectra.

The spectrum of light scattered from a molecule generally contains an elastic contribution, where the emitted frequency equals the incident frequency (Rayleigh scattering), together with several spectral components for which these frequencies differ (Stokes and anti-Stokes scattering), as illustrated in Figure 1. One source of this frequency-shifted light is a sequence of processes known as relaxed fluorescence, in which the frequency of the incident light falls within an electronic absorption band of the interacting molecule. The molecule is raised to an excited state as it absorbs an incident photon and, after losing some energy by making non-radiative molecular transitions, re-emits light at a different frequency.

Raman scattering is another source of frequency-shifted light. To Raman scatter, the incident light frequency need not be within the absorption band of the scattering molecule. The frequency difference between the incident and scattered light, which is commonly expressed in units of inverse wave length or wave numbers (cm^{-1}), corresponds to vibrational state transitions in the scattering molecule. During Raman scattering, a molecule changes state from one vibrational energy level to another. To conserve energy and

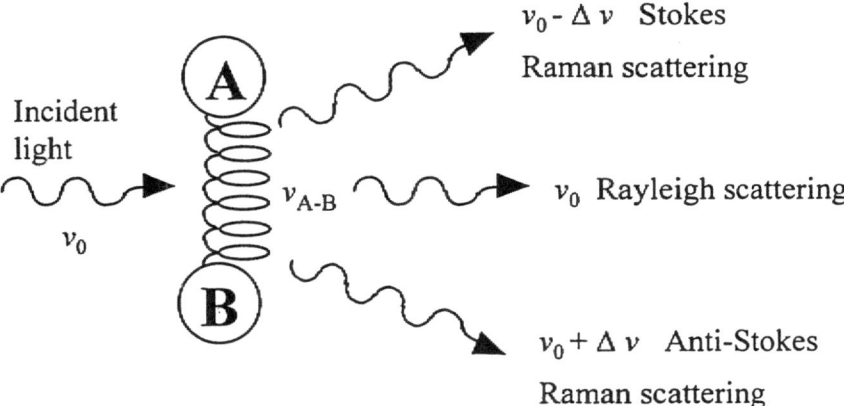

Figure 1. A schematic illustration of Raman and Rayleigh scattering. The scattered photon is like the incident photon in Rayleigh scattering, but in Raman scattering the scattered photon has a lower or higher frequency (v_0). The difference in energy between the incident and scattered photons is the same as the change in molecular vibrational energy.

momentum, the energies of the scattered photons are different from the incident photon energy by an amount equal but opposite to the molecular energy change.

Rayleigh scattering can be looked on as an elastic collision between the incident photon and the molecule and is by far the strongest component of the scattered radiation. Since the rotational and vibrational energy of the molecule is unchanged in an elastic collision, the wavelength of the scattered photon is the same as that of the incident photon. When an incident photon interacts with a molecule in the lowest vibrational state of the molecule, the molecule absorbs the photon energy and is raised momentarily to some high level of energy which is not stable (a virtual state). The molecule immediately loses energy and returns to the lowest vibrational level, as it emits a photon at a wavelength which is the same as that of the incident photon.

The Raman effect can be viewed as an inelastic collision between the incident photon and the molecule, where, as a result of the collision, the vibrational or rotational energy of the molecule is changed. In some instances after a molecule absorbs a photon and enters an unstable state, it may fall to an excited vibrational state of the molecule and not to the lowest vibrational level (Figure 2). In this case, the scattered photon has less energy than the exciting photon and gives rise to a so-called Stokes line in the Raman spectrum, which is at a wavelength longer than that of the incident photon. If the molecule was initially in an excited vibrational state

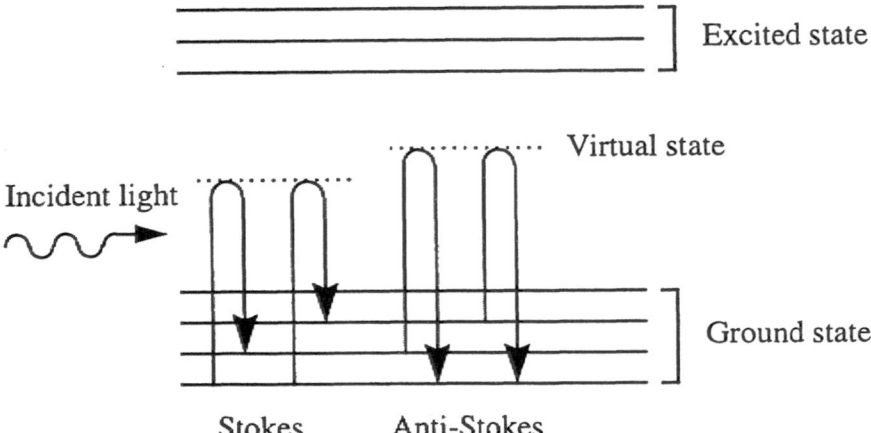

Figure 2. *A schematic illustration of the molecular energy levels and transitions between them during Raman scattering. With near infrared incident light, the energy of the virtual state is well below that of the first excited electronic state. After a Raman event, the molecule has changed vibrational state, but remains in the electronic state.*

before it absorbed an incident photon and entered the virtual state, so-called anti-Stokes Raman scattering can occur where the emitted photon is at a wavelength shorter than that of the incident photon. This effect is usually much weaker than Stokes scattering and was not studied by us.

For illustration, we picture an imaginary compound with a single vibrational state. If this compound is illuminated with 850 nm light, a spectrum of the scattered light may contain a Rayleigh line at 11,765 cm^{-1} (850 nm) and a Stokes line at say 10,165 cm^{-1} (984 nm). The frequency difference between the incident and emitted photons (1600 cm^{-1}) would correspond to the vibrational energy change in the molecule. A Raman spectrum of a compound usually has several spectral peaks, and their positions and intensities can be used as a molecular fingerprint. For more information about the basic principles of Raman spectroscopy and its biological applications, the reader is referred to the book written by Anthony T. Tu.[16]

Prof. C.V. Raman

In 1888 C.V. Raman was born in Thiruvanaikkaval, Southern India, as one of seven children. He graduated in Physics at the University of Madras and went to Calcutta, in 1907 where he became Professor and Head of the Department of Physics of the Calcutta University of Science in 1917.[32]

Before he detected the phenomenon that bears his name, he published more than 50 papers on light scattering and magnetism of liquid and solid media. With a quartz mercury lamp as light source, a simple set of lenses and filters, and a pocket spectroscope, he observed by eye that highly purified organic liquids, which were positioned in an incident light beam path, generated weak frequencies in the scattered light not present in the original incident light. He exposed photographic plates for hours, even days, to obtain his spectra.

Prof. Raman first announced his discovery in an inaugural lecture entitled "A New Radiation" at a meeting of the South Indian Association in 1928.[33] He was very confident of his new finding and predicted the usefulness of this new type of radiation by stating: "We are obviously at the fringe of a fascinating new region of experimental research which promises to throw light on diverse problems relating to radiation and wave theory, x-ray optics, atomic and molecular spectra, fluorescence and scattering, thermodynamics and chemistry. It all remains to be worked out".[33] Also in 1928, he published two papers in Nature about the phenomenon, which made it known throughout the world.[34,35] He received the Nobel prize for his work in 1930.[36] At present, numerous publications on Raman spectroscopy have been published. Prof. Raman died in 1970, just before the wide exploration of biological applications of Raman spectroscopy started.[16]

Raman spectroscopy instrumentation

The methods used to collect Raman spectra are relatively easy to follow. Basically, light of a single wavelength is directed onto a sample, and then light scattered from the sample is collected and launched into a spectrometer. The spectrometer separates the light according to its wavelength, like a prism spreads sunlight into a rainbow. This rainbow of light is projected onto a detector which can record the intensities of each color of light. A plot of these intensities as a function of wavelength (or frequency) is called a spectrum.

In our laboratory studies, we irradiated coronary artery samples with near infrared laser light of ~850 nm (sometimes ~830 nm) and collected the scattered light with a lens (Figure 3). Special optical filters were used to remove the intense Rayleigh scattered light from the collected light before it was launched into a high-efficiency spectrometer. In the spectrometer, the light was collimated, separated spatially by wavelength with a diffraction grating, and imaged onto a charge coupled device (CCD) camera. We could collect Raman spectra in a few seconds with a signal-to-noise ratio sufficiently high to calculate chemical information about the artery wall (see

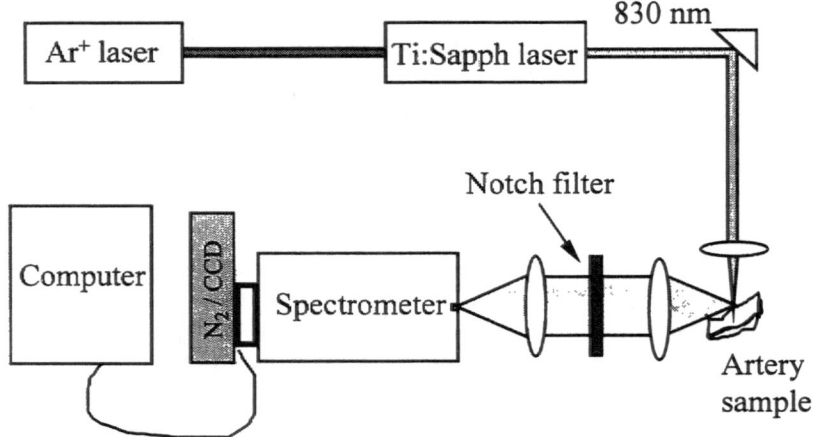

Figure 3. Schematic diagram of Raman instrumentation.

below).

We also designed an exploratory clinical system to collect real-time Raman spectra in hospital clinical settings. Infrared light was delivered to and collected from tissue via a 5 F (˜1.7 mm diameter) 3-m-long optical fiber probe consisting of six 200-μm-core diameter collection fibers surrounding a central delivery fiber. The distal tip of the optical fiber probe was brought into contact with the tissue to be spectroscopically examined. The collection fibers were arranged in a line at the proximal end of the probe and coupled into the spectrometer.

The present clinical system can detect the presence of hydroxyapatite in calcified coronary artery in a 0.01 s signal collection time, but fiber background is currently the most significant limitation to the spectral quality. Typically, the fiber background at ˜1000 cm^{-1} is >30 times larger than the Raman spectral features of cholesterol. Reduction of this fiber background signal in future optical fiber probes will greatly improve the clinical system performance. Data from the clinical system will not be presented in this chapter. Interested readers are directed to the references.[10,37]

Raman spectra of coronary artery

For most studies, we obtained coronary artery samples from explanted recipient hearts within one hour of heart transplantation. The artery samples were snap frozen in liquid nitrogen and stored at -80 °C until spectroscopic

examination.
NIR Raman spectra measured from three different types of human coronary
artery are shown in Figure 4.

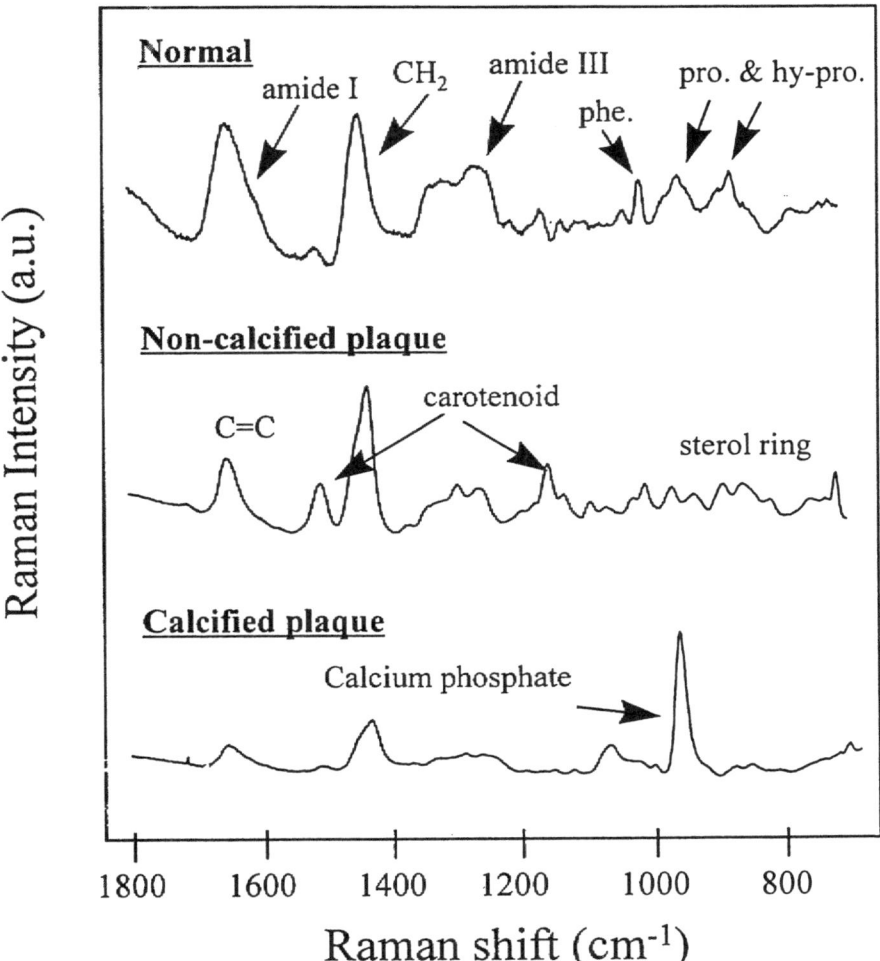

*Figure 4. Raman spectra of three different types of coronary artery. Spectral features can be
assigned to specific molecular vibrations.*

The top spectrum was obtained from a sample of nonatherosclerotic
coronary artery; the middle from a noncalcified atheromatous plaque; and
the bottom from a calcified plaque. The spectra from these different artery
types are distinct and provide clear features for determining the chemical
composition and histological classification of the arterial wall. For example

the normal coronary artery spectrum is dominated by protein features such as the amide I and III modes at ˜1650 and 1250 cm⁻¹, respectively, and the CH_2 bending modes at ˜1450 cm⁻¹. In noncalcified atheromatous plaques, spectral features of cholesterol and cholesterol esters constitutes the major part of the spectrum. The symmetric stretch at 960 cm⁻¹ of phosphate, which is a constituent of calcium hydroxyapatite, dominates the spectrum of calcified plaques.

Artery chemistry with Raman spectra

We examined hundreds of coronary artery samples that represented various pathological states and obtained their spectra. In this study, our objective was to determine the chemical compositions of the artery samples from these spectra. To achieve this, we developed a model that viewed a coronary artery spectrum as a linear superposition of spectra of individual chemical components. We found that spectra of seven arterial components were needed to model adequately all of the measured coronary artery spectra. These components were free cholesterol (FC), cholesterol esters (CE), calcium salts (CS), triglycerides (TG), two delipidized artery segments (DA) and β-carotene.

The contribution of some components in a coronary artery's spectrum, such as triglycerides and proteins, is difficult to model with spectra obtained from commercially available chemicals, because these components in the artery contain mixtures of related molecules in the class. Therefore, these components were extracted from the artery wall itself. The TG spectra were obtained from triglycerides isolated from adventitial fat. The individual DA spectra were obtained from delipidized artery samples, one which appeared to be non-atherosclerotic tissue (DA I) and another which appeared to be non-calcified atherosclerotic tissue (DA II) by visual inspection. The DA spectra were used to model the spectral contribution of all non-lipid, non-mineral components of arterial wall. Four of the seven spectra were measured from mixtures directly extracted from coronary artery samples (DA I and II, TG and CS). Linear superpositions modeled the measured coronary artery spectra well, judging by the residuals of the fit that are obtained by subtracting the model fit from the artery spectrum.

The spectra of the seven model compounds were obtained and a scaling factor determined so that a linear combination of the individual spectra could be used to estimate the amount of each component in an examined artery. Mixtures of compounds were prepared, and their spectra measured, in order to infer how the seven model spectra should be scaled. The overall spectral model was then validated by comparing chemical concentrations in the

185

coronary artery minces calculated from the Raman spectra to the actual concentrations measured with standard assay techniques. Artery segments obtained from nine explanted hearts and exhibiting various stages of atherosclerosis were selectively combined and finely ground to produce a set of nine minces containing varying amounts of lipids, lipid classes and calcium salts. Raman spectra were obtained from each of these minces at ten different sites on the mince and used to calculate the relative weights of the major chemical components of the tissue. Excellent agreement was reached between the relative weights calculated with Raman spectroscopic techniques and those determined with standard assays conducted on the minces (Figure 5).

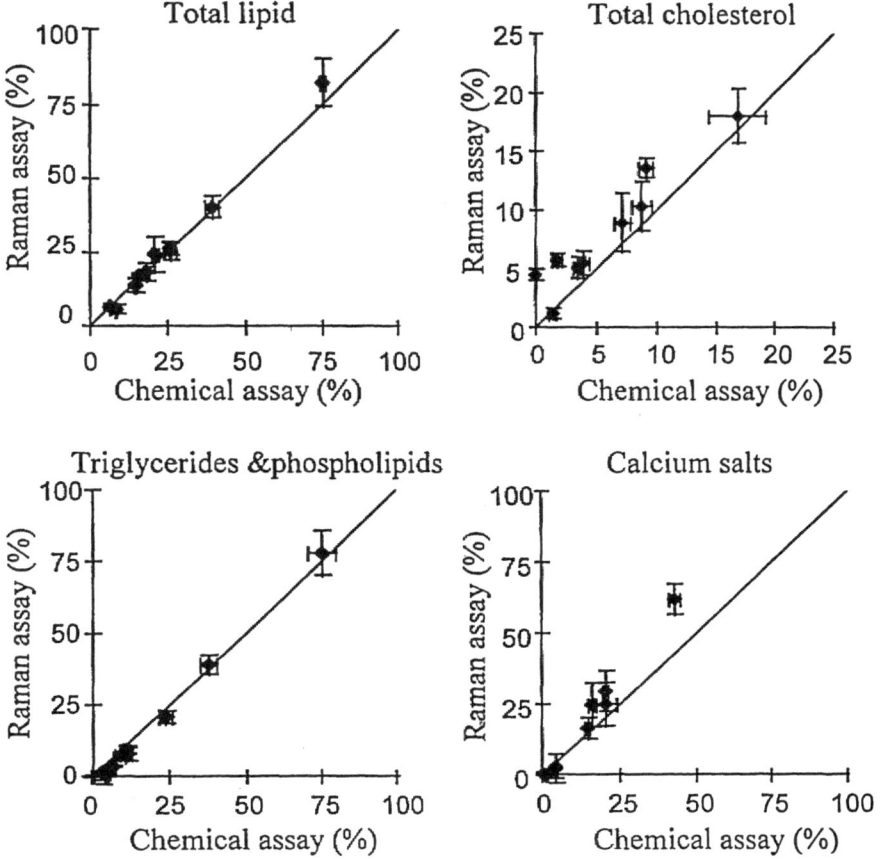

Figure 5. Comparison of the percentage weights of lipids and calcium salts measured in coronary artery minces by Raman spectral analysis and standard chemical assay techniques. (Adapted from Reference 13 with permission from Circulation.)

The amounts calculated with Raman spectroscopy agreed with standard chemical assays for lipids (± 3 %) and calcium salts (± 2 %). Details of the model and its validation with standard chemical assays have been described previously.[12,13,37]

Histopathology with Raman spectra of coronary artery

In this study, we extracted quantitative chemical information from Raman spectra obtained from coronary artery in different stages of atherosclerois and correlated this information with standard histological tissue diagnosis. To improve clinical utility, we developed an algorithm based on these chemical parameters that allows the classification of coronary artery atherosclerosis *in situ*, according to standard pathological classification schemes. This technique, when applied in a percutaneous setting, may give the clinician not only access to information which has been unavailable for evaluating the type and degree of severity of the disease, but it may also provide the clinician with a new and more definitive basis for guiding treatment.

In Figure 6, Raman spectra (dots) of intimal fibroplasia, non-calcified atheromatous plaque and calcified atheroscleromatous plaque are modeled with the previously described model (line). The curve below each spectrum and model fit is the residual, obtained by subtracting the fit from the artery spectrum. Figure 6A shows a spectrum of intimal fibroplasia, which is dominated by protein and TG features visible at about 1650, 1250 and 1450 cm^{-1}. The TG's located in the adventitial layer are stronger Raman scatterers than the proteins in the intima and media, so the TG spectral features dominate the artery spectrum although the relative weight of TG is lower than that of proteins. In the spectrum of an atheromatous plaque shown in Figure 6B, spectral features from the sterol rings of FC and CE are visible below 1000 cm^{-1}. The Raman spectral model calculated a 13 % relative weight of FC and a 6 % relative weight of CE. Raman spectra obtained from calcified plaque are distinguishable by the symmetric stretch vibration of phosphate (960 cm^{-1}) found in calcium salts, mainly calcium hydroxy-apatite. A large relative weight of CS was calculated from the spectrum of a highly calcified atheromatous plaque shown in Figure 6C.

As shown, Raman spectra of coronary artery are fingerprints of the tissue's molecular composition. Figure 7 shows that the quantification of the chemical composition calculated from artery spectra correlates with standard histologic tissue classification. We found that an artery's cholesterol and calcium salts content is useful for classifying the artery as either non-atherosclerotic tissue, non-calcified plaque, or calcified lesion. Using these

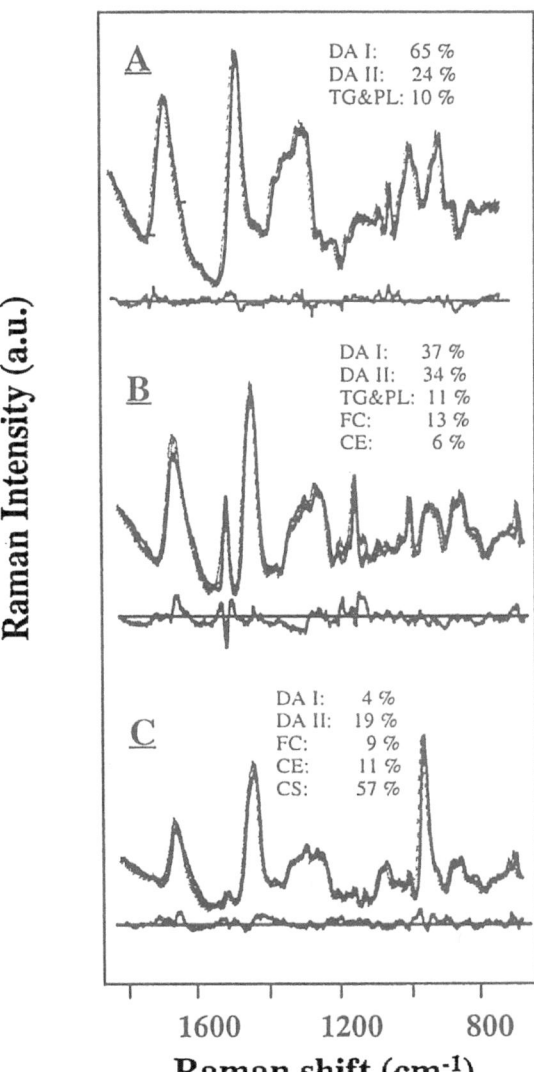

Figure 6. *Raman spectra (dotted line) of intimal fibroplasia (6A), atheromatous plaque (6B) and calcified plaque (6C) modeled with the set of spectra from individual components (line) to quantify the chemical composition of the artery wall. The curve under each spectrum shows the difference of the spectrum and the model fit.*

188

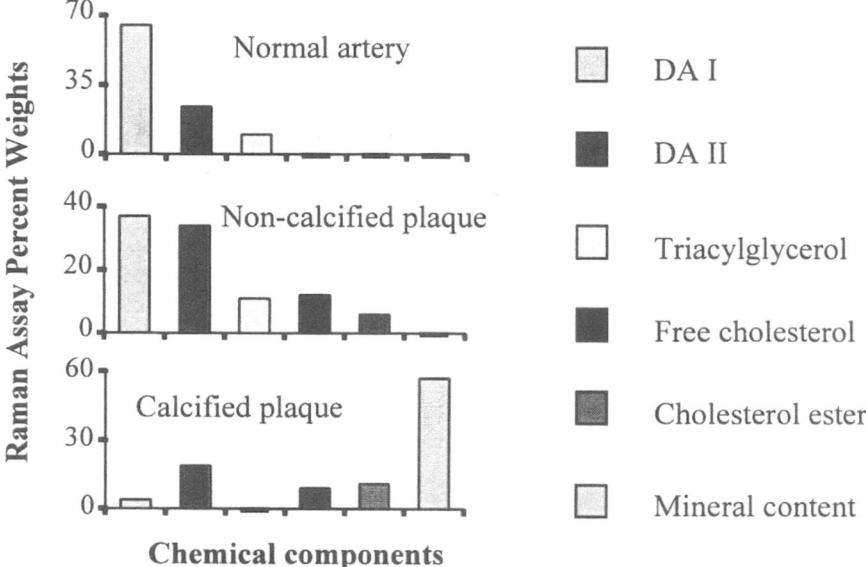

Figure 7. Quantitative chemical information provided by Raman spectroscopy correlates to histopathology. DA indicates delipidized artery (see text).

two chemical parameters, we made diagnostic algorithms that could calculate the probability that an area of interest in a coronary artery is in one of these three categories. These algorithms were successful in separating ~170 samples into their proper diagnostic categories, as determined by the pathologist, to an accuracy of a few percent. This study suggests that the pathological state of a coronary artery site can be assessed successfully from its chemical composition determined with Raman spectra.[14]

Raman spectroscopic analysis of tissue shows certain advantages over microscopic examination. A pathologist needs to observe lipid-bearing morphological structures, such as cholesterol crystals and foam cells, and calcification remnants in tissue sections to diagnose a given artery sample, but these telling structures may be missed on microscopic examination due to sampling error during tissue sectioning. Raman spectroscopy examines a large volume of tissue (about a cubic mm in this study), so it is not subject to this type of sampling error. To examine the same volume of tissue, a pathologist would need to inspect hundreds tissue sections.

As discussed, the detection of individual structures and chemical components is crucial for the diagnosis of artery wall, but individual chemical components are difficult to quantify by light microscopy. Special stains are needed to visualize accurately fine lipid droplets and small calcifications, but the opacity and extent of the stain must be quantified to objectively determine the compound's presence. Unless a technique such as digital microscopy is used, this visual quantification is qualitative (or, at best, semi-quantitative) and subject to variability between observers and even within the same observer. Raman spectroscopic techniques can non-destructively detect and objectively quantify these chemical amounts regardless of tissue handling.

Sampling depth

We also investigated how deeply Raman spectroscopy could detect subsurface lesions in an arterial wall. When we validated the previously-discussed spectral model, we obtained spectra from homogeneous minces of coronary artery where the amount of a chemical compound was uniformly distributed throughout the sample. Chemical amounts calculated by processing Raman spectra collected from intact, inhomogeneous plaques are more difficult to interpret than those obtained from homogeneous samples. The strength and shape of a spectrum measured at the surface of an artery wall is determined by a complex interaction between the compound's scattering cross-section, the depth of the scattering center into the arterial wall, the excitation / collection geometry of the spectroscopic system, and the light absorption and scattering properties of the intervening tissue. We studied how the relative weight of cholesterol calculated with Raman spectra is related to the depth of the cholesterol deposit into an arterial wall.[38]

The attenuation of a cholesterol deposit's contribution to a Raman spectrum seems to decrease roughly exponentially as a function of distance from the artery surface. We found that a 300 μm layer of non-atherosclerotic intima / media attenuates the Raman signal of plaque cholesterol by ~50 % at 850 nm excitation. Other researchers found similar results in calcified aortic media using 1024 nm excitation light.[9] These results indicate that NIR Raman spectroscopy can detect subsurface structures that are ~1-1.5 mm beneath the artery surface and therefore should be capable of detecting atherosclerotic deposits under thick fibrous caps. Atherosclerotic plaques in coronary arteries vary in thickness and may reach a fibrous cap thickness of 200-300 μm and an underlying core thickness of ~400 μm.[39]

We compared cholesterol amounts calculated with Raman spectra of intact plaques to those calculated with quantitative absorption microscopy of tissue sections from these plaques that were specially stained to visualize cholesterol. If one properly accounts for the depth of a cholesterol deposit into an arterial wall, we showed that cholesterol amounts calculated with spectra correlate strongly to amounts determined with quantitative microscopy. These results suggest that one may map *in vivo* chemical concentrations throughout the thickness of an arterial wall by combining Raman spectroscopic techniques with a non-destructive depth-sensing tool, such as intravascular ultrasound or optical coherence tomography.

Raman spectroscopy combined with intravascular ultrasound

Coronary intravascular ultrasound (IVUS) imaging provides tomographic information about vessel wall structure. Previous studies demonstrated that IVUS can detect intimal thickening, lipid deposits and calcific deposits.[40-43] For instance, the presence of a calcific deposits corresponds with an echodense area and the presence of lipid deposits with an echolucent area. However, studies in which IVUS is compared with histologic examination under high-power magnification demonstrated that IVUS can detect these deposits only if they are at least 0.25 mm in diameter.[40] In addition, accurate determination of the size of calcific deposits was impossible with IVUS, since ultrasound waves are reflected mostly at the particle surface. The sensitivity in detecting lipid and calcific deposits was found to be low, 46% and 77% respectively.[40,44]

Future catheters could be designed to collect simultaneously Raman spectra via optical fibers and IVUS images. This powerful diagnostic tool would combine the quantitative chemical information provided by Raman spectroscopy and the morphologic information provided by IVUS. This combination would give the clinician unprecedented capabilities that could serve many purposes, such as monitoring the effects of lipid lowering therapies, locating rupture-prone lesions, and identifying lesions likely to restenose following angioplasty.

We explored the feasibility of combining IVUS and Raman spectroscopy technologies. IVUS images were collected from intact coronary artery segments (a few cm long) in different stages of atherosclerois. Before collecting the images, a steel needle was positioned in the adventitia as an angular bearing for future comparisons. The arteries were opened longitudinally, and Raman spectra were collected at 0.5 mm interval steps over the circumference of the locations marked with a needle, as shown in Figure 8A.

Figures 8B-D reveal the results of examining a calcified plaque with both IVUS and Raman spectroscopy. The IVUS image (Figure 8B) shows a shadow, directly behind an echodense area, opposite the location of the needle, indicating the presence of a calcified deposit. The calcium salts amounts determined with Raman spectra indicate clearly the presence of calcified tissue in this region (Figure 8C), and elevated cholesterol amounts (Figure 8D) are present in the non-calcified regions that are not plainly visible in the IVUS image. Histologic sections, which were made through this circumferential cross-section and stained specifically for cholesterol, confirmed that an elevated level of cholesterol was present in these areas.

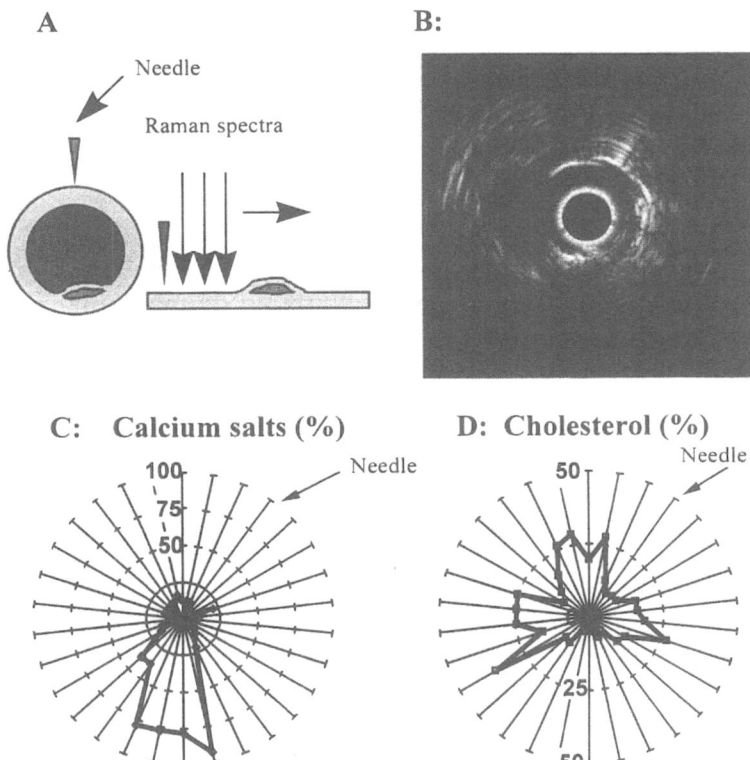

Figure 8. IVUS images were obtained from an intact artery segment, which were marked by a needle. The artery was opened, and Raman spectra were collected from the artery's inner circumference (8A). The IVUS image shows a calcification (8B), in agreement with the CS detected with Raman spectroscopy (8C). In addition, cholesterol is detected with Raman spectroscopy but cannot be seen in the IVUS image (8D). (Note the difference in scale.)

Chemical mapping of transgenic mice aortas

Our model of Raman spectra developed on human coronary artery can be altered easily to quantify the chemical composition of aortas from APOE*3 Leiden transgenic mice. After they are fed with a high fat / cholesterol (HFC) diet, these mice are highly susceptible to diet-induced atherosclerosis and develop human-like atherosclerotic plaques within six months.[45] This animal model may be ideal to monitor and evaluate the effects of hypolipidemic, antithrombogenic and other drugs on plaque progression and regression.[46] The lipids in these plaques can be visualized with standard light microscopy after Oil Red O staining of ~10 μm thick sections. Raman spectroscopy adds an extra dimension to the assessment of atherosclerosis by quantifying the chemical composition of the plaque *in situ*. This information cannot be obtained with any other available technique.

We fed groups of these mice with a HFC diet for 1 to 6 months. We followed the development of plaques in these mice with Raman spectroscopy, as illustrated in Figure 9. To create this chemical map, a mouse that received the HFC diet for 6 months was sacrificed, and its aorta (~4 mm circumference) was flushed, prepared and cut open for spectroscopic examination. Raman spectra were obtained in 0.5 mm steps over the width and length of the aorta, starting from the aortic valve until ~8 mm distally. The Raman spectra were processed to quantify the relative amounts of cholesterol and calcium salts. As shown in Figure 9, a cholesterol-rich plaque with calcium salts deposits in its center developed just distally of the aortic valve at the inner circle of the arch. The relative weight of this calcified deposit amounted to > 70 % of the volume examined spectroscopically at that location. Aortas of mice that received normal chow did not exhibit elevated levels of cholesterol or calcium salts deposits.

As this study suggests, Raman spectroscopy can map the chemical composition of atherosclerotic plaques from transgenic mice, which could aid the study of atherogenesis and help assess hypolipidemic and anti-atherosclerotic therapies.

Conclusion

Since its discovery in the 1920s, Raman spectroscopy has been widely explored and utilized. Over the last decade, technological advances have made Raman spectroscopy suitable for cardiac studies. In our studies, we modeled coronary artery spectra with spectra of arterial compounds and used the results of the model to quantify the chemical composition of arterial wall. The amounts of lipids and calcium salts were seen to vary with the type and extent of atherosclerotic disease in the arterial wall, which illustrated that Raman spectroscopy can provide *in situ* histopathology. Our results also indicated that NIR Raman spectroscopy can detect subsurface structures that are ~1-1.5 mm beneath the artery surface and therefore should be capable of detecting atherosclerotic deposits under thick fibrous

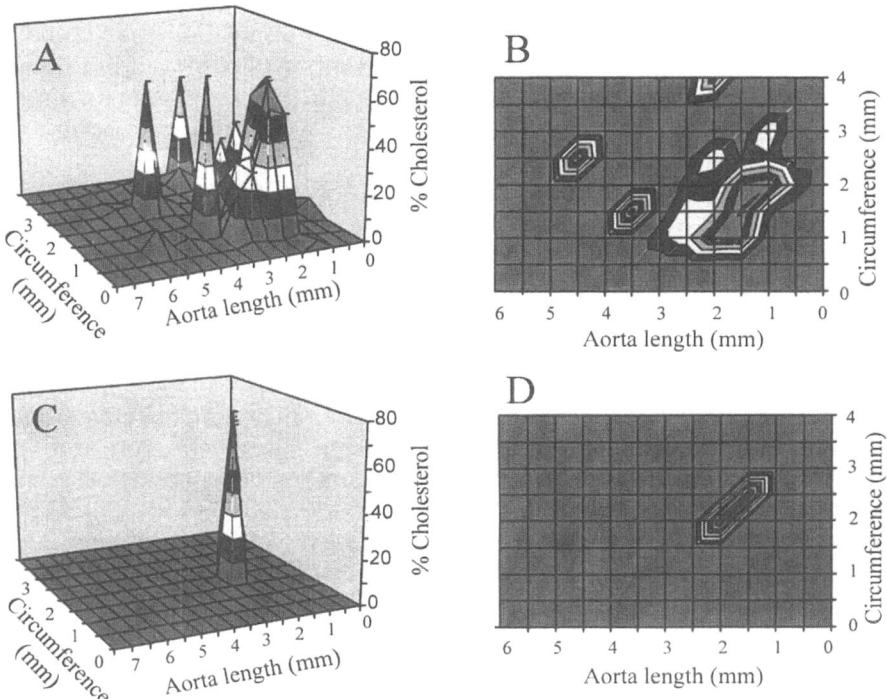

Figure 9. *Accumulation of cholesterol in the aorta of a APOE*3-Leiden transgenic mouse, just distally of the aortic valve, quantified with Raman spectroscopy. (9A, and top view 9B). In the centre of the plaque, a calcium salts deposit was found and quantified with Raman spectroscopy (9C and top view 9D).*

caps.

The applications in cardiology of Raman spectroscopy techniques will be probably widespread, and we discussed some exploratory studies to illustrate its potential. This technique, combined with intravascular ultrasound, may be used to map the chemical composition of an arterial wall. Raman spectroscopy can provide a detailed chemical map of atherosclerotic lesions developed in transgenic mice, which may be used to monitor and evaluate the effects of lipid lowering agents on plaque progression and regression.

Raman spectroscopy is reproducible, objective and thus independent of intra- and inter-observer variability. Cardiovascular studies with Raman spectroscopy have been performed *in vitro* with arterial tissue, but successful *in vivo* measurements have been impeded by the high background noise generated by scattering within the optical fibers used to construct

194

intravascular Raman probes. Once *in vivo* measurements are possible, the clinician will be provided with unprecedented capabilities that could serve many purposes, such as monitoring the effects of lipid lowering therapies, locating rupture-prone lesions, and identifying lesions prone to restenosis following angioplasty.

Acknowledgement

The Raman spectroscopy model development and histological comparison studies were done at the MIT Spectroscopy Laboratory (Cambridge, MA, U.S.A.) with financial support from the National Institutes of Health (NIH R01-HL51265 & NIH P41-RR02594). The remaining work was done at the Cardiology department and Gaubius Laboratory / TNO-PG at the Leiden University Medical Center, Leiden, The Netherlands, and Laboratory for Intensive Care Research and Optical Spectroscopy at the Dijkzigt Hospital, Rotterdam, The Netherlands, with financial support from the Netherlands Heart Foundation (R93.310 and 95.134). Many collaborators were involved in this work, but we wish to thank Michael Feld, John Kramer, Gerwin Puppels, Arnoud van der Laarse and Albert Bruschke in particular.

References

1. Small DM. George Lyman Duff memorial lecture. Progression and regression of atherosclerotic lesions. Insights from lipid physical biochemistry. Arteriosclerosis 1988;8:103-29.
2. Steinberg D, Witztum JL. Lipoproteins and atherogenesis. JAMA 1990;264:3047-52.
3. Stary HC. Composition and classification of human atherosclerosis. Virchows Archiv A Pathol Anat 1992;421:277-90.
4. Loree HM, Tobias BJ, Gibson LJ, Kamm RD, Small DM, Lee RT. Mechanical properties of model atherosclerotic lesion lipid pools. Arterioscler Thromb 1994;14:230-4.
5. Libby P. Molecular bases of the acute coronary syndromes. Circulation 1995;91:2844-50.
6. Manoharan R, Baraga JJ, Rava RP, Dasari RR, Fitzmaurice M, Feld MS. Biochemical analysis and mapping of atherosclerotic human artery using FT-IR microspectroscopy. Atherosclerosis 1993;103:181-93.
7. Manoharan R, Baraga JJ, Feld MS, Rava RP. Quantitative histochemical analysis of human artery using Raman spectroscopy. J Photochem Photobiol B 1992;16:211-33.
8. Baraga JJ, Feld MS, Rava RP. Rapid near-infrared Raman spectroscopy of human tissue with a spectrograph and a CCD detector. Appl Spectrosc 1992;46:187-90.
9. Baraga JJ, Feld MS, Rava RP. In situ optical histochemistry of human artery using near infrared Fourier transform Raman spectroscopy. Proc Natl Acad Sci USA 1992;89:3473-7.

10. Brennan III JFB, Wang Y, Dasari RR, Feld MS. Near-infrared Raman spectrometer systems for human tissue studies. Applied Spec 1997:201-8.
11. Kramer JR, Brennan III JF, Römer TJ, Wang Y, Dasari RR, Feld MS. Spectral diagnosis of human coronary artery: A clinical system for real time analysis. Proc. BIOS/SPIE 1995(2305):376-82.
12. Brennan III JF, Römer TJ, Tercyak AM et al. In situ histochemical analysis of human coronary artery by Raman spectroscopy compared with biochemical assay. Proc. BIOS/SPIE 1995(2388):105-9.
13. Brennan III JF, Römer TJ, Lees RS, Tercyak AM, Kramer JR Jr., Feld MS. Determination of human coronary artery composition by Raman spectroscopy. Circulation 1997:In press.
14. Römer TJ, Brennan III JF, Fitzmaurice M et al. Histopathology of human coronary atherosclerosis by quantifying its chemical composition with Raman spectroscopy. Circulation 1997:In press.
15. Carey PR. Biochemical applications of Raman and resonance Raman spectroscopy. New York: Academic press, 1982.
16. Tu AT. Raman spectroscopy in biology. New York: John Wiley and Sons, 1982.
17. Fehrmann A, Franz M, Hoffmann A, Rudzik L, Wust E. Dairy product analysis: identification of microorganisms by mid-infrared spectroscopy and determination of constituents by Raman spectroscopy. J AOAC Int 1995;78:1537-42.
18. Nave SE, O'Rourke PE, Toole WR. Sampling probes enhance remote chemical analysis. Laser Focus World 1995;12:83-8.
19. Yaroslavsky IV, Yaroslavsky AN, Otto C et al. Combined elastic and Raman light scattering of human eye lenses. Exp Eye Res 1994;59:393-9.
20. Duindam HJ, Vrensen GF, Otto C, Puppels GJ, Greve J. New approach to assess the cholesterol distribution in the eye lens: confocal Raman microspectroscopy and filipin cytochemistry. J Lipid Res 1995;36:1139-46.
21. Thomas GJ Jr., Agard DA. Quantitative analysis of nucleic acids, proteins, and viruses by Raman band deconvolution. Biophys J 1984;46:763-8.
22. van der Veen MH, ten Bosch JJ. The influence of mineral loss on the auto-fluorescent behaviour of in vitro demineralised dentine. Caries Res 1996;30:93-9.
23. Tsuda H, Ruben J, Arends J. Raman spectra of human dentin mineral. Eur J Oral Sci 1996;104:123-31.
24. Puppels GJ, de Mul FF, Otto C et al. Studying single living cells and chromosomes by confocal Raman microspectroscopy. Nature 1990;347:301-3.
25. Bakker Schut TC, Puppels GJ, Kraan YM, Greve J, van der Maas LL, Figdor CG. Intracellular carotenoid levels measured by Raman microspectroscopy: comparison of lymphocytes from lung cancer patients and healthy individuals. Int J Cancer 1997;74:20-5.
26. Egeberg KD, Springer BA, Martinis SA, Sligar SG, Morikis D, Champion PM. Alteration of sperm whale myoglobin heme axial ligation by site-directed mutagenesis. Biochemistry 1990;29:9783-91.
27. Peticolas WL. Raman spectroscopy of DNA and proteins. Methods Enzymol 1995;246:389-416.
28. Lewis IR, Griffiths PR. Raman spectrometry with fiber-optic sampling. Applied Spec 1996;50:12A-30A.
29. Loudon. The quantum theory of light. (2nd ed.) Oxford: Oxford Science Pub., 1991.
30. Marcuse. Principles of quantum electronics. New York: Academic Press, 1980.
31. Yariv A. Quantum electronics. (3rd ed.) New York: John Wiley & Sons, 1975.

32. Chakravarti RN. Fifty years of Raman effect: 1928-1978. J Inst Chem (India) 1978.
33. Raman CV. A new radiation. Indian J Phys 1928;2:387-98.
34. Raman CV, Krishnan KS. A new type of secondary radiation. Nature 1928;121:501-2.
35. Raman CV. A change of wave-length in light scattering. Nature 1928;121:618.
36. Raman CV. The molecular scattering of light. Nobel Lecture. Stockholm: Imprimerie Royale, P.A. Norstedt, 1930.
37. Brennan III JF. Near infrared Raman spectroscopy for human artery histochemistry and histopathology . Cambridge: Massachusetts Institute of Technology, 1995.
38. Römer TJ, Brennan III JF, Bakker Schut TC et al. How deeply can near-infrared Raman spectroscopy detect cholesterol deposits in coronary arteries? Manuscript in preparation 1997.
39. Tracy RE, Kissling GE. Age and fibroplasia as preconditions for atheronecrosis in human coronary arteries. Arch Pathol Lab Med 1987;111:957-63.
40. Peters RJG, Kok WEM, Havenith MG, Rijsterborgh H, van der Wal AC, Visser CA. Histopathologic validation of intracoronary ultrasound imaging. J Am Soc Echocardiography 1994;7:230-41.
41. Mintz GS, Popma JJ, Pichard AD et al. Patterns of calcification in coronary artery disease. A statistical analysis of intravascular ultrasound and coronary angiography in 1155 lesions. Circulation 1995;91:1959-65.
42. Nissen SE, Gurley JC, Booth DC, De Maria AN. Intravascular ultrasound of the coronary arteries: current applications and future directions. Am J Cardiol 1992;69:18H-29H.
43. Nissen SE, De Franco AC, Tuzco EM, Molitherno DJ. Coronary intravascular ultrasound: diagnostic and interventional applications. Coronary artery disease 1995;6:355-67.
44. Benkeser PJ, Churchwell AL, Lee C, Abouelnasr D. Resolution limitations in intravascular ultrasound imaging. J Am Soc Echocardiogr 1993;6:158-65.
45. Groot PH, van Vlijmen BJ, Benson GM et al. Quantitative assessment of aortic atherosclerosis in APOE*3 Leiden transgenic mice and its relationship to serum cholesterol exposure. Arterioscler Thromb Vasc Biol 1996;16:926-33.
46. Jukema JW, Zwinderman AH, van Boven AJ et al. Evidence for a synergistic effect of calcium channel blockers with lipid-lowering therapy in retarding progression of coronary atherosclerosis in symptomatic patients with normal to moderately raised cholesterol levels. The REGRESS Study Group. Arterioscler Thromb Vasc Biol 1996;16:425-30.

MODULATION OF ARTERIOSCLEROSIS BY GENE-THERAPY

Theo J.C. van Berkel, Miranda van Eck, Nicole Herijgers,
Peter M. Hoogerbrugge, Pieter H.E. Groot

Summary

Abnormalities in plasma lipoprotein metabolism are mostly based upon
specific gene defects. Gene therapy forms the ultimate treatment of these
disorders. The present data, focused upon the treatment of apolipoprotein
E (ApoE) and LDL-receptor deficiency are the first examples of and analysis
of gene-replacement on the development atherosclerotic lesions.
Inactivation of the apoE gene in mice leads to a prominent increase in serum
cholesterol and triglyceride levels and the development of premature
atherosclerosis. The role of monocyte/macrophage-derived apoE in
atherogenesis was assessed by bone marrow transplantation in apoE-
deficient mice, using donor bone marrow of wild-type mice. Quantitation of
atherosclerotic lesions in the aortic root, after 4 months of "Western-type"
diet, revealed that the mean lesion area was approximately 10-fold smaller
in mice transplanted with bone marrow from wild-type donors as compared
to control apoE-deficient mice.
The influence of apoE gene-dosage on serum lipid concentrations was
determined by transplantation with homozygous apoE-deficient,
heterozygous apoE-deficient and wild-type bone marrow. The concentration
of apoE, detected in serum, was found to be gene-dosage dependent, being
$3.52 \pm 0.74\%$, $1.87 \pm 74\%$ and 0% of normal in transplanted mice receiving
either wild-type, heterozygote apoE-deficient, or homozygous apoE-deficient
bone marrow, respectively. These low concentrations of apoE nevertheless
reduced serum cholesterol levels dramatically due to a reduction of VLDL,

E.E. van der Wall et al. (eds.), Vascular Medicine, 197-218.
© 1997 *Kluwer Academic Publishers.*

and to a lesser extent, of LDL, while HDL levels were slightly raised.

The relative importance of the LDLR on macrophages for lipoprotein metabolism and atherogenesis was assessed by transplantation of LDLR knockout (-/-) mice with bone marrow of normal C57Bl mice. The transplantation resulted in a decrease of total serum cholesterol of maximally 27% when compared to LDLR-/- mice which were transplanted with LDLR-/- bone marrow. This decrease can almost completely be attributed to a decrease in LDL-cholesterol. The specific lowering of LDL-cholesterol was more pronounced 4 weeks after transplantation than 12 weeks after transplantation.

Quantitation of atherosclerotic lesions of mice fed a 1% cholesterol diet for 6 months, revealed that there were no differences in mean lesion area between mice transplanted with wild-type bone marrow or LDLR-/- bone marrow. We anticipate that in the LDLR-/- mice transplanted with wild-type bone marrow, the LDLR is down-regulated by the relatively high concentrations of circulating cholesterol. *In vitro* incubations of peritoneal microphages with ^{125}I-LDL indicated that the LDLR of these cells could be downregulated by 25-OH cholesterol. Peritoneal macrophages isolated from LDLR-/- mice transplanted with wild-type bone marrow, in contrast to those transplanted with LDLR-/- bone marrow, were able to degrade ^{125}I-LDL, indicating that the capacity to express functional LDLR was achieved. In conclusion, introduction of the LDLR in LDLR-/- mice via bone marrow transplantation resulted in a relatively modest decrease of LDL-cholesterol, while apoE expressing bone marrow dramatically reduced serum cholesterol levels in apoE-deficient mice. Atherosclerotic lesions in apoE deficient mice were 10-fold smaller in mice transpanted with bone marrow from wild-type donor, establishing the anti-atherogenic role of macrophage-associated apoE production.

Introduction

Abnormalities in plasma lipoprotein metabolism are mostly based upon specific gene defects. The ultimate treatment is clearly related to correction of the specific gene by gene-therapy protocols. Initial experiments are establishing that more fundamental and basic research is needed to understand the persistence and regulation of gene expression before clinical protocols can be developed. The present data, focused upon the treatment of apoE and LDL-receptor deficiency, are the first examples of an analysis of the effect of gene replacement on the development of atherosclerotic lesions.

Abnormalities in plasma lipoprotein metabolism, including defects in the gene encoding for apoE, form a well-defined risk factor for atherosclerosis. Apo E, a 34 kDa arginine-rich protein, plays an important role in lipoprotein metabolism. It serves as a high affinity ligand for several receptor systems in the liver, including the low density lipoprotein (LDL) receptor, LDL receptor-related protein (LRP), remnant receptor, and/or proteoglycans[1-3]. Structural mutations in the apoE gene, associated with a loss in binding affinity for lipoprotein receptors, can result in the development of type III hyperlipoproteinemia (HLP)[4-6]. Type III HLP is characterized by elevated serum cholesterol levels and premature coronary heart disease due to accumulation of atherogenic, apoE containing lipoproteins, such as chylomicron remnants and very low density lipoprotein (VLDL) remnants (ßVLDL). Compared to VLDL remnants and chylomicron remnants, ßVLDL is relatively enriched in apoE and cholesteryl esters and does exert ß-electrophoretic mobility on agarose gels. A rare genetic disorder also leading to the development of type III HLP, is the complete deficiency in apoE[7-10]. Mice, deficient in apoE, have been generated by targeted inactivation of the apoE gene in mouse embryonic stem cells[11-13]. Inactivation of the apoE gene in these mice is associated with a prominent increase in serum cholesterol levels and the development of premature atherosclerosis. ApoE-deficient mice provide a unique model to study the relation between apoE production and atherogenesis.

The role of macrophage apoE synthesis in the clearance of cholesterol from the circulation can be studied using bone marrow transplantation (BMT). BMT can be used to introduce wild-type haematopoietic stem cells into an apoE-deficient recipient. In this animal model, apoE synthesis will be limited to haematopoietic cells of the monocyte/macrophage lineage. Therefore, using this highly specialised technique, it is possible to study specifically the role of apoE secretion by these cell types in lipoprotein metabolism.

The aim of the present study was to determine the effect of apoE gene-dosage in cells of monocyte/macrophage cell lineage on hypercholesterolemia and to delineate the mechanism of the highly efficient lowering in serum cholesterol levels after BMT. To attain this, bone marrow of wild-type, heterozygous and homozygous apoE-deficient donors was transplanted into irradiated apoE-deficient mice. Our results indicate that macrophage-derived apoE can reduce cholesterol and triglyceride levels dose-dependently by increasing the uptake of (ß)VLDL by parenchymal cells of the liver.

Familial hypercholesterolemia (FH) is a common hereditary disorder, which is characterized by the absence or decrease of active LDL receptors[14,15]. The plasma levels of LDL in these patients are elevated, resulting in hypercholesterolemia and premature atherosclerosis. Recently, Herz and co-workers developed a mouse model for homozygous FH through targeted disruption of the LDL receptor gene: the LDL receptor knockout (LDLR-/-) mouse[16]. The total plasma cholesterol levels in these mice appeared to be twofold higher than those of wild-type littermates, mainly as a consequence of an increase in IDL and LDL, while the clearance of VLDL, IDL and LDL from the plasma was delayed. On a cholesterol-rich diet, these mice exhibit massive xanthomatosis and atherosclerosis[17]. Therefore, they form an excellent model to investigate the role of the LDL receptor in lipoprotein metabolism.

Uptake of LDL by Kupffer cells does not result in intracellular accumulation of cholesterol esters, because it is coupled to transport to liver parenchymal cells and biliary secretion[18,19]. These cells, thus, can form a potentially important target for the treatment of FH. Bone marrow transplantation thereby allows the specific study of the role of the LDL receptor on Kupffer cells and other macrophages in the clearance of cholesterol from the circulation. Introduction of wild-type hematopoietic stem cells into irradiated LDLR-/- mice may lead to the appearance of cells of hematopoietic origin with an intact LDL receptor gene.

Results

Effect of bone marrow transplantation on serum cholesterol in apo E-deficient mice

The effect of bone marrow transplantation (BMT) of apoE-deficient mice with marrow from wild-type mice (apoE$^{+/+}$ $^{-/-}$) or apoE-deficient animals (apoE$^{-/-}$ $^{-/-}$) on serum lipids is shown in Figure 1. Even on a normal chow diet apoE-deficient mice demonstrate a marked hyperlipidemia, and transplantation with apoE$^{+/+}$ bone marrow decreases serum cholesterol levels by more than 75% over a 4 week period.

Observing the dramatic specific decrease in cholesterol levels upon apoE$^{+/+}$ $^{-/-}$ BMT, we also incorporated studies on the transplantation of bone marrow from heterozygous apoE deficient mice. Thus, either apoE$^{-/-}$, apoE$^{+/-}$, or apoE$^{+/+}$ bone marrow was transplanted into apoE^{-} recipients. Heterozygous apoE$^{+/-}$ as well as wild-type apoE$^{+/+}$ bone marrow was very efficient in lowering cholesterol and triglyceride levels. Four weeks after transplantation, the control transplantation apoE$^{-/-}$ $^{-/-}$ induced a decrease of 13.4% and 35.8% for total cholesterol and triglyceride levels, respectively. ApoE$^{+/-}$ bone marrow induced decreases of 81.6% and 51.9%, respectively, while apoE$^{+/+}$ bone marrow induced decreases of 90.8% and 72.3%, respectively. Serum cholesterol and triglyceride levels remained lowered over the period of 4-10 weeks following transplantation, suggesting that the chimeric status in the transplanted animals is stable (Figure 1).

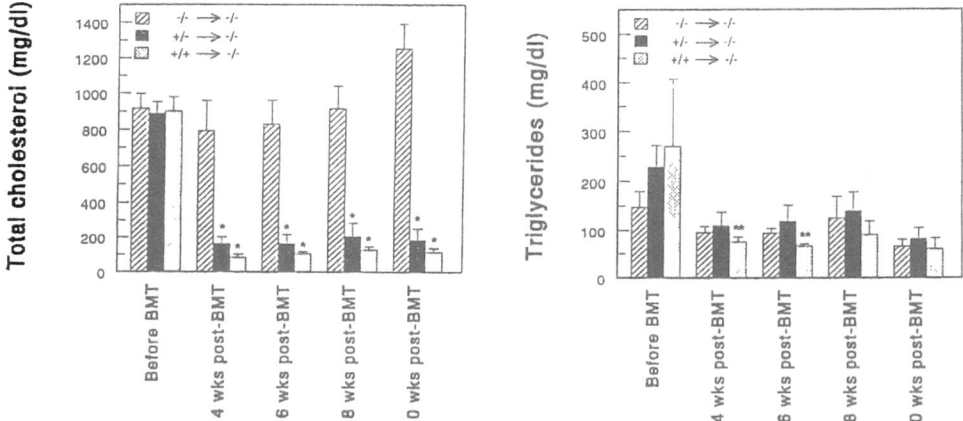

Figure 1. Effect of apoE gene-dosage in BMT of ApoE-deficient mice on total serum cholesterol (A) and triglyceride levels (B). Female apoE$^{-/-}$ mice were transplanted with apoE$^{-/-}$ (hatched bars), apoE$^{+/-}$ (closed bars) or apoE$^{+/+}$ (dotted bars) bone marrow. Values are means ± sd of at least five mice. *P < 0.001 versus control. **P < 0.05 versus apoE$^{+/-\ to\ -/-}$.

Effect of BMT in apo E-deficient mice on serum lipoproteins

The effect of BMT on serum lipoprotein profiles was analyzed 5 weeks after transplantation. Serum lipoproteins were fractionated for each animal by liquid chromatography. The lowering of serum cholesterol levels upon BMT was mainly due to a dramatic decrease in cholesterol, associated with the VLDL fraction, while LDL levels were lowered to a lesser extent (Figure 2). This effect was accompanied by a small increase in HDL levels. The lowering of triglyceride levels was solely caused by a decrease in VLDL levels (data not shown).

The concentration of apoE measured in serum of apoE$^{+/+\ -\ -/-}$ mice was 3.52 ± 0.74% of the concentration from wild-type mice, whereas the concentration was approximately 2-fold lower (1.87 ± 0.37%) if apoE$^{+/-}$ bone marrow was used (mean ± sd; n = 5-6). To illustrate the effect of gene-dosage further, the apoE levels in the three transplantation groups are plotted against the corresponding cholesterol concentration in VLDL, LDL, and HDL for each individual mouse (Figure 3). A marked reciprocal lowering of cholesterol, associated with VLDL and LDL, with increasing serum apoE concentrations was evident, while HDL demonstrated a dose dependent increase. A serum concentration of 3.52 ± 0.74% of that from normal C57Bl/6 mice, induced approximately a 25-fold decrease in VLDL cholesterol and a 5-fold decrease in LDL cholesterol. In addition, HDL cholesterol increased 2.5-fold.

202

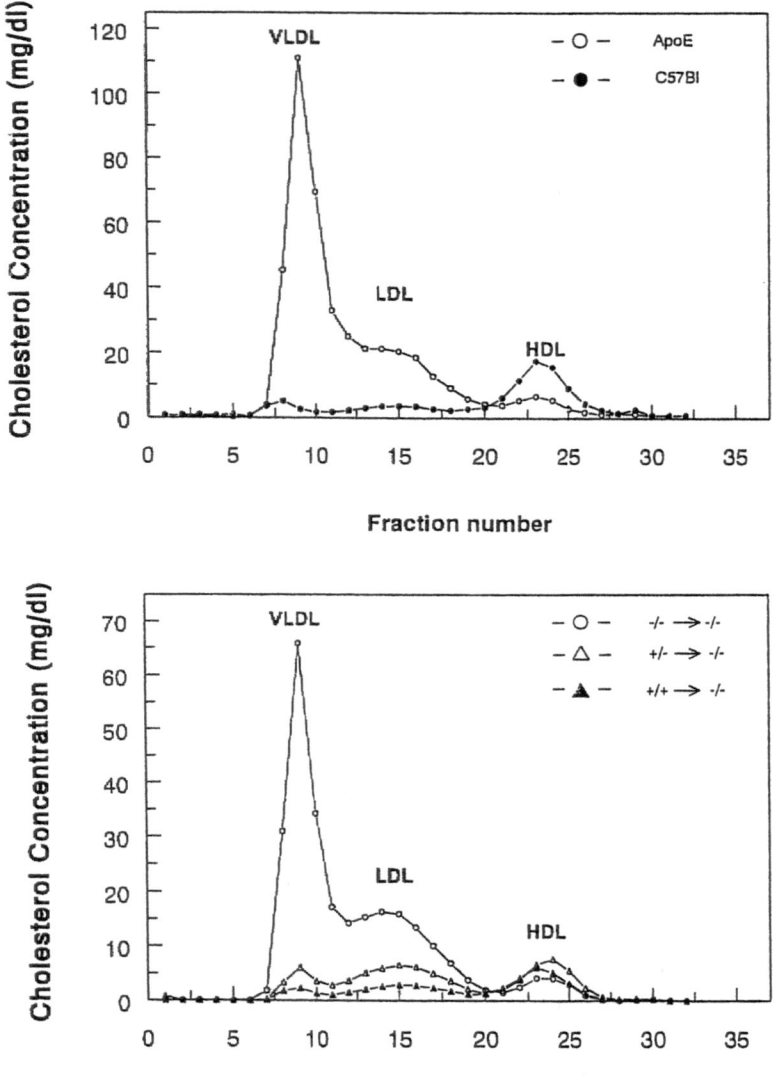

Figure 2. Effect of apoE gene-dosage in BMT on the distribution of serum lipoprotein cholesterol in apoE-deficient mice. Blood samples were drawn by tail bleeding after an overnight fasting period. A 30 μl aliquot of serum of each individual mouse was loaded onto a Pharmacia Smart column and fractions were collected. Fractions 7-12 represent VLDL and chylomicrons, fractions 13-20 LDL, and fractions 21-27 HDL. Panel A shows the distribution of cholesterol over lipoproteins in control apoE-deficient (○; n = 4) and C57Bl/6 (●; n = 2) mice. Panel B shows the distribution in transplanted apoE-deficient mice (n = 5-6) 5 weeks after BMT. Open circles represent transplantation with apoE$^{-/-}$ bone marrow (○), open triangles apoE$^{+/-}$ bone marrow (△) and closed triangles apoE$^{+/+}$ bone marrow (▲).

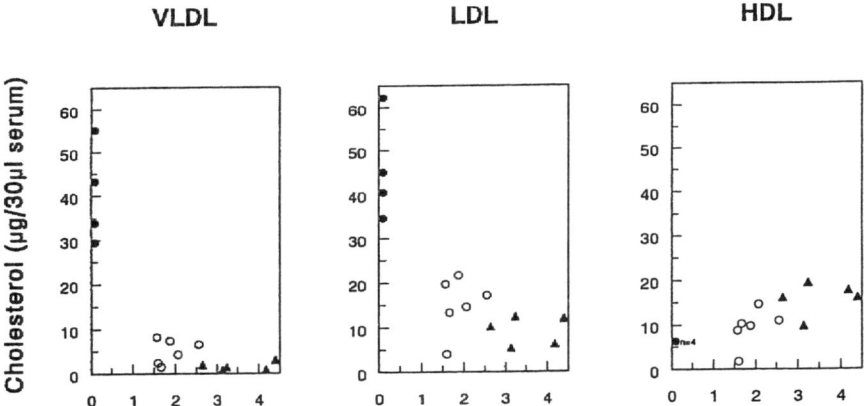

Figure 3. *Effect of the apoE concentration in mouse serum on the amount of cholesterol in VLDL, LDL and HDL. Serum was isolated 5 weeks after transplantation from apoE-deficient mice with either apoE⁻/⁻, apoE⁺/⁻ or apoE⁺/⁺ bone marrow. An aliquot of 30 μl was analysed by gel filtration on a Pharmacia Smart column and cholesterol distribution over the lipoproteins was determined. The amount of cholesterol in the different lipoprotein fractions was calculated from the area under the curve. Closed circles (●) represent cholesterol levels in the different lipoprotein fractions for apoE⁻ ⁻ ⁻/⁻, open circles (O) for apoE⁺/⁻ ⁻ ⁻/⁻ and closed triangles (▲) for apoE⁺/⁺ ⁻ ⁻/⁻.*

Effect of BMT in apo E-deficient mice on atherosclerosis

To assess the effect of transplantation of wild-type bone marrow into apoE⁻/⁻ mice on atherosclerosis, transplanted mice, control apoE⁻/⁻ and C57Bl/6 mice were fed a "Western-type" diet. After 4 months, the hearts and aortas were perfused, fixed and examined histologically. Representative photomicrographs of lesions in cross sections of the aortic root are shown in Figure 4 and the measured mean lesion area is shown in Figure 5. Cross sections of control apoE⁻/⁻ and apoE⁻ ⁻ ⁻/⁻ mice showed extensive lipid-rich lesions (Figures 4B,C), whereas hardly any lesions could be demonstrated in the sections of C57Bl/6 mice (Figure 4A). The mean lesion area in apoE⁺/⁺ ⁻ ⁻/⁻ mice (Figures 4D) was approximately 10-fold reduced in size compared to control apoE⁻/⁻ and apoE⁻ ⁻ ⁻/⁻ mice. Atherosclerosis was also visualised throughout the aortic tree by staining with Sudan IV, a lipid stain. In accordance with the results obtained in cross sections at the aortic root, extensive lesions were seen in apoE⁻ ⁻ ⁻/⁻ mice, whereas only a few fatty streaks can be seen in apoE⁺/⁺ ⁻ ⁻/⁻ mice (Figure 6). In apoE⁻ ⁻ ⁻/⁻ mice, lesions were observed in the aortic arch and coronary arteries, as well as at branch sites along the whole aorta, while in the apoE⁺/⁺ ⁻ ⁻/⁻ mice these sites were relatively unaffected.

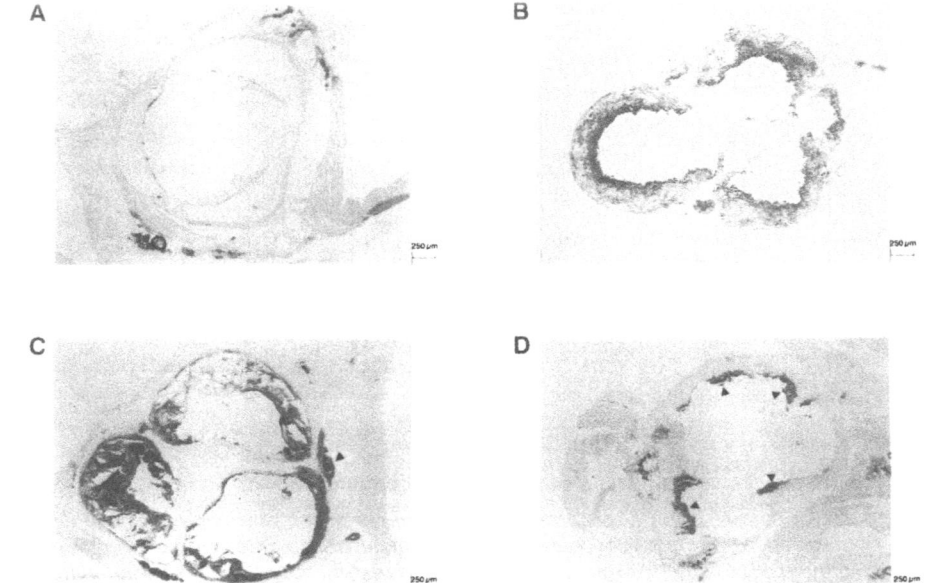

Figure 4. *Visualization of atherosclerosis in cross-sections at the aortic sinuses on the level of the three cups of control C57Bl/6, apoE$^{-/-}$ and transplanted mice, fed a "Western-type" diet for 4 months. Sections are stained with oil red O to visualize lipid rich lesion areas. Panel A shows a section from a control C57Bl/6 mouse without lesions. Panel B shows severe lipid-rich lesions in an apoE$^{-/-}$ mouse. Panel C shows a section from an apoE$^{-/- \to -/-}$ mouse with extensive lipid-rich lesions in both the aortic sinus and in a coronary artery (arrow). In panel D it is demonstrated that transplantation with wildtype bone marrow into an apoE$^{-/-}$ animal (apoE$^{+/+ \to -/-}$) results in a large reduction of the lesion area. Arrows indicate the localization of lesions in apoE$^{+/+ \to -/-}$ mice (D) and lesions in the coronary artery in apoE$^{-/- \to -/-}$ mice (C). Magnification x40.*
(For colour plate of figure 4 see page 222)

Effect of BMT in LDL-receptor deficient mice on total serum cholesterol level
During the weeks after BMT the total serum cholesterol levels of the transplanted mice were determined repeatedly. The results are shown in Figure 7. Four weeks after BMT, the cholesterol level decreased in both the (+/+ to -/-) transplanted mice and the (-/- to -/-) transplanted mice as compared to the non-transplanted LDLR-/- mice. Because the decrease was present in both transplanted groups it suggests an effect of BMT itself. The decrease in the (-/- to -/-) group, however, lasted only till week 6 after BMT and was maximally 26% (p≤0.05) compared to the untreated group. In contrast, in the (+/+ to -/-) group the effect continued throughout the experiment (12 weeks) and reached a maximum decrease in week 6 of 42% (p≤0.001) in comparison with the control group. When compared to the (-/-

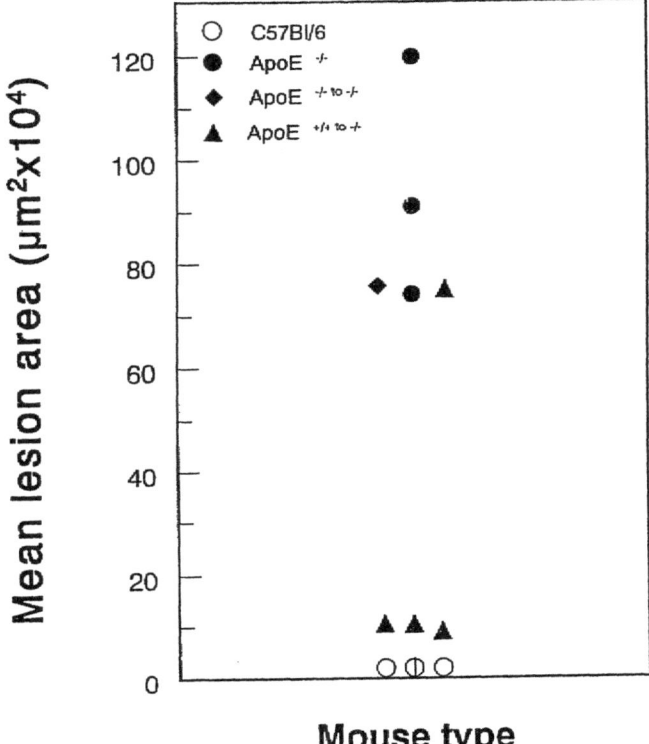

Figure 5. Areas of atherosclerotic lesions at the aortic root C57Bl/6 mice, in apoE-deficient mice, and mice transplanted with either apoE$^{/-}$ or apoE$^{+/+}$ bone marrow, after 4 months of feeding a "Western type" diet. The mean lesion area was calculated from 10 oil red O stained sections per mouse.

to -/-) group, the (+/+ to -/-) group has lower total cholesterol values, which were significant in week 6 and 12 after BMT. The decrease was maximally 27% (p≤0.001).

These data, thus, show that introduction of the LDLR in Kupffer cells and other macrophages in LDLR-/- mice results in a decrease of total serum cholesterol, although this is not sufficient to normalize the cholesterol levels.

Effect of BMT in LDL-receptor deficient mice on the distribution of serum lipoprotein cholesterol

The effect of BMT on the distribution of serum cholesterol over the different lipoproteins was analyzed by liquid chromatography. Four weeks after BMT the (+/+ to -/-) group showed a considerable decrease in LDL-cholesterol; this decrease was 46% (p≤0.001) compared to the non-transplanted LDLR-/-

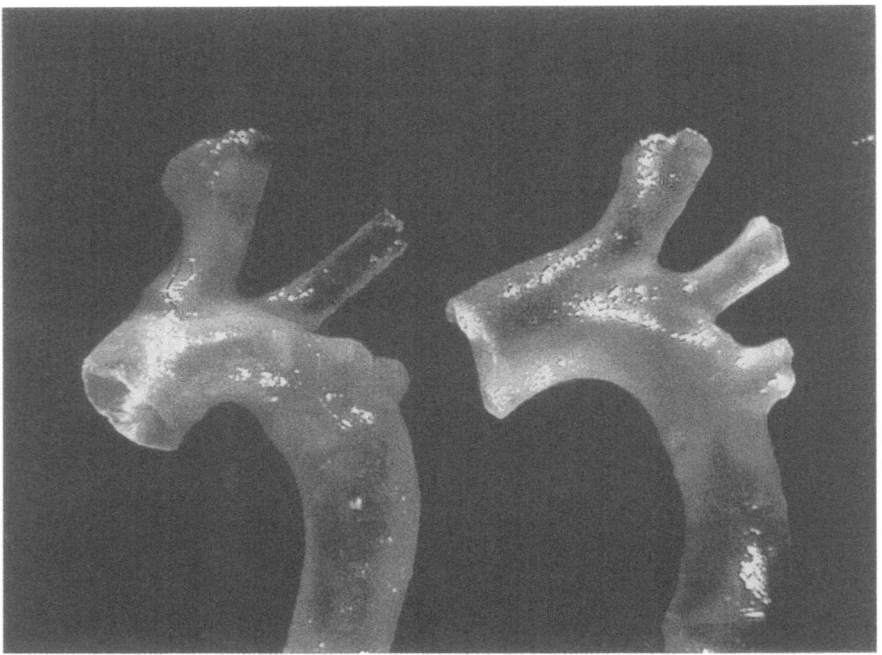

Figure 6. *Atherosclerotic lesions in aortas in apoE$^{/-}$ mice, transplanted with apoE$^{/-}$ or apoE$^{+/+}$ bone marrow, both fed a "Western-type" diet for 4 months. Aortas were perfusion-fixed with neutral-buffered formalin and stained with Sudan IV to visualize lipid rich lesions. An enlargement of the aortic arch of apoE$^{/-}$ mice transplanted with apoE$^{/-}$ (left) or apoE$^{+/+}$ (right) bone marrow is shown. Magnification x15.* (For colour plate of figure 6 see page 221)

mice and 37% (p≤0.01) compared to the (-/- to -/-) group (Figure 8A). Although the decrease in LDL-cholesterol of the (+/+ to -/-) group is evident, the level still remains higher than that of the control C57Bl/6J mice (Figure 8B). The amount of cholesterol in HDL remained unchanged after BMT.

Twelve weeks after BMT, the (+/+ to -/-) group showed a decrease of 22% in LDL cholesterol (p≤0.05) in comparison to the control LDLR-/- mice and 19% (p≤0.05) in comparison to the (-/- to -/-) group (Figure 8C). When compared to 4 weeks after BMT, the (+/+ to -/-) group, however, had a less pronounced decrease in LDL-cholesterol. Again, no significant difference in HDL-cholesterol was observed.

These lipoprotein profiles, thus, show that introduction of the LDLR in hematopoietic cells of LDLR-/-mice lower cholesterol content of LDL and that this lowering was more pronounced at 4 weeks after BMT than at 12 weeks after BMT.

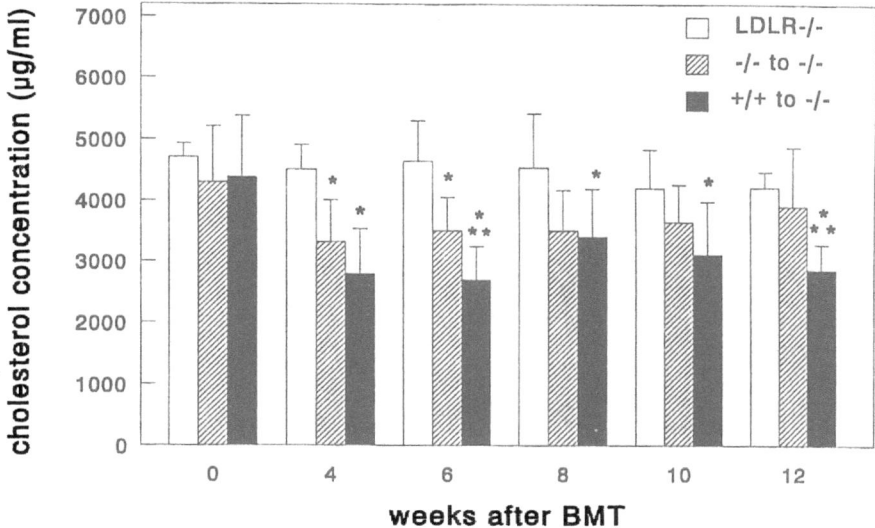

Figure 7. *Effect of BMT on total serum cholesterol levels in LDLR-/- mice. Cholesterol levels were measured at the indicated time points after transplantation of LDLR-/- bone marrow (hatched bars; n = 14) or wild-type bone marrow (closed bars; n = 20) into female LDLR-/- mice, or non-transplanted control LDLR-/- mice (open bars; n = 4). Values are means ± SD. * indicates significant differences vs. non-transplanted control LDLR-/- mice (p≤0.001). ** indicates significant differences vs. (-/- to -/-) transplanted mice (p≤0.05).*

Effect of BMT in LDL-receptor deficient mice on ^{125}I-LDL metabolism by peritoneal macrophages

Synthesis of the LDL receptor is susceptible to feedback inhibition by intracellular cholesterol[20]. Since LDLR-/- mice have elevated serum cholesterol levels[16] it might be possible that the LDLR that has been introduced in LDLR-/- mice by BMT is (partially) downregulated. It is therefore of interest to investigate whether macrophages in LDLR-/- mice which are transplanted with wild-type bone marrow potentially have obtained the capacity to express functional LDLR, and whether this LDLR can be down-regulated by cholesterol. To address this question, peritoneal macrophages were isolated from mice at 20-25 weeks after BMT and these cells were cultured for two days in medium containing lipoprotein deficient serum to induce a maximal expression of LDLR.

In Figure 9A the degradation of ^{125}I-LDL is shown. The degradation by macrophages of the (-/- to -/-) group is comparable to that by the macrophages of the LDLR-/- mice. Macrophages of the (+/+ to -/-) group show a 6 fold increase in degradation, although it is not as high as that of the macrophages of C57Bl6 mice (88%). When preincubated with increasing

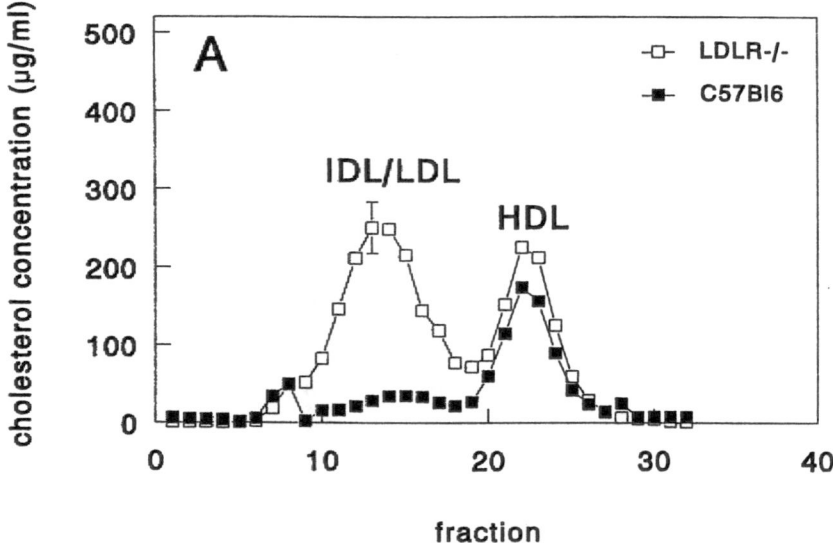

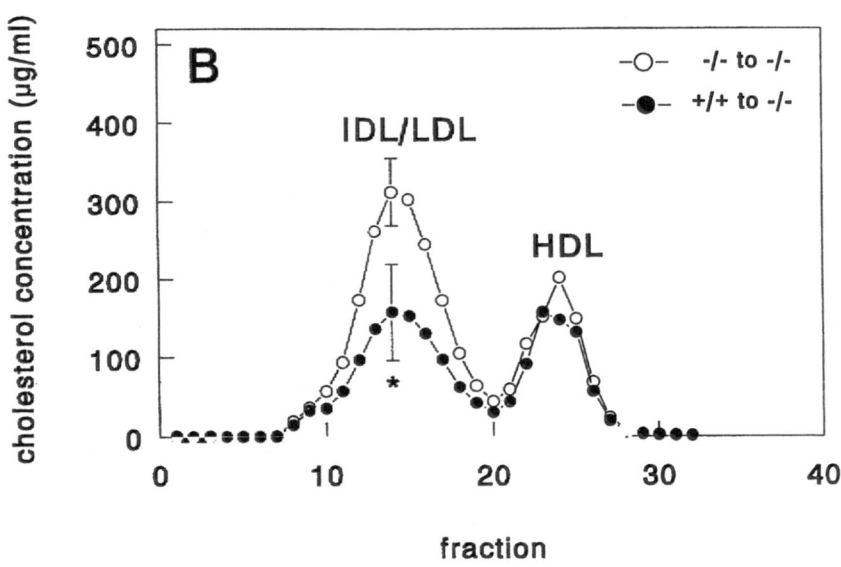

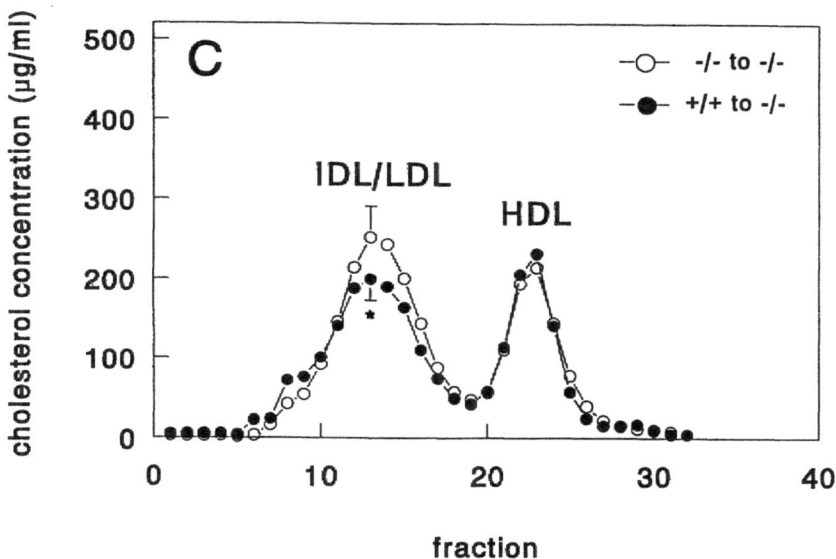

Figure 8. *Effect of BMT on the distribution of serum lipoprotein cholesterol over various lipoprotein fractions in control and transplanted LDLR-/- mice. Sera of individual mice were analysed on a Pharmacia Smart column. Fraction 7 to 12 represent VLDL and chylomicrons, fraction 13 to 20, IDL and LDL, and fractions 21 to 27, HDL. Panel A shows the distribution of cholesterol in control C57Bl6 and LDLR-/- mice. Panels B and C show the distribution in transplanted mice at 4 [B] and 12 [C] weeks after transplantation, respectively. Open squares represent LDLR-/- mice (□; n = 4), closed squares represent C57Bl/6J mice (■; n = 2), open circles represent LDLR-/- mice transplanted with LDLR-/- bone marrow (O; n = 6) and closed circles represent LDLR-/- mice transplanted with wild-type bone marrow (●; n = 5). For clarity reasons, only the SD of the fraction containing the top of the IDL/LDL cholesterol peak is given. * indicates significant differences vs. (-/- to -/-) transplanted mice (p≤0.01 [fig. 4B]; p≤0.05 [fig. 4C]).*

concentrations of 25-OH cholesterol, the degradation of ^{125}I-LDL by macrophages of C57Bl6 mice was decreased (Figure 9B), whereas the degradation by macrophages of LDLR-/- mice remained constantly low. This indicates that the LDLR on peritoneal macrophages is susceptible to downregulation by 25-OH-cholesterol. It thus appears that peritoneal macrophages of (+/+ to -/-) transplanted mice, in contrast to (-/- to -/-) transplanted mice, do have the capacity to express functional LDLR and that this LDLR can be down regulated by 25-OH-cholesterol.

Effect of BMT in LDL-receptor deficient mice on atherosclerosis
To investigate the effect of introduction of the LDL receptor in LDLR-/- mice on the development of atherosclerotic lesions via bone marrow transplantation, transplanted mice, control LDLR-/-, and C57Bl/6J mice were

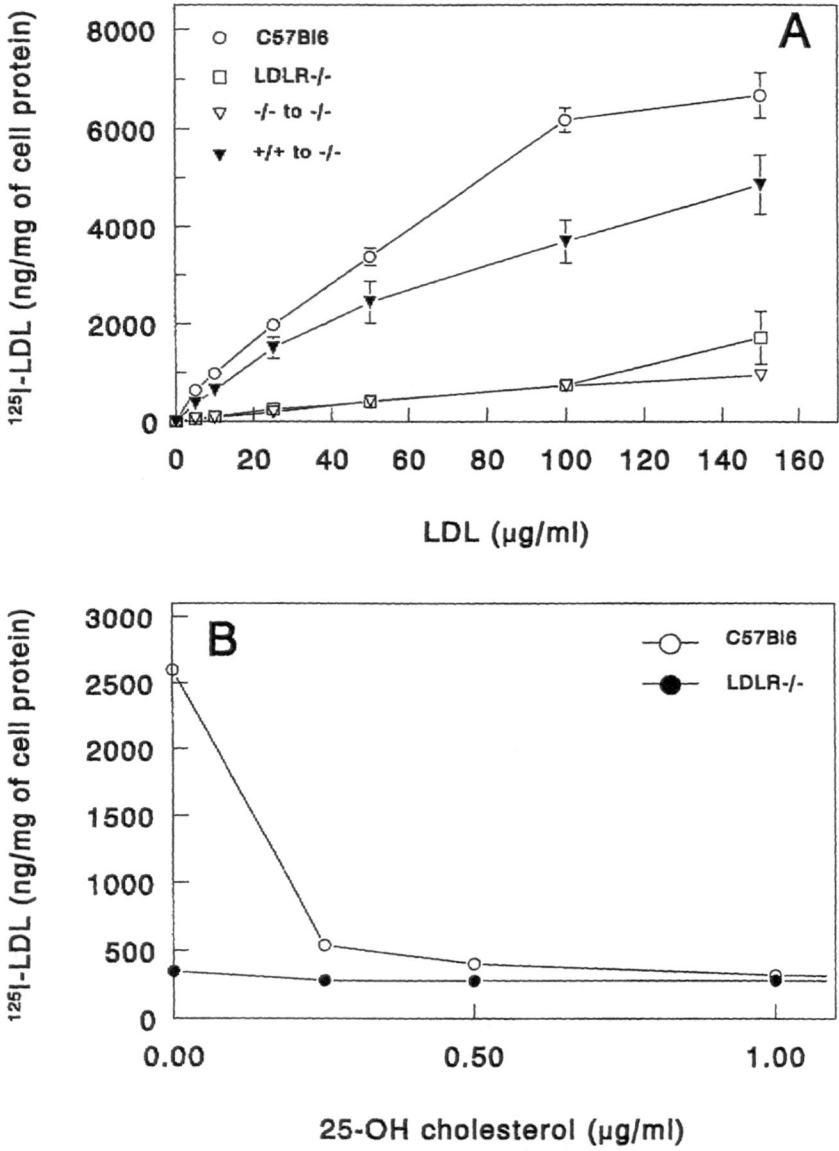

Figure 9. Effect of BMT on ^{125}I-LDL metabolism of peritoneal macrophages. Peritoneal macrophages of C57Bl/6J mice (O; n = 2), LDLR-/- mice (□; n = 2), (+/+ to -/-) transplanted mice (▾; n = 4) and (-/- to -/-) transplanted mice (▿; n = 2), were isolated and cultured in lipoprotein deficient medium for 2 days. Panel A shows the degradation of ^{125}I-LDL by the macrophages (3h, 37°C). Panel B shows the degradation of ^{125}I-LDL (25 μg/ml) by macrophages of C57Bl/6J (O; n = 3) and LDLR-/- (●; n = 3) mice that were preincubated with 25-OH-cholesterol for 20 hours. Values are means ± SD.

fed a 1% cholesterol diet for 6 months. The cholesterol levels of the LDLR-/-
mice, (-/- to -/-) transplanted mice, and (+/+ to -/-) transplanted mice
increased about 4-fold, whereas the cholesterol level of C57Bl/6J mice did
not change significantly by the diet (Figure 10).

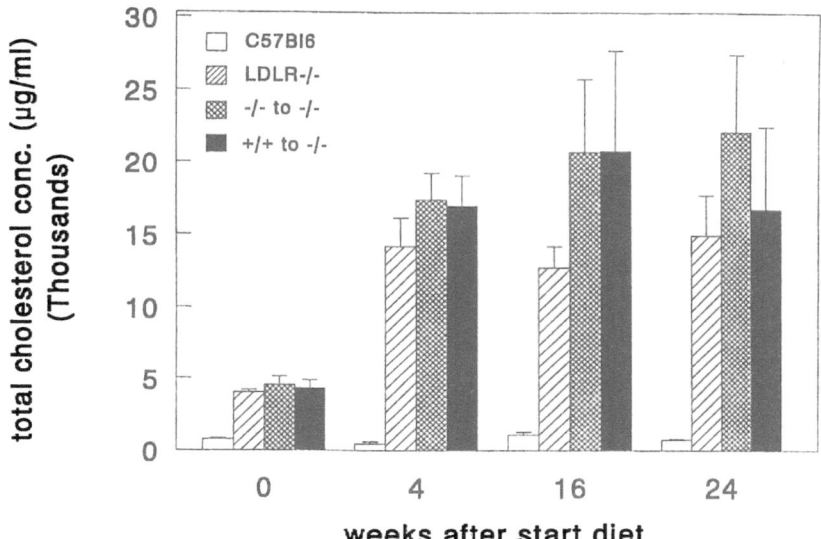

Figure 10. *Effect of 1% cholesterol diet, fed during 6 months, on serum total cholesterol
levels. C57Bl/6J mice (n = 4) are indicated with open bars, LDLR-/- mice (n = 5) with hatched
bars, (-/- to -/-) transplanted mice (n = 4) with chequered bars and (+/+ to -/-) transplanted
mice (n = 3) with closed bars. The transplanted mice were put on the diet 5 months after BMT.
Before the start of the diet, the mice were fed standard chow diet (SMR-A). Values are means
± SD. No significant differences between the total serum cholesterol values of the LDLR-/-
mice, (-/- to -/-) transplanted mice, and (+/+ to -/-) transplanted mice were observed at the
different time points.*

Tangirala et al.[21] found a comparable increase of cholesterol levels in LDLR-/-
mice that were fed the same diet. No significant differences in total serum
cholesterol values between the LDLR-/- control and transplanted mice were
observed at the indicated time points. After 6 months of diet, the hearts and
aortas were perfused and fixed. Cross sections of the aortic root were
examined and representative photomicrographs of the aortic valves are
shown in Figure 11. The mean lesion area in the aortic root was calculated
and is presented in Figure 12. The cross sections of C57Bl/6J mice showed
hardly any lesions, whereas extensive lipid-rich lesions could be demonstrated in LDLR-/- mice. The increase in mean lesion area in LDLR-/- mice was
approximately 7-fold (p≤0.001). Cross sections of the transplanted LDLR-/-
mice, both (-/- to -/-) and (+/+ to -/-), showed lesions that were even more

advanced than that of the LDLR-/- control mice, because of the presence of calcified areas in these sections (Figures 11C and D). The mean lesion area was increased approximately 1.5-fold (p≤0.05 in case of LDLR-/- vs. +/+ to -/-; p≤0.01 in case of LDLR-/- vs. -/- to -/-) (Figure 12). The bone marrow transplantation procedure itself, thus, aggravates atherosclerosis. No statistically significant differences in mean lesion area could be demonstrated between the (-/- to -/-) and (+/+ to -/-) transplanted mice.

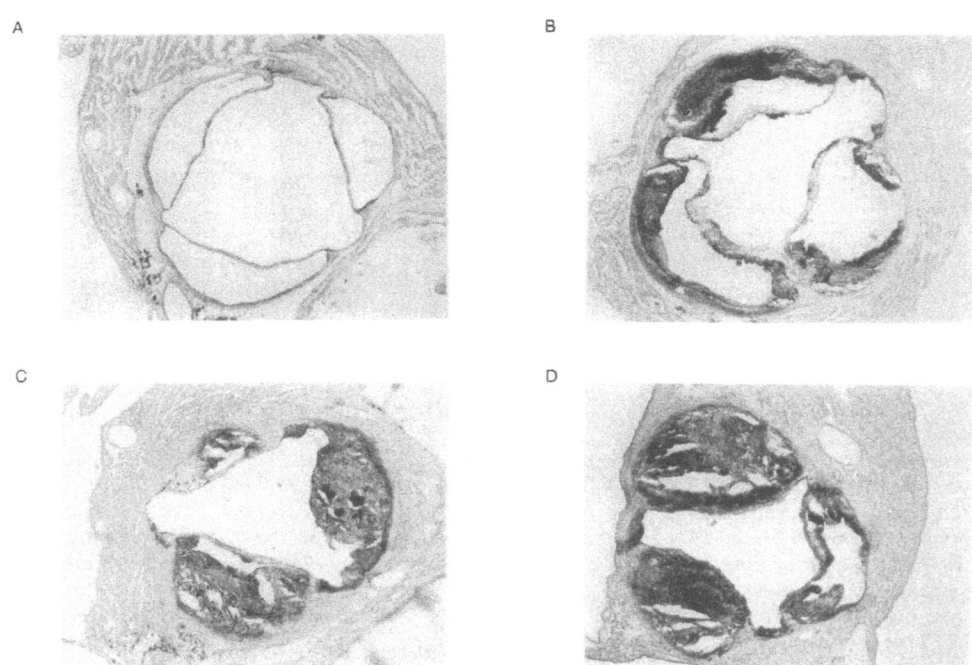

Figure 11. Photomicrographs of cross sections of aortic root of C57Bl6, LDLR-/- and transplanted LDLR-/- mice. These mice were fed a 1% cholesterol diet during 6 months. The sections were stained with oil red O (lipids) and hematoxylin (contrastaining). Representative sections of C57Bl6 mice [A], LDLR-/- mice [B], (-/- to -/-) transplanted mice [C], and (+/+ to -/-) transplanted mice [D] are shown. Magnification x40.
(For colour plate of figure 11 see page 223)

Discussion

Several functions have been proposed for the role of macrophage apoE synthesis in cholesterol homeostasis and its relation to atherosclerosis, including either pro- or anti-atherosclerotic functions. The present study confirms that hypercholesterolemia in apoE-deficient mice can be markedly

Lesion area x 100000 (um2)

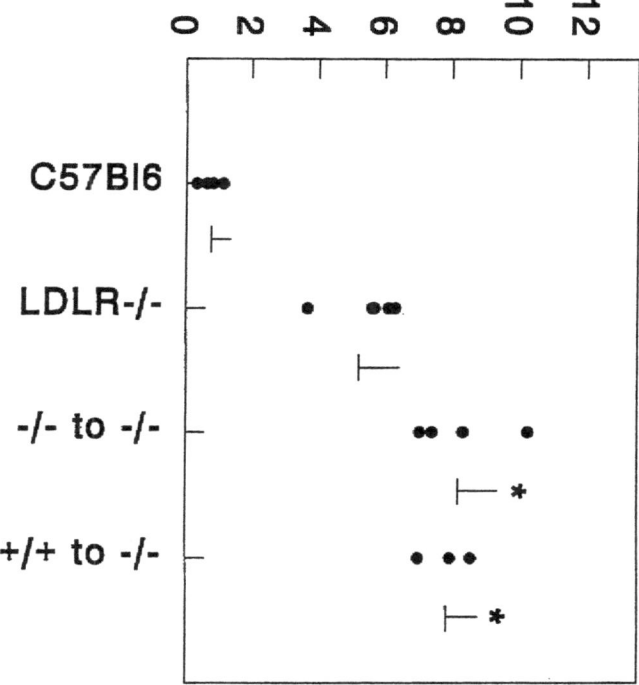

Figure 12. Effect of BMT on mean atherosclerotic lesion area. C57Bl6 (n = 4), LDLR-/- (n = 5), [-/- to -/-] (n = 4) and [+/+ to -/-] (n = 3), transplanted LDLR-/- mice were fed a 1% cholesterol diet during 6 months. The mean lesion area was calculated from cross sections of the aortic root that were stained with oil red O. Values are means ± SD. * indicates signifiant differences vs. non-transplanted LDLR-/- mice (p≤0.01).

reduced by transplantation with wildtype bone marrow, while heterozygous apoE-deficient bone marrow appeared to be nearly equally effective.

Following total body irradiation, aplasia of bone marrow develops within 2 to 3 days. Bone marrow transplantation will lead to recovery of haematopoietic tissues after two distinct phases of engraftment. In the first, unsustained phase, monocytes and macrophages are derived from committed progenitors. In the second, sustained phase, these cells are derived from pluripotent stem cells in the bone marrow. Transplantation of apoE-deficient mice with either heterozygous apoE-deficient (apoE$^{+/-}$ $^{-/-}$) or wild-type (apoE$^{+/+}$ $^{-/-}$) bone marrow resulted in a dramatic drop of cholesterol by 4 weeks after transplantation. It is thus the initial phase of engraftment by committed progenitors and the subsequent appearance of apoE producing mononuclear cells in the circulation by 4 weeks after transplantation that is responsible for this effect.

ApoE was found to be extremely efficient in lowering serum cholesterol levels, as at a steady state concentration as low as $1.89 \pm 0.37\%$ of the apoE concentration from normal C57Bl/6 mice, an almost complete normalization of cholesterol levels was found. This decrease in cholesterol levels in transplanted mice is mainly caused by a decrease in (ß)VLDL (25-fold) and to a lesser extent in LDL (5-fold), implying that apoE is more important for the clearance of VLDL than of LDL. This can be explained by the fact that the affinity of apoE for the LDL-receptor is higher than the affinity of apoB100, the apolipoprotein responsible for the recognition of LDL by the LDL-receptor. In addition, the decrease in LDL can be explained by the fact that VLDL is a precursor for LDL and a reduction of the VLDL pool will lead to reduced competition with LDL for the LDL receptor, resulting in lowering of LDL levels. The reduction of VLDL and LDL, and the increase in HDL, are apoE concentration dependent. However, with only a small increase in the apoE concentration an already dramatic decrease in VLDL and LDL levels is achieved. Cholesterol levels remained constant in the weeks following transplantation, suggesting that the chimeric status in the transplanted animals is stable.

Transplantation of wild-type bone marrow into apoE-deficient mice protected these mice from developing atherosclerosis on a "Western-type" diet. This protection against atherogenesis after transplantation is probably a combined effect of both the dramatic lowering of serum cholesterol levels and an apoE-mediated enhanced efflux of cholesterol from the arterial wall.

The present data indicate that macrophage-derived apoE normalizes hypercholesterolemia by an apoE gene-dosage dependent reduction of cholesterol, due to an increased recognition and uptake of cholesterol-rich lipoproteins by parenchymal liver cells. It is suggested that pharmacological approaches to increase macrophage apoE synthesis in the arterial wall may be specifically useful in the treatment of atherosclerosis.

Transplantation of LDL-receptor positive haematopoietic stem cells into LDL-receptor deficient mice resulted in a moderate decrease of total serum cholesterol, while especially LDL-cholesterol was lowered. The decrease, however, was not sufficient to normalize the serum cholesterol levels. In the weeks after transplantation total serum cholesterol levels were determined frequently. Four weeks after BMT in LDL-receptor deficient mice the cholesterol levels dropped in both the (+/+ to -/-) group as the (-/- to -/-) group. This drop in cholesterol, independent of the type of bone marrow, is probably caused by the irradiation and/or transplantation procedure itself.

During the repopulation of the hematopoietic system the macrophages may be activated, which could result in a stimulation of the LDLR-independent uptake of cholesterol. On the other hand the influx into plasma of cholesterol may also be influenced by the irradiation and/or transplantation procedure, as we also observed in apoE knockout mice. In the weeks after the initial drop in cholesterol, its level in the (-/- to -/-) mice returned to that of the control LDLR-/- mice, whereas the levels in the (+/+ to -/-) group remained lower (Figure 7). Introduction of the LDLR in LDLR-/- mice, therefore, can result in a decrease of total serum cholesterol levels, although this is clearly not sufficient to normalize the levels.

From *in vitro* studies with cultured human fibroblasts it is known that LDLR down-regulation by cholesterol can occur within one day. *In vivo*, however, a longer time is needed. In our study we demonstrate that the LDLR on murine peritoneal macrophages can be down-regulated by 25-OH-cholesterol. 25-OH-cholesterol is an oxysterol and is, like LDL itself, a known potent inhibitor of LDLR synthesis in cultured cells. Our studies on the catabolism of LDL by peritoneal macrophages isolated from the (+/+ to -/-) group indicated that the LDLR is functionally present in these macrophages when cultured in lipoprotein-deficient serum, i.e. under conditions that the LDLR is upregulated. This is in contrast to peritoneal macrophages of the control (-/- to -/-) transplanted group which hardly show any catabolism of LDL. These results, therefore, support the suggestion that the LDLR in the transplanted LDLR-/- mice may be subject to downregulation *in vivo*.

Transplantation of wild-type bone marrow into LDLR-/- mice will not only result in the introduction of the LDLR in liver Kupffer cells, but it also leads to the presence of the LDLR gene in macrophages that are located in the arterial wall. The role of the LDLR on these arterial wall macrophages in mediating foam cell formation is still unclear; controversy exists whether the expression of the LDLR in these arterial wall macrophages does mediate an increase in foam cell formation. We quantified the aortic atherosclerotic lesions in control and transplanted mice. The mean lesion areas of the control LDLR-/- mice largely corresponded to earlier publications of Tangirala et al.[21] The (-/- to -/-) transplantation itself, however, already caused a 1.5 fold increase in mean lesion area when compared to the LDLR-/- control mice. This effect cannot be attributed to a change in serum cholesterol concentration, because the cholesterol level of the transplanted mice did not differ significantly from that of the non-transplanted LDLR-/- mice. No statistically significant differences in mean lesion area could be observed between the (-/- to -/-) and the (+/+ to -/-) transplanted group. Thus, under the present conditions the absence or presence of the gene for the LDLR on macrophages does not influence the overall atherosclerotic process.

In future studies we want to overexpress the gene for the LDLR in macrophages in order to lower LDL-levels to a larger and more benificial extent. Several studies have been performed in which the LDLR was being overexpressed in parenchymal liver cells. In Watanabe heritable hyperlipidemic rabbits[22,23], FH patients [24], and LDLR-/- mice [16] this gene transfer resulted in a correction of the LDLR deficiency. Also in normal mice, adenovirus-mediated transfer of LDLR accelerated cholesterol clearance[25], demonstrating the important role of the LDLR for LDL-turnover. So far, no reports have been published in which the effects of overexpression of LDLR gene in macrophages are described.

Conclusion

We showed that transplantation of wildtype bone marrow into LDLR-/- mice does result in a lowering of serum cholesterol, especially IDL/LDL-cholesterol. This effect is not sufficient to normalize the cholesterol levels and it appears to be temporary. No differences in atherosclerosis were observed in mice transplanted with wildtype bone marrow and LDLR-/- bone marrow. We suggest that the LDLR introduced in LDLR-/- mice via bone marrow transplantation is down regulated by the sustained increased serum cholesterol levels. Further studies with macrophages overexpressing the LDLR, or expressing the LDLR in a cholesterol-insensitive way, may lead to a more beneficial effect on cholesterol levels and possibly atherosclerosis. In contrast, macrophage-derived apoE can normalize hypercholesterolemia dose-dependently in apoE-deficient mice due to increased recognition and uptake of ßVLDL by parenchymal liver cells. These changes are associated with a major decrease in susceptibility for atherosclerotic lesion development.

References

1. Mahley RW. Apolipoprotein E: cholesterol transport protein with expanding role in cell biology. Science. 1988;240:622-30.
2. Moestrup SK. The α2-macroglobulin receptor and epithelial glycoprotein-330: two giant receptors mediating endocytosis of multiple ligands. Biochim Biophys Acta. 1994;1197:197-213.
3. Krieger M, Herz J. Structures and functions of multiligand receptors: macrophage scavenger receptors and LDL receptor-related protein (LRP). Annu Rev Biochem. 1994;62:601-37.
4. Rall jr SC, Mahley RW. The role of apolipoprotrein E genetic variants in lipoprotein disorders. J Int Med. 1992;231:653-9.
5. Havekes L, De Wit E, Gevers Leuven J et al, Beisiegel U. Apolipoprotein E3-Leiden. A new variant of human apolipoprotein E, associated with familial type III

hyperlipoproteinemia. Hum Genet. 1986;73:157-63.

6. Horie Y, Fazio S, Westerlund JR, Weisgraber KH, Rall SC Jr. The functional characteristics of a human apolipoprotein E variant (cysteine at residue 142) may explain its association with dominant expression of type III hyperlipoproteinemia. J Biol Chem. 1992;267:1962-8.

7. Ghiselli G, Schaefer EJ, Gascon P, Brewer HB Jr. Type III hyperlipoproteinemia associated with apolipoprotein E deficiency. Science. 1981;214:1239-41.

8. Schaefer EJ, Gregg RE, Ghiselli G, Forte TM, Ordovas JM, Zech LA, Brewer jr HB. Familial apolipoprotein E deficiency. J Clin Invest. 1986;78:1206-19.

9. Cladaras C, Hadzopoulou-Cladaras M, Felber BK, Pavlakis G, Zannis VI. The molecular basis of familial apoE deficiency. An acceptor splice site mutation in the third intron of the deficient apoE gene. J Biol Chem. 1987;262:2310-5.

10. Lohse P, Brewer III HB, Meng MS, Skarlatos SI, LaRosa JC, Brewer HB Jr. Familial apolipoprotein E deficiency and type III hyperlipoproteinemia due to a premature stop codon in the apolipoprotein E gene. J Lipid Res. 1992;33:1583-90.

11. Zhang SH, Reddick RL, Piedrahita JA, Maeda N. Spontaneous hypercholesterolemia and arterial lesions in mice lacking apolipoprotein E. Science. 1992;258:468-71.

12. Plump AS, Smith JD, Hayek T et al. Severe hypercholesterolemia and atherosclerosis in apolipoprotein E-deficient mice created by homologous recombination in ES cells. Cell. 1992;71:343-53.

13. Van Ree JH, Van den Broek WJAA, Dahlmans VEH et al. Diet-induced hypercholesterolemia and atherosclerosis in heterozygous apolipoprotein E-deficient mice. Atherosclerosis. 1994;111:25-37.

14. Hobbs HH, Brown MS, Goldstein JL. Molecular genetics of the LDL receptor gene in familial hypercholesterolemia. Hum Mutat. 1992;1:445-66.

15. Goldstein JL, Brown MS. Familial hypercholesterolemia. In: Stanbury JB, Wyngaarden JB, Frederickson DS, Goldstein JL, Brown MS, ed. The metabolic basis of inherited diseases. New York: McGraw-Hill;1983:622-730.

16. Ishibashi S, Brown MS, Goldstein JL, Gerard RD, Hammer RE, Herz J. Hypercholesterolemia in low density lipoprotein receptor knockout mice and its reversal by adenovirus-mediated gene delivery. J Clin Invest. 1993;92:883-93.

17. Ishibashi S, Goldstein JL, Brown MS, Herz J, Burns DK. Massive xanthomatosis and atherosclerosis in cholesterol-fed low density lipoprotein receptor-negative mice. J Clin Invest. 1994;93:1885-93.

18. Nagelkerke JF, van Berkel ThJC. Rapid transport of fatty acids from rat liver endothelial to parenchymal cells after uptake of cholesterylester labeled acetylated LDL. Biochim Biophys Acta. 1986;875:593-8.

19. Pieters MN, Esbach S, Schouten D, Brouwer A, Knook DL, van Berkel ThJC. Cholesterylesters from oxidized LDL are in vivo rapidly hydrolysed in rat Kupffer cells and transported to liver parenchymal cells and bile. Hepatology. 1994;19:1459-67.

20. Goldstein JL, Brown MS. Progress in understanding the LDL receptor and HMG-CoA reductase, two membrane bound proteins that regulate the plasma cholesterol. J Lipid Res. 1984;1450-61.

21. Tangirala RK, Rubin EM, Palinski W. Quantitation of atherosclerosis in murine models: correlation between lesions in the aortic origin and in the entire aorta, and differences in the extent of lesions between sexes in LDL receptor-deficient and apolipoprotein E deficient mice. J Lipid Res. 1995;35:385-98.

22. Wilson JM, Johnston DE, Jefferson DM, Mulligan RC. Correction of the genetic

defect in hepatocytes from the Watanabe heritable hyperlipidemic rabbit. Proc Natl Acad Sci USA. 1988;85:4421-5.

23. Kozarsky KF, McKinley DR, Austin LL, Raper SE, Stratford-Perricaudet LD, Wilson JM. In vivo correction of low density lipoprotein receptor deficiency in the Watanabe heritable hyperlipidemic rabbit with recombinant adenoviruses. J Biol Chem. 1994;18:13695-702.

24. Grossman M, Raper SE, Kozarsky K et al. Successful ex vivo gene therapy directed to liver in a patient with familial hypercholesterolaemia. Nature Genet. 1994;6:335-41.

25. Herz J, Gerard RD. Adenovirus-mediated transfer of low density lipoprotein receptor gene acutely accelerates cholesterol clearance in normal mice. Proc Natl Acad Sci USA. 1993;2812-6.

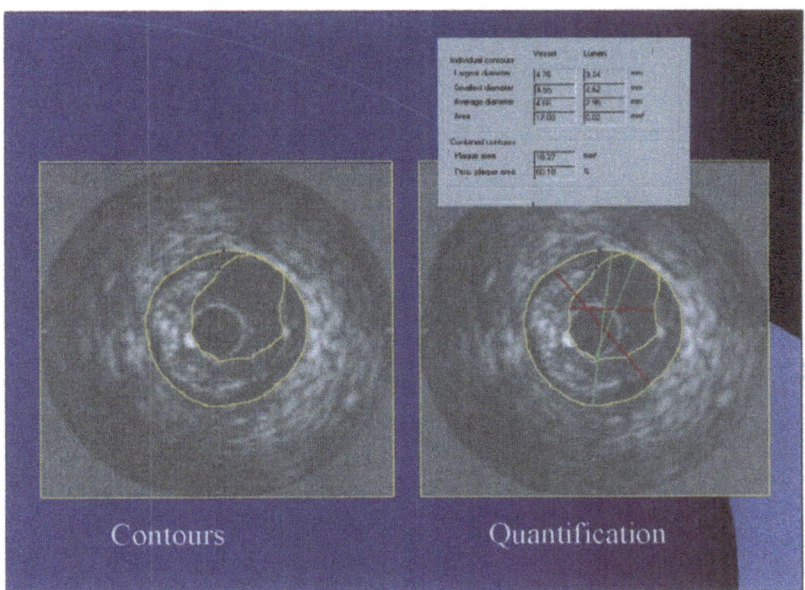

Figure 3. *(Chapter 8) First results of our automated contour detection approaches for the luminal and vessel boundaries in IVUS images.*

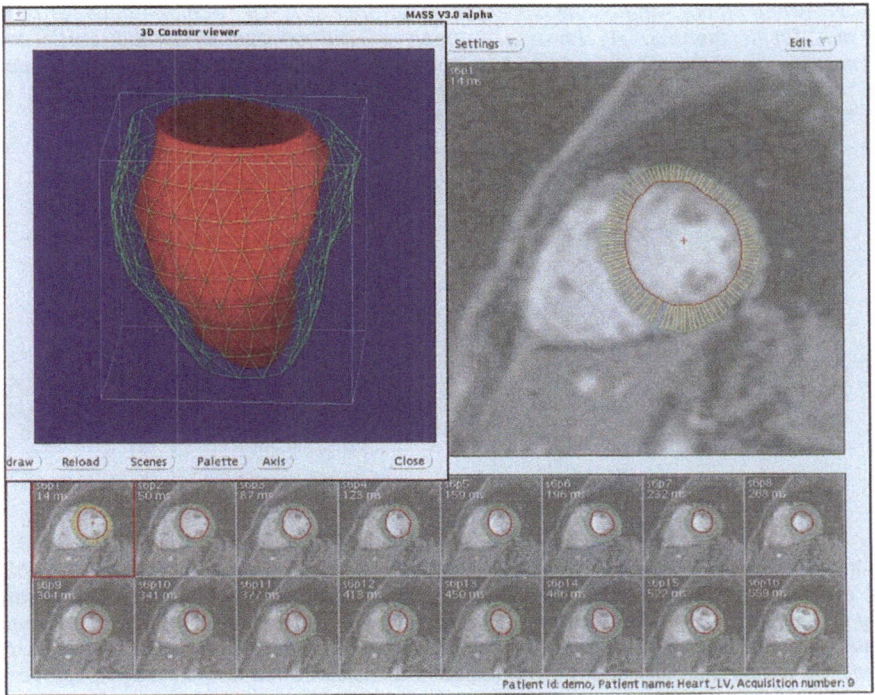

Figure 5. *(Chapter 8) Computer display of the MASS analytical software package. The small images along the bottom represent the individual frames over a cardiac cycle at a certain anatomic level. The endo- and epicardial contours were detected automatically. From the contours in all the frames and slices, a 3D model can be reconstructed that can also be used as a functional display representing e.g. regional wall thickening/thinning.*

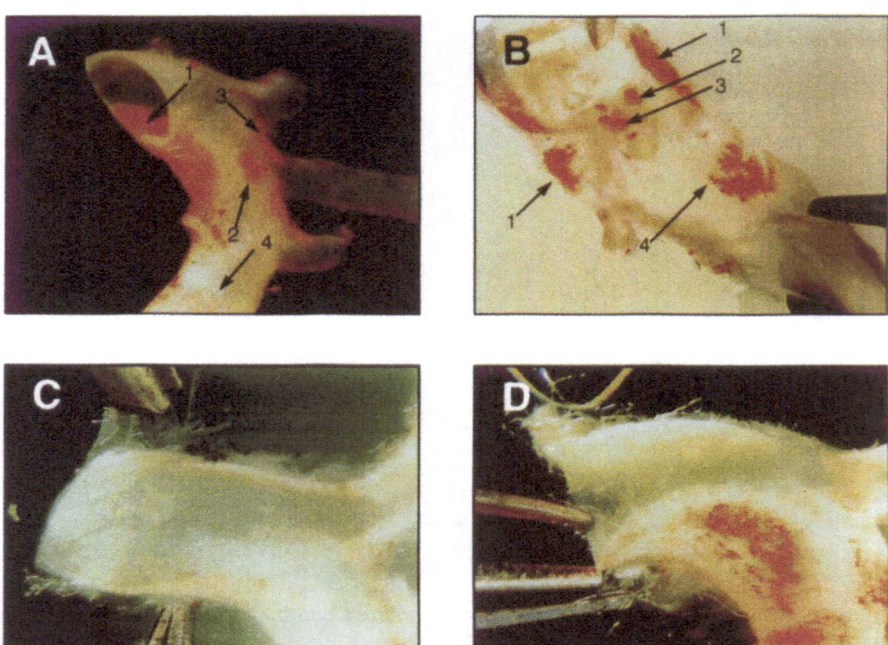

Figure 1. (Chapter 10) Atherosclerosis in the aortic arch of APOE*3Leiden mice, after feeding HFC diet for 3 months. A, Photomicrograph of the oil red O-stained aortic arch. B, Photomicrograph of the same aortic arch as shown in A, after opening longitudinally along the inner curvature. C and D, En face view of the aortic arch of a control mouse and an APOE*3Leiden mouse, respectively, after 3 months of feeding HFC diet.

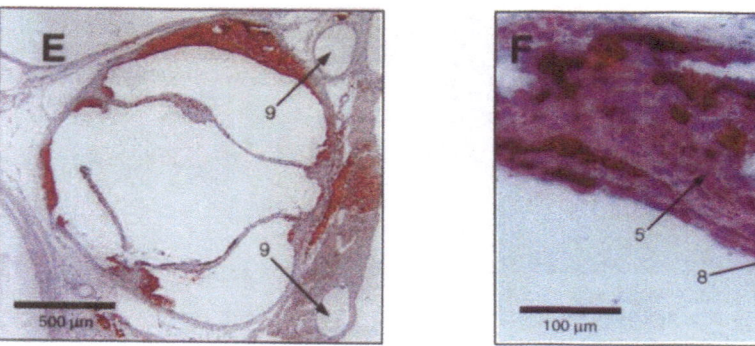

Figure 2. (Chapter 10) Photomicrographs of a cross section of the aortic root of APOE*3Leiden mice, after feeding HFC diet for 3 months. Slide was stained with oil red O and hematoxylin. F, higher magnification of the lesion shown in E. Note the presence of many lipid foam cells (arrow 5), as well as large amounts of extracellular lipid in the core of the lesion (arrow 6). Also note the dark blue deposits (arrow 7), indicative of calcification and oil red O-positive spindle shaped cells (arrow 8). Note also that the proximal coronary arteries do not show any sign of lesion development (arrows 9).

1mm

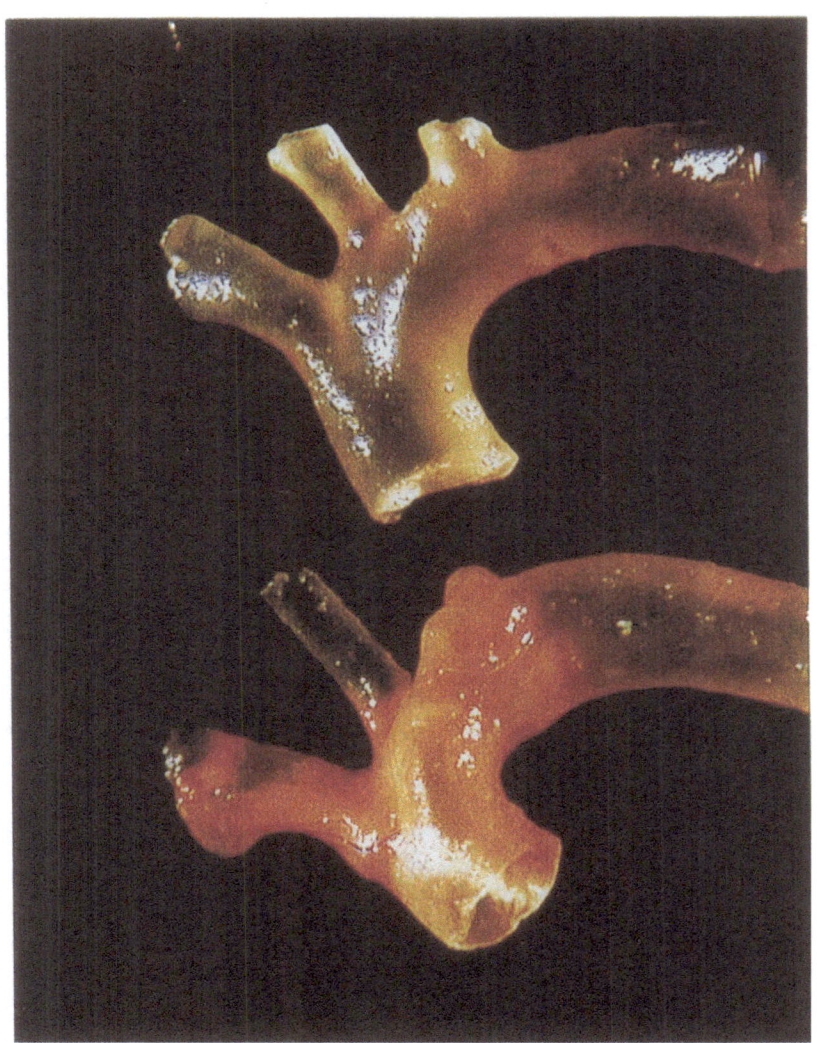

Figure 6. (Chapter 12) *Atherosclerotic lesions in aortas in apoE⁻ mice, transplanted with apoE⁻ or apoE⁺/⁺ bone marrow, both fed a "Western-type" diet for 4 months. Aortas were perfusion-fixed with neutral-buffered formalin and stained with Sudan IV to visualize lipid rich lesions. An enlargement of the aortic arch of apoE⁻ mice transplanted with apoE⁻ (left) or apoE⁺/⁺ (right) bone marrow is shown. Magnification x15.*

222

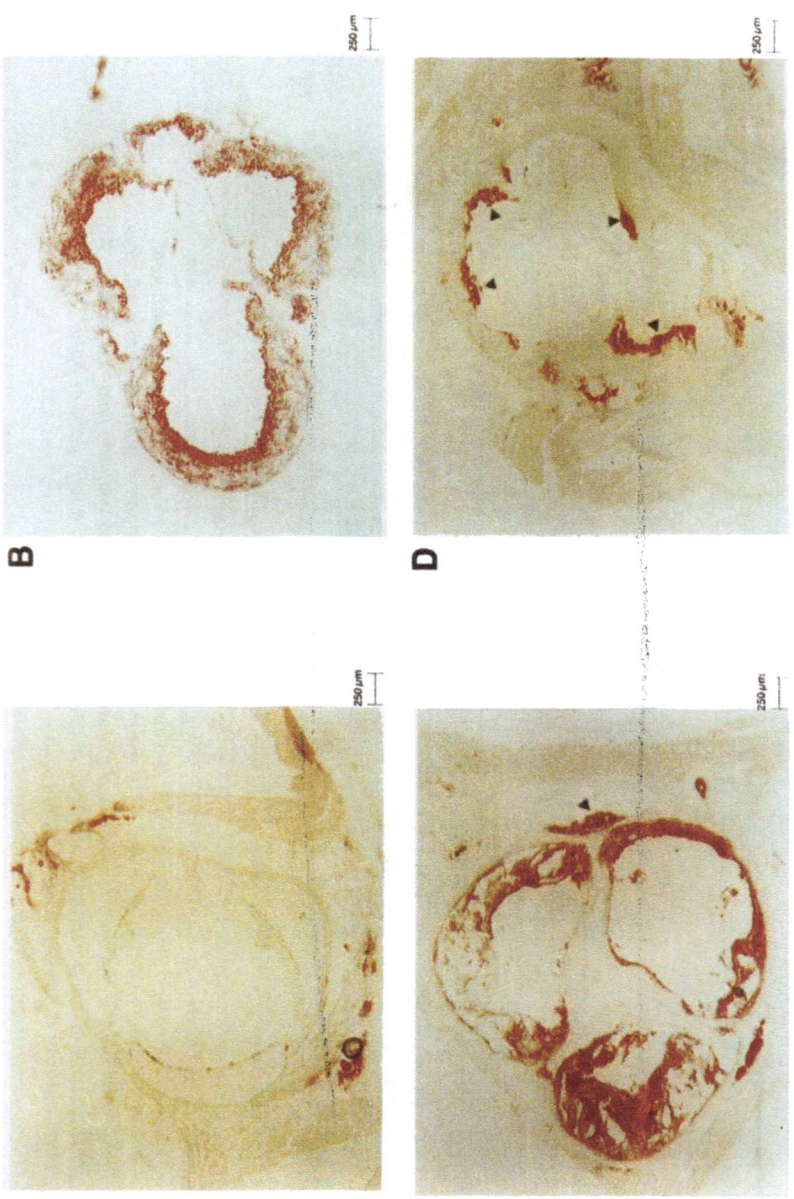

Figure 4. *(Chapter 12) Visualization of atherosclerosis in cross-sections at the aortic sinuses on the level of the three cups of control C57Bl/6, apoE[-/-] and transplanted mice,[1] fed a "Western-type" diet for 4 months. Sections are stained with oil red O to visualize lipid rich lesion areas. Panel A shows a section from a control C57Bl/6 mouse without lesions. Panel B shows severe lipid-rich lesions in an apoE[-/-] mouse. Panel C shows a section from an apoE[+/- -/-] mouse with extensive lipid-rich lesions in both the aortic sinus and in a coronary artery (arrow). In panel D it is demonstrated that transplantation with wildtype bone marrow into an apoE[-/-] animal (apoE[+/+ - -/-]) results in a large reduction of the lesion area. Arrows indicate the localization of lesions in apoE[+/+ - -/-] mice (D) and lesions in the coronary artery in apoE[-/- -/-] mice (C). Magnification x40.*

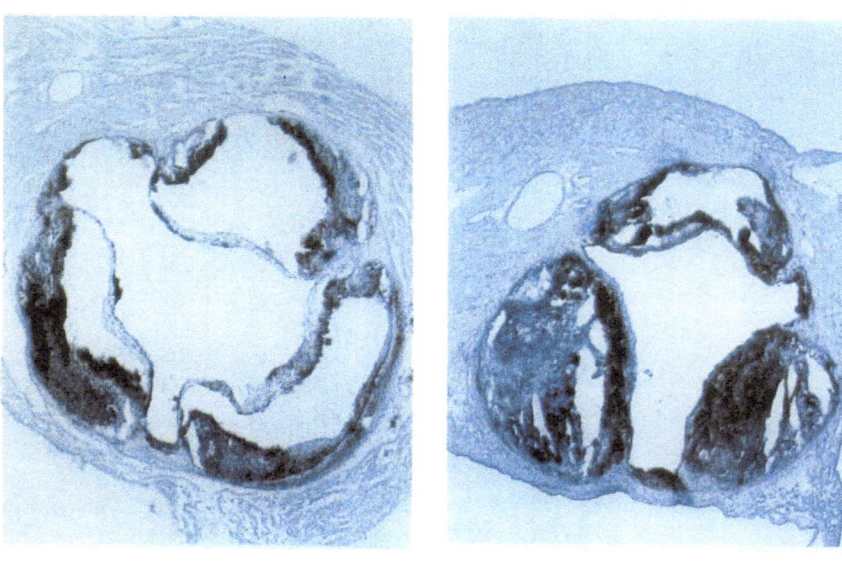
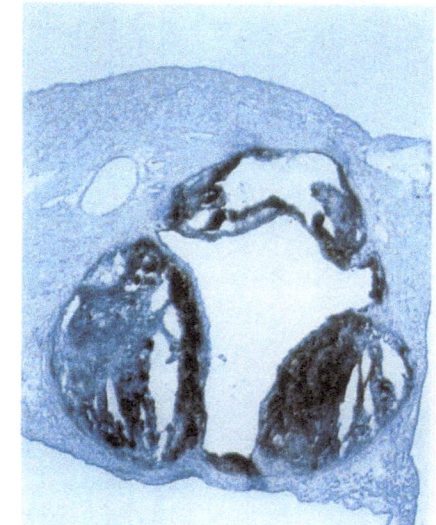
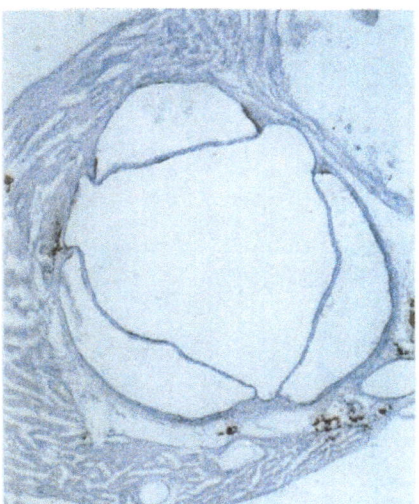
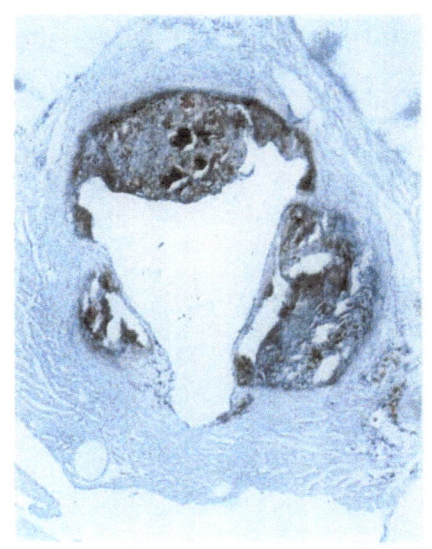

Figure 11. *(Chapter 12) Photomicrographs of cross sections of aortic root of C57Bl6, LDLR-/- and transplanted LDLR-/- mice. These mice were fed a 1% cholesterol diet during 6 months. The sections were stained with oil red O (lipids) and hematoxylin (contrastaining). Representative sections of C57Bl6 mice [A], LDLR-/- mice [B], (-/- to -/-) transplanted mice [C], and (+/+ to -/-) transplanted mice [D] are shown. Magnification x40.*

INDEX